Parsley, Sage, Rosemary and Thyme . . .

and so much more!

Herbs are so much more than a dash of flavor in your food . . . they're gentle, natural cosmetics; beautiful additions to your garden and home; essential ingredients in simple home remedies . . . The uses and varieties of herbs are surprising, and this clear, simple guide will show you . . .

- **How to grow an herb garden**
- **How to add a new dimension to your cooking**
- **How to create crafts with herbs**
- **How to prevent seasickness and so much more!**

THE COMPLETE HERB BOOK

Berkley Books by Maggie Stuckey

THE HOUSEPLANT ENCYCLOPEDIA

THE COMPLETE HERB BOOK

THE COMPLETE SPICE BOOK

the COMPLETE HERB BOOK

MAGGIE STUCKEY

Produced by The Philip Lief Group, Inc.

BERKLEY BOOKS, NEW YORK

Most Berkley Books are available at special quantity discounts for bulk purchases for sales promotions, premiums, fund-raising, or educational use. Special books, or book excerpts, can also be created to fit specific needs.

For details, write: Special Markets, The Berkley Publishing Group, 375 Hudson Street, New York, New York 10014.

A Berkley Book
Published by The Berkley Publishing Group
A division of Penguin Putnam Inc.
375 Hudson Street
New York, New York 10014

When using herbs for medicinal purposes, the reader should bear in mind that this book is intended to serve as a general reference only, and should not be used to replace the advice of a physician. For cautionary advice concerning the use of herbs described in this book, see the What About Safety section in the preface. Responsibility for any adverse effects or unforeseen consequences of the applications, preparations, or recipes contained in this book is expressly disclaimed by the author and publisher.

Copyright © 1994 by The Philip Lief Group, Inc.
Produced by The Philip Lief Group, Inc.
Book design by Tiffany Kukec
Cover design by Erika Fusari
Cover photographs by Faune Yerby

All rights reserved.
This book, or parts thereof, may not be reproduced in any form without permission. BERKLEY and the "B" design are trademarks belonging to Penguin Putnam Inc.

PRINTING HISTORY
Berkley mass market edition / May 1994
Berkley trade paperback edition / July 2001

The Penguin Putnam Inc. World Wide Web site address is
www.penguinputnam.com

Library of Congress Cataloging-in-Publication Data

Stuckey, Maggie.
The complete herb book / Maggie Stuckey.
p. cm.
Includes bibliographical references (p.).
ISBN 0-425-17969-9
1. Herbs. 2. Herb gardening. 3. Cookery (Herbs) 4. Herbs—Therapeutic use. I. Title.

SB351.H5 S77 2001
635'.7—dc21

2001025641

PRINTED IN THE UNITED STATES OF AMERICA

10 9 8 7 6 5 4 3 2 1

Contents

Preface

The main text of this book tries hard to avoid the pronoun *I* or any other forms of the first person. The goal of the book is to provide you with usable information, not personal reminiscences or homespun philosophy.

In the preface, I get to speak for myself.

Some Personal Comments

First, you should probably know that I majored in history in college. To this day I love reading about how people in earlier times managed the business of daily living. I find myself trying to picture what their life was like, how they coped, how they went about the multiple undertakings, great and ordinary, that defined their civilization.

In this regard, the study of herbs is for me a sheer delight. It is not too much to say that the entire story of humankind can be found there, for in the use and culture of herbs we can trace the thread of history all the way back to the first written records (even earlier, if you count archaeological evidence).

Herbs were used for healing, for religious ceremony, for magic, for protection against each generation's awesome calamities. The accumulated knowledge about them was written down, to be passed to the next generation. Along the way, people discovered homelier ways to use herbs, and noted their contribution to the taste of foods. These, too, were written down.

And so in reading what people from these earlier centuries had to say about herbs, we can discern much about the totality of their lives. And when we use those same herbs today, often in the same ways, we feel a very real link with the people of long ago.

It is my hope that you too will find pleasure in learning some of the old traditions and legends that herbs have birthed. But if you are not much for history, I hope you will not be offended if I take the time to share some of these old stories with readers who are.

Second, I might as well confess right now that I have two "pet" herbs, one for cooking and one for fragrance—basil and lavender. Fresh basil is my candidate for the eighth wonder of the world, and I absolutely swoon over the smell of fresh lavender. Later on in this book, in general discussions on gardening, cooking, or crafts, whenever I need an example to clarify the point at hand, I probably use one of those two.

Notice I say "fresh" in both cases. This is the third, and last, personal comment, and it's a pet peeve. Sometimes people who write about, talk about, teach about, or otherwise work with herbs get a bit carried away with themselves and their subject. If the instructor in a cooking demonstration insists, "oh my dears you just *must* use fresh herbs for this dish," I start looking for a back door to slip out of. Yes, fresh herbs are nice to cook with, but it's not always possible, or practical. Implying that fresh herbs are somehow morally superior to dried is pretentious. Good cooks use what they have—including common sense.

However . . . fresh basil is simply *different* from dried, not only in taste but in how it feels and smells on your fingers, and that difference is the very quality that I enjoy. And with lavender: if you have it growing fresh in your garden, you can revel in its haunting scent just by running your hand across the top, and the flower head remains on the plant to provide you that same pleasure another day.

In this book, the situations that depend on using fresh herbs are noted as such: for example, herbal vinegars, some floral crafts, and those culinary herbs that are simply not available in the market.

Comments About the Book

What Is an Herb?

Every definition that has ever been devised to explain exactly what makes a plant an herb has enough exceptions to render it imperfect. The best all-around definition I have found (and it is not perfect) is this.

> An herb is any plant that is used for meat (that is, flavoring), texture, fragrance, or dyeing and that grows in the temperate zone.

In the final analysis, definitions don't really matter. What matters is your success and your pleasure in the gentle adventure we are about to undertake together.

Why These Herbs in Particular?

The encyclopedia section contains individual profiles of fifty-some herbs. That is not, by a long shot, all the herbs known to man or woman. The ones included here were chosen because they are

- important in at least one usage category
- reasonably easy to find—either in the supermarket spice section, in the plant store, or in seed catalogs
- not tricky to grow
- not esoteric; all these herbs are ones that an average person could actually use

What About Safety?

First of all, the herbs in this book are things you would buy from some source: either a manufacturer of commercial seasonings, or a greenhouse, or a seed company. We are not talking about plants that you find growing in the wild and decide to bring home and throw into the stewpot. If you don't know what you're doing, that is one good way to get yourself seriously sick.

Second, this book takes a quite conservative position on plants that may be potentially harmful. If there is *any* reported suspicion about its safety, the text will say so. Until we know for certain, let's use something else. Working with herbs, cooking with them, growing them, smelling them, fondling them—this is all too much fun to risk spoiling the whole endeavor with a negative physiological reaction.

This book aims to introduce you to the joys of herbs. It's rather like an old-fashioned sampler, except that it uses words instead of embroidery stitches. It contains a bit about gardening, a bit about cooking, a bit about crafts, a bit about herbal medicine. Each one of these topics could be a book in itself—and is, as a casual glance in any bookstore will show.

Obviously, then, in one book it is not possible to treat all those areas in detail; instead, each main section presents the basics of that area and a few samples: sample craft projects, sample recipes, sample garden designs, and so on.

It is my hope that you will find here two things: (1) the fundamental information you need on whatever area interests you, and (2) the inspiration to delve further into those areas. Toward that end, in the back of the book you will find a highly opinionated listing of other good books.

Maggie Stuckey
Portland, Oregon

PART ONE

The Herb Encyclopedia

In this section are profiles of fifty-some herbs, chosen for their value in cooking, in the garden, in crafts, homemade cosmetics, or home remedies—or some combination. Each writeup begins with the basics: common and scientific names, primary uses, whether you can buy it readily at the supermarket or have to grow it in your garden, and three important things you will need to know if you decide to grow it: whether it's annual, perennial, or biennial; how tall it gets; and what gardening conditions it requires.

Each profile then includes:

- A verbal description of what the plant looks like (although in this case a picture is definitely worth a few thousand words)
- Brief information about growing, propagating, and harvesting the herb if you choose to grow it in your garden
- Description of the ways the plant is most commonly used today

- A collection of traditions, legends, and folklore associated with the herb, along with medicinal and household applications it may have had in past centuries

You may, as you browse through this section, come across some terms that are new to you, and you will find yourself wondering, What is a strewing herb? What does *biennial* mean? And what the heck is a tussy-mussy? Rather than burden this section by explaining those terms every time one is used, which would be extraordinarily cumbersome, I decided to save the definitions for later. Have faith; they are all explained in other parts of the book.

Angelica *Angelica archangelica*

BIENNIAL (APPROXIMATELY)

SIZE: 5 to 8 feet

GARDEN: Shade or partial shade; moist, rich soil

USED FOR: Cooking, tea, cosmetics, potpourri

AVAILABLE COMMERCIALLY: No (except the stem, in gourmet sections very occasionally)

Description: This is a *big* plant; by its second year it can be well over 6 feet high. Overall, it looks something like a giant celery and gives a lush, tropical look to your garden. The stems are as much as 3 inches across, and hollow. The bright apple-green leaves look much like celery leaves; individual leaflets, about 2 inches long, are set in pairs from a central stem. The white flower is a flattish cluster, like a dill flower, and blooms in early summer. Bees love it.

Gardening: Unlike most herbs, this plant prefers shady spots and loves soil that is moist and rich; it is at home along stream banks and marshy areas. It is a native of northern regions, and grows wild in Iceland and Lapland.

Angelica is usually started from seed. The first year, the plant sends up leaves directly from the ground. The second year, the tall, hollow stem develops and usually the flower stalk, although sometimes it doesn't flower until the third year. If you leave the flower head on the plant, it will make seeds that fall to the ground and you will have a large supply of baby plants. If you cut the flower stalk off before it seeds, the original plant will live for many years.

Because it gets so very tall, this plant should be at the back of your herb bed.

Uses: Every single part of the plant is useful, and every part has a sweet aroma and flavor like a mild licorice. The root is dried and

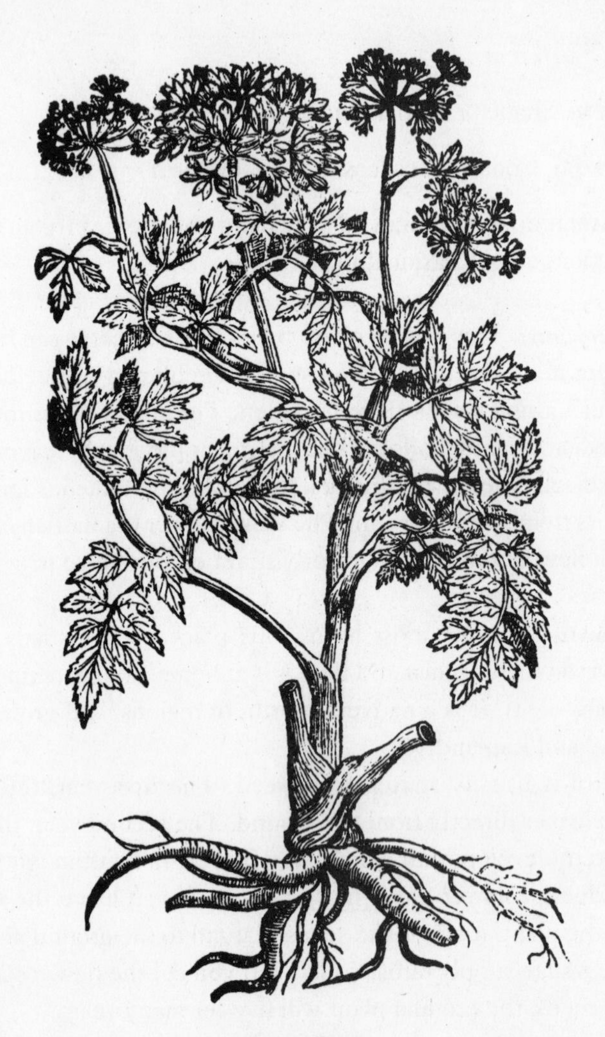

Angelica

ground up as sweet-smelling fixative for potpourri; dried leaves are also used in potpourri. Oil distilled from the roots is used in vermouth, Benedictine, and other liqueurs and in some perfumes.

The lightly sweet leaves can be used in fruit salads or desserts, either fresh or dried. And they make a delicious tea. Angelica tea has a calming effect, whether you drink it or take a bath in it. Make a strong infusion and add it to your bath water to unwind after a stressful day. The seeds, dried and ground, are used in baking cookies and sweet breads.

But mostly, angelica is known for its stem, which is used in two main ways: candied, and cooked with tart fruits. Earlier in this century candied angelica was a popular sweet treat, and it is still used in cake decorations as the "stems" of floral creations. The fresh stem is often stewed with tart fruits, especially rhubarb, to reduce the quantity of sugar needed. For a delicious rhubarb jam, substitute angelica for one-fourth of the total quantity of fruit.

In the past angelica has been used for medicinal purposes, especially to treat colds and bronchial infections, but its value has not been proved, and currently there is some debate about possible toxicity in very large quantities or strong concentrations. So, while angelica is safe for food consumption, it is not recommended as a medicine.

Traditions: This is one of the herbs closely associated with Christianity; indeed it is named for an archangel. The legend is that in the Middle Ages, during the time of a terrible plague, the Archangel Michael appeared in a dream to a monk and told him how to use this particular herb to cure the disease. From that time onward, angelica bloomed each year on May 8, the feast day of St. Michael. It came to be known as "Holy Ghost root," and it was believed to have very strong powers against witches, pestilence, and all sorts of evil.

Anise *Pimpinella anisum*

ANNUAL

SIZE: 1 to 2 feet high

GARDEN: Full sun; light, well-drained soil

USED FOR: Flavoring, tea, medicine

AVAILABLE COMMERCIALLY: Yes

Description: A dainty, rather fragile-looking plant, with clusters of tiny white flowers in late summer and two very different kinds of leaves. The lower leaves (formed when the plant is very young) are bright green and round, with scalloped edges; the upper leaves (formed as the plant matures) are very feathery and frilly, and have a gray-green tinge. The flowers dry into the familiar brown seeds that commercial spice companies sometimes call "aniseed."

Gardening: Anise is a native of hot, dry Mediterranean countries, and grows best in garden conditions that mimic that climate. Plant the seeds directly into the garden where they will grow, for they do not transplant successfully. If you live in cold regions, start peat pots indoors. Germination can be slow; some gardeners mix the seeds with radish seeds, which sprout quickly, to keep the soil loose and mark the spot.

To harvest the seeds, wait till the stalks are yellow and the seeds have turned gray-green. Cut off the entire flower head and hang it upside down in a paper bag until the seeds dry and fall off.

Uses: Anise is what gives a licorice flavor to cookies, cakes, candy, liqueurs—even cough syrup and toothpaste. Mostly it is the seeds that are used, but if you grow anise in your garden, you can also use the leaves. The flavor is less concentrated than in the seeds, but the leaves add color and make a very pretty garnish. French cooks add anise leaves to baby carrots, soups, and salads. Add a

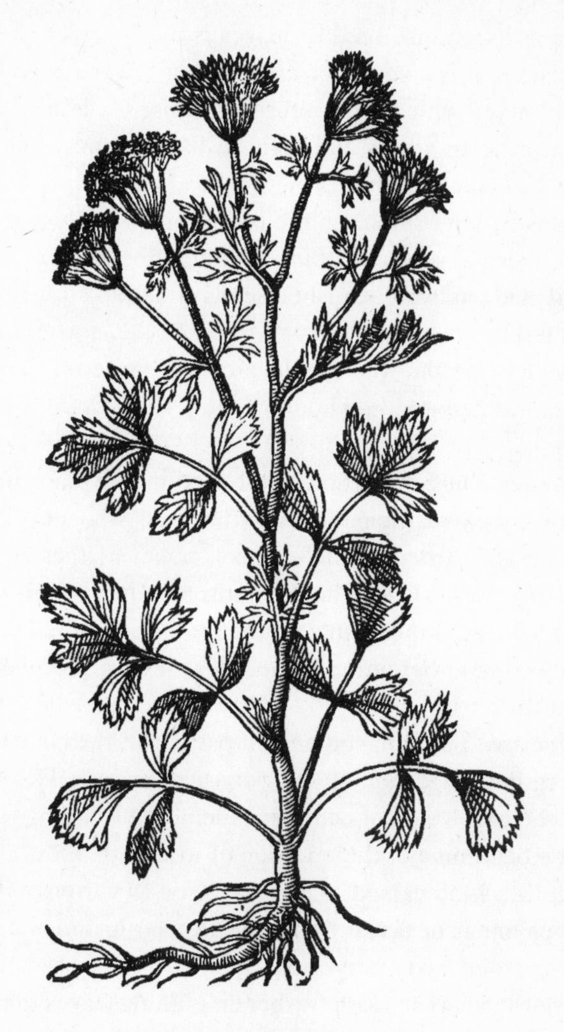

Anise

handful to the water when you boil shrimp. The seeds, traditionally used in anise cookies and spice cake, also go well in applesauce and apple pie.

Tea made from anise seed or leaves is mildly sweet; because it helps digestion, it is a very nice after-dinner beverage. At bedtime, warm milk mixed with anise is soothing. Anise tea is an old remedy for stomachache in adults and colic in babies, and some think it helps cure headaches.

Chew anise seed to sweeten the breath or to stop hiccups. Soak a handful of crushed seeds in a pint of brandy for six weeks, and you have homemade anisette. Crushed seeds added to a facial pack will fade freckles.

Dogs love anise the way cats love catnip; anise oil is applied to the mechanical rabbit in greyhound racing.

Traditions: Anise was known and used in very ancient civilizations. The Greek mathematician Pythagoras, who developed the theorem we all learned in high school, believed that anise could cure epilepsy if the patient held a sprig of it in his left hand long enough. That was in the sixth century B.C. One hundred years later, Hippocrates, the father of medicine, prescribed it for coughs (as do modern herbalists).

The Romans used it in cooking; in particular, they created a special cake to help digestion after a very heavy meal. This cake was served at the conclusion of banquets, including wedding feasts, and may be the beginning of the tradition of wedding cakes.

This herb was so valued that it was used as currency in biblical times, in payment of taxes. Pliny, the Roman historian of the first century, recorded sixty ways that the herb was used, including chewing the seeds as a breath freshener, pinning leaves to the pillow to prevent bad dreams, and bathing with it to give a youthful appearance to the skin.

Artemisia, Silver King *Artemisia ludoviciana*

PERENNIAL

SIZE: 1 to 3 feet

GARDEN: Full sun, well-drained soil

USED FOR: Crafts; garden ornamental

AVAILABLE COMMERCIALLY: No

Description: *Artemisia* is the name of a genus, and in that genus are included southernwood, wormwood, and tarragon—each of which is described in its own entry later in this book.

Artemisia is also sometimes used, rather confusingly, as the name of a particular group within that genus, with several varieties, including Silver Queen and Silver King. Both have long, narrow leaves that are a beautiful silvery gray color. Silver Queen is somewhat smaller overall, and the leaves are lacier. A variety called Silver Mound is very fine and lacy and grows in a perfectly rounded mound about 12 inches high.

Gardening: A very hardy plant that is easy to grow. It spreads by underground runners, like mint, and so needs either lots of room or lots of pruning.

The artemisias, with their lustrous gray foliage, make good accent plants for any garden. They form an attractive contrast border with green-leaved plants, and a dramatic backdrop for flowers of any color.

Uses: Aside from their ornamental beauty, artemisias are grown for their use in floral crafts. Silver King or Silver Queen (your choice) is probably the single most important herb for wreath makers, and that is why it is included in this book.

If you are interested in making wreaths or dried arrangements, and have any kind of garden space, plant lots of artemisia, and you

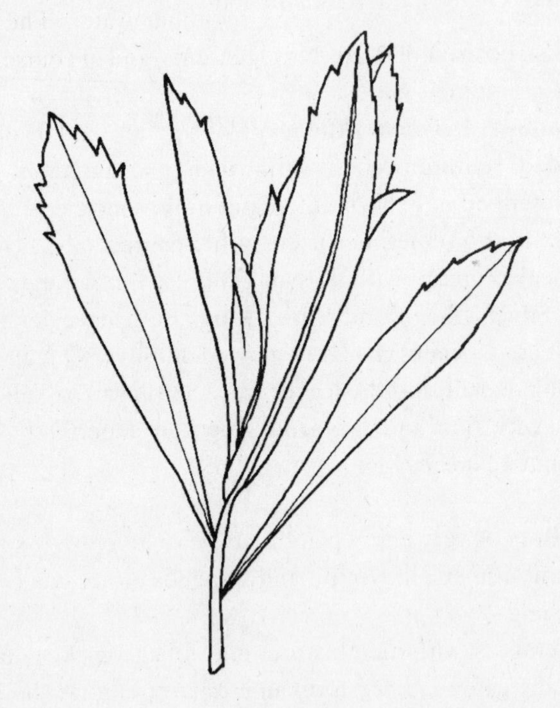

Artemisia

won't be sorry. It is much easier to work with fresh rather than dried plant material, for the stems are flexible and can be twisted and formed easily.

In the summer, artemisias form curled and twisted flower stalks that eventually blossom into tiny yellow buttons. For an all-white look, cut branches before the flower buds open. The dried leaves retain their silver color well. To dry, hang in bunches or simply place in a vase without water. The dried foliage is handsome in flower arrangements, and of course is the basis for many dried wreaths.

Basil *Ocimum basilicum*

ANNUAL

SIZE: 1 to 2 feet

GARDEN: Sun; rich, moist soil

USED FOR: Seasoning, cosmetics

AVAILABLE COMMERCIALLY: Yes (dried, and fresh in season)

Description: The common species of basil is a smallish plant with rich green leaves, oval-shaped, about 1½ inches long. Deep veins in the leaves give the surface a crinkled look. By midseason, a spike containing small white flowers appears above the foliage.

Other varieties: Because basil has become so popular in recent years, seeds and seedlings of many exotic varieties are commonly available. In addition to the very familiar sweet basil, *O. basilicum*, you may find:

- Lettuce-leaf basil (leaves up to 5 inches long) and mammoth (8-inch leaves).
- Dwarf basil, also called bush or Greek basil, a group of very small and compact plants with tiny but richly flavored leaves.
- Scented basils: a group with unusual aromatic leaves, such as cinnamon, anise, and lemon.
- Opal or purple basil, which has less pronounced flavor but makes beautiful vinegar and is stunning as an ornamental plant.

Gardening: Two things to remember about growing basil: (1) It needs hot weather, and (2) you need to keep pinching off the flower heads before they form.

Start basil from seed indoors and set out in the garden when you

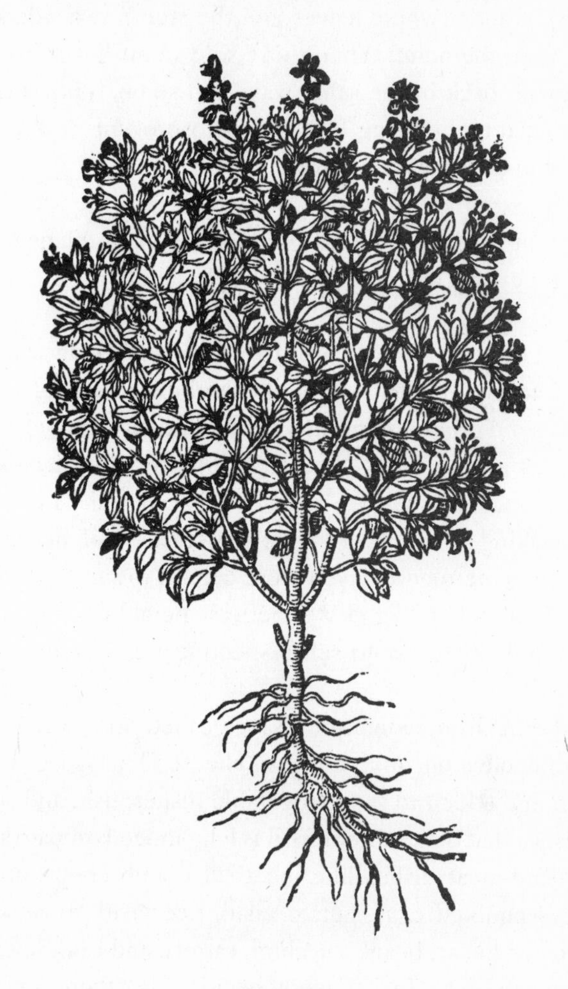

Basil

are certain the ground is thoroughly warm. Or sow seed directly in the ground when it is warm, if your growing season is long.

When the plant has three or four sets of leaves, cut the stem off just above a node (where leaves join the stem); two side stems will develop from the node. When those side stems have several sets of leaves, pinch back in the same way. And so on. This is the way to keep the plant producing leaves and to prevent flowering, which will result in bitter-tasting leaves.

Basil is extremely sensitive to cold. When the weather report even *hints* at frost, go out and pull up the whole plant for one last harvest, for even a touch of frost will kill the plant.

Uses: The main use of basil, by a long shot, is in cooking. The spicy sweet smell and flavor is like nothing else, and it has been known to send otherwise normal people into ecstasy.

Basil has always been popular in Mediterranean cuisines and, because it goes so well with tomatoes, is especially identified with Italian cooking. Until recently, when fresh basil became readily available in supermarkets, you were certain to see a pot of basil on every windowsill in big-city American neighborhoods with large Italian populations, for no self-respecting Italian family would be without it.

It is the main ingredient of a sauce called *pesto*, a thick blend of basil, garlic, olive oil, and parmesan cheese. The sauce is used with spaghetti and added to soup, vegetable dishes, fish, and stews. The list of dishes that benefit from basil is long indeed: tomato soup, bean soup, spiced-meat dishes like meatballs, lamb chops, any kind of chicken, scrambled eggs, potato salad, rice salad, many vegetables (including eggplant, beans, zucchini, carrots, and cauliflower), and of course tomato sauce. In fact, many people think there is nothing that basil doesn't go with.

The scented basils lend an extra note to cooking: lemon basil with fish, cinnamon basil in fruit desserts, anise basil in Oriental dishes. And, if you can bear to part with them, they add an exotic richness and depth to potpourri mixtures.

Other uses tend to be overshadowed by basil's reputation as a culinary herb, but we should not forget to try an herbal bath with basil, or adding it to a hair rinse for luster. Tea made from basil helps with digestion, and it is surprisingly tasty. At a barbecue, throw some basil on the coals after your meal is cooked; the fumes help keep mosquitoes away.

Traditions: In India, basil is sacred. The legend is that the wife of the god Vishnu came to earth in the form of this plant, and prayers of apology are offered whenever it is necessary to cut the plant. Basil water is used to prepare bodies for burial, and a branch of this revered herb is laid on the corpse to ease the travel to the next life. The Egyptians apparently used basil in burial ceremonies also, for wreaths of it have been found in the pyramids. In ancient Greece, basil was well known as a medicine (Hippocrates described how to use it), but it also was believed to have sinister powers, and for a time only the king was allowed to pick the plants grown in the royal garden. The word *basil* comes from the Greek word for king.

There is an old story about basil and scorpions, which probably has its base in the fact that both the plant and the creature thrive in hot, dry climates, and the scorpion would rest during the heat of the day in the shade of the plant. In sixteenth-century Europe, snuff made of dried, powdered basil was a common indulgence, and it was said that a certain Italian gentleman, so fond of the aroma of basil that he used snuff every day, went mad and died, and doctors found a nest of scorpions in his brain. This fable may be the reason that Europeans believed that basil seeds would not germinate unless the gardener cursed vigorously while sowing them.

Bay *Laurus nobilis*

PERENNIAL

SIZE: To 5 feet in container, 10 feet in garden

GARDEN: Sun; rich, well-drained soil; protect from wind; not cold-hardy

USED FOR: Cooking, crafts, fragrance, cosmetics

AVAILABLE COMMERCIALLY: Yes

Description: The true laurel (known as bay or sweet bay) is an evergreen tree that is native to the warm, dry climate of the Mediterranean. The leaves are elongated ovals, about 2 inches long, rich dark green. Leaves of true laurel have slightly wavy edges; if you buy a spice with smooth edges it is probably California laurel, which has much less flavor. Also, be aware that some ornamental plants called laurel, such as mountain laurel in the eastern United States, are poisonous. Only *Laurus nobilis* is appropriate for cooking.

Gardening: Starting bay from seeds or a cutting is tedious and frustrating; much better to buy a small plant at your local nursery. In the warm southern areas of the country, plant bay in a sunny spot that has some protection from wind. Elsewhere, you're better off to plant a young bay in a container so that you can move it indoors during the winter; a semiheated porch is ideal. Leaves can be harvested any time of year.

Uses: Today we think of bay primarily as a cooking herb. It is one of three ingredients of the classic bouquet garni of French cuisine, and it goes well with hearty soups, stew, pot roast, and tomato-based spaghetti sauce. Put a leaf in the water you use for poaching fish, or boiling potatoes for salad; put several whole leaves in the cavity of a chicken to be roasted.

Unlike most leafy herbs, which give up their flavor quickly, bay

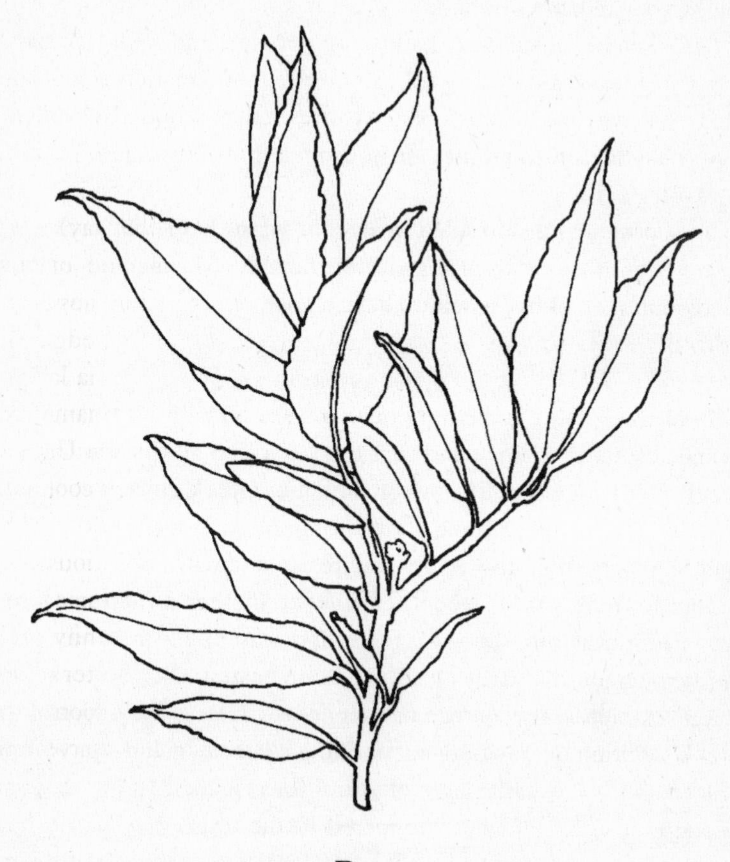

Bay

releases its oil over a long time, and so goes into the saucepan at the start of cooking. Dried bay leaves have more flavor than fresh. But whatever you do, **do not crumble** bay leaves into a dish you're cooking. The leaves are very tough and could cause someone to choke, so you need to remove them before serving the food. If they're in small pieces, they're harder to find.

Bay branches make very handsome wreaths, and a sprig of bay is pretty in a tussy-mussy. In prewar America, homemakers sometimes put bay leaves in the wash water to freshen bed linens, and many kept a bay leaf in the flour canister to ward off bugs; both customs are worth reviving.

To soothe aching muscles, soak in a warm bath that contains a strong bay infusion; it's also good for the skin. Massage oil containing essential oil of bay is said to have a good effect on sore joints and arthritis.

Traditions: Bay is the herb most associated with nobility (notice its species name *nobilis*), and that can be traced all the way back to Greek mythology. Apollo, one of the chief Greek gods, was in love with the beautiful Daphne, but she spurned his attentions. The more he persisted, the more she resisted; finally she asked her mother for help, and to keep her safe the mother turned her into a tree. From that time onward, the laurel was Apollo's favorite tree, and he decreed that its leaves were to be bestowed on any who displayed extraordinary courage or excellence. That is the origin of the Greek tradition of crowning outstanding citizens, including Olympic athletes, with a wreath made of laurel (bay) leaves. In our day, this recognition of excellence is reflected in the terms *poet laureate* and *baccalaureate.*

For many centuries, the noble bay was thought to have magical qualities; people believed it would protect them from witches, evil spirits, and lightning. During the time of plagues in Europe, people carried a sprig of bay in their mouths when they had to be out in the streets.

Bergamot/Bee balm *Monarda didyma*

PERENNIAL

SIZE: 2 to 3 feet

GARDEN: Sun to partial shade; light, rich, moist soil

USES: Tea, crafts, cooking, ornamental

AVAILABLE COMMERCIALLY: Occasionally, in natural food stores (dried for tea)

Description: Bergamot has a shallow root system and sends up single stems straight from the ground, with leaves in opposite pairs and the flower at the top. Leaves are about 3 inches long, oval shaped with a pointy end. The flower is very unusual: individual narrow flowerlets set in a circle around a brown button center; the entire flower head, about the size of a golf ball, has a shaggy, unkempt look—but what a color!

There are more than a dozen varieties of bergamot, and the main difference is in the color of the flowers. The main species is a true cardinal red; varieties are soft pink, mauve, lavender, deep pink, magenta, even white.

Both the leaves and flowers have a lemony-orange fragrance that is very attractive to both hummingbirds and bees. The herb, native to North America, was given the common name *bergamot* because its fragrance resembles the bergamot orange of the Mediterranean, an entirely different plant.

Gardening: Bergamot likes rich soil and lots of water, and will reward your efforts with its stunning flowers. If you cut the flower stalks as soon as they open, often you will get a second flowering later in the season. In the fall, cut the stems off close to the ground.

By the third year, the plant will need to be divided, which is easy to do. Dig up the clump, pull the new plants from around the worn-

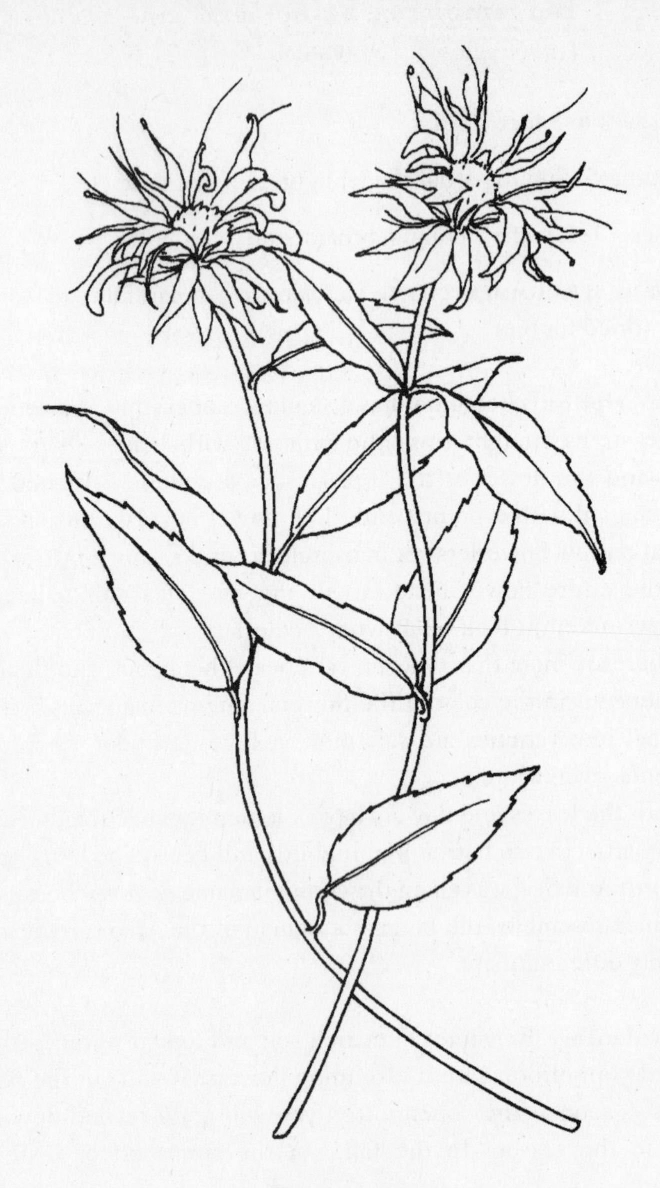

Bergamot

out center, and throw the center away. Plant the babies about a foot apart in soil to which you have added compost or light manure.

Uses: One of the chief reasons people grow bergamot is for its very showy flowers; few herbs have flowers so large or so richly colored. As a bonus over most ornamental flowers, these blossoms are edible. Sprinkle bergamot flowers over a tossed salad for a pretty contrast with the greens; to create a truly spectacular salad, combine the bright red bergamot flowers with the intense blue flowers of borage, another herb.

Bergamot leaves have a light, citrusy sweetness that goes well in fruit salads and jellies, and gives a very intriguing flavor to pork dishes.

Both leaves and flowers retain something of their aroma when dried, and so are a good addition to potpourri. The color of the dried flowers is a bit softer than when fresh, but still remarkable. They make dramatic accent points in wreaths and dried floral arrangements. And of course they are very noteworthy in fresh arrangements and growing in the garden.

Aside from the flowers, the main use of bergamot is for tea, which is described below.

Traditions: Bergamot grows wild in the northeastern United States, and Native Americans brewed its leaves into a tea as both beverage and medicine. During the American Revolution, when colonists boycotted imported—and heavily taxed—tea from England as a symbol of protest, colonists were introduced to this native tea by the Oswego Indians of New York State. The beverage became known as Oswego tea, and today the plant still has that common name.

During the Revolution, a British general named Earl Grey became so fond of Oswego tea that he added bergamot leaves to China tea, creating the blend that bears his name (although the modern product is flavored with essential oil of the bergamot orange).

Bergamot tea is orange-scented and very fragrant, and still makes a delicious blend when brewed with regular black tea.

Borage *Borago officinalis*

ANNUAL

SIZE: 1½ to 3 feet

GARDEN: Full sun; light, well-drained soil

USED FOR: Cooking, crafts, ornamental

AVAILABLE COMMERCIALLY: No

Description: Borage has two characteristics that make it unmistakable: the leaves and stems are covered with stiff hairs that give the whole plant a fuzzy look, and it produces exquisite blue flowers. The stems produce many branches, with heavy flower clusters at the ends of each, so that overall the plant has a sprawling look. The flowers have five petals, shaped like a perfect star that is just a bit smaller than an inch across; the center is black. The plant produces lots of flowers, and the buds are heavy, so the outer ends are always nodding down. Leaves are oval shaped, 3 to 4 inches long, and hairy.

Gardening: The first year, you must plant seeds; ever after, the plant reseeds itself and you don't have to do a thing. In fact, you'll have to be vigilant about pulling up seedlings or you'll be swamped. Plant near strawberries; each helps the other grow. Honeybees love the flowers. Small plants can be grown indoors, and will flower in good light.

Uses: Both the leaves and stems have a cucumber taste. You can use either one to give a light cucumber flavor to cooked dishes to which you wouldn't usually add cucumbers themselves: tomato soup, pea soup, vegetable stews, and so on. Fresh leaves can be added to a salad, cream cheese spreads, or a sour cream dip. For cooking, take the youngest leaves and stems, before the hairs become tough.

But mostly, cooks are interested in the flowers. They too have a

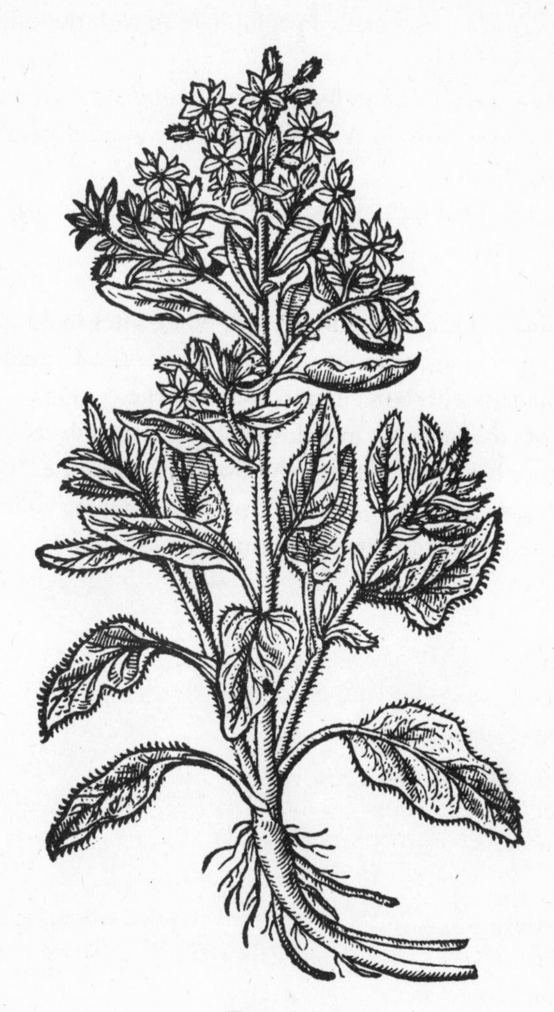

Borage

slight cucumber taste, and can be floated in almost any cool drink or punch. In England they are used to flavor—and to beautify—the mixed drink known as Pimm's Cup. Sprinkle a few flowers over the top of a green salad, especially in combination with the brilliant red flowers of bergamot.

Flowers are easy to crystallize: dip in beaten egg white, then in sugar, dry on paper towel. A very beautiful way to decorate cakes, ice cream, or fruit trays.

The flowers dry nicely, for a color accent to both potpourri and wreaths.

Traditions: Since the earliest days, borage has had the reputation of giving courage; before they left home, the Crusaders were given a wine cup with borage in it. Whether the courage came from the alcohol or the herb is a matter of debate, although there is some evidence that borage stimulates the flow of adrenaline. It was also thought to erase sadness and lift the spirits, and young ladies bathed with borage waters to soften their skin.

Calendula/Pot Marigold *Calendula officinalis*

ANNUAL

SIZE: 12 to 18 inches

GARDEN: Full sun; light, well-drained soil

USED FOR: Cooking, medicine, ornamental

AVAILABLE COMMERCIALLY: No

Description: A small, shrubby plant with long, rather narrow leaves; both leaves and stem are lightly fuzzy. Flowers are orange or rich yellow, 2 to 3 inches wide, and have one layer of petals, like a daisy. This plant is sometimes called pot marigold, but herb gardeners usually use *calendula*, to distinguish from the familiar garden flower known as marigold.

Gardening: Because this is an annual, it must be grown from seed every year, but often it reseeds itself after the first year. If you plant seeds, be sure to thin seedlings. An extremely easy plant to grow, it tolerates almost any kind of soil except a swamp and blooms all summer long and through the cool days of autumn, especially if you keep cutting the flowers. The flowers open in the morning and close at night. To retain color, dry individual petals, spreading out well on screen or drying rack so they do not touch.

Uses: Many people grow calendula just for the cheerful orange flowers, and don't even think of it as an herb. It has an old-fashioned look that goes well in almost any flower garden.

But the flowers are very useful. They can be used in cooking as a substitute for saffron (color, not taste), for example in rice dishes, custards, breads, and cookies. A few fresh petals sprinkled in a green salad make a pretty color combination. The petals turn a rich deep gold color when dried, and add strong color to potpourri.

Calendula contains ingredients that help rough and irritated skin

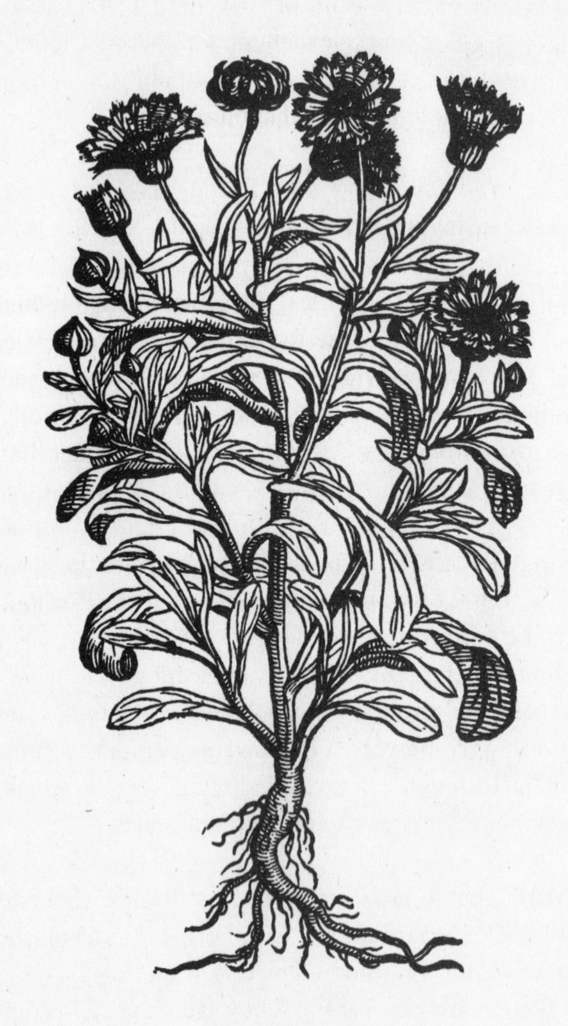

Calendula

to heal, and cosmetics manufacturers add it to many skin creams. Make a strong herbal water from either fresh or dried petals, and add to your bath for smoother skin, or soak tired feet in it. Lotion or salve containing calendula is excellent for chapped hands or sunburn, and calendula vinegar (petals soaked and then strained out) eases toothache when rubbed on the gums.

Traditions: Calendula was used by the ancient Egyptians, the Greeks, and by the Romans, who introduced it into the British Isles and thus eventually to the British colonies in the New World. Throughout those many centuries, it has been used much as we do today: to add color to foods, and to heal wounds and damaged skin. In the Civil War and World War I, it was used to stop bleeding and dress wounds, and patriotic gardeners grew masses of the flowers to be shipped to the battlefront.

One legend that remains unsubstantiated concerns stolen goods. It was said that if a person who had suffered a theft would sleep with calendula under his pillow, he would have a dream in which he would see the face of the thief and the location of his stolen possessions.

Caraway *Carum carvi*

BIENNIAL

SIZE: 1 foot first year; 2 feet second year

GARDEN: Tolerates some shade, but full sun is best; moist but well-drained soil

USED FOR: Flavoring

AVAILABLE COMMERCIALLY: Yes

Description: The foilage is fine and feathery, and very much resembles carrot tops. Umbrella-shaped flower clusters with tiny white blossoms sit at the end of a long stalk. Overall, the plant has a dainty, airy look.

Gardening: Start seeds in early spring, in the place they will stay, for caraway doesn't transplant well. The first year, you'll get only the feathery leaves and a very long taproot; that winter, the foliage will die back, unless the weather is mild. The next year, new leaves will develop and the plant sends up the tall flower stalks. Flowers turn to seeds, which—unless you harvest them all—drop to the ground and start new plants the following year.

Why bother, when caraway seed is so readily available in the supermarket? Because you get to use the leaves, because the plant is a pretty little thing, and because if you really get hungry, Scarlett, you can eat the root.

Uses: Every part of the plant is edible, but primarily it's the seed we use in cooking. It's most familiar in baking: cookies, cakes, and particularly rye bread; also customary in split pea soup, Hungarian goulash, sauerkraut, and pork sausage. Cooked with cabbage, it reduces the cabbage-y smell. It adds a nice touch to apple pie and applesauce, and goes well with many vegetables.

The root can be peeled and cooked like a parsnip. The leaves

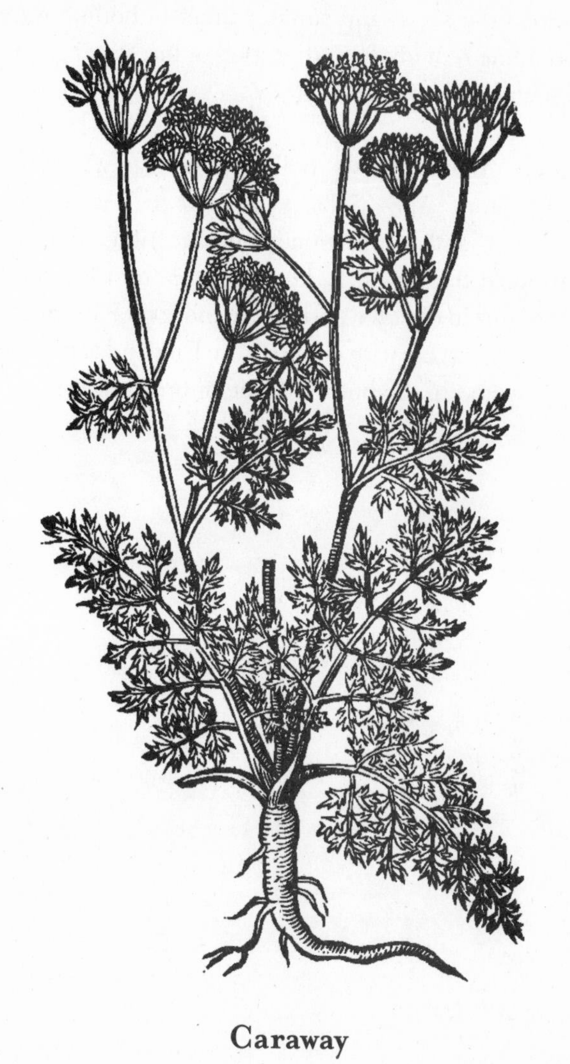

Caraway

have the caraway flavor, but milder; use them in a salad, or to garnish fish. Essential oil distilled from the plant is an ingredient in aquavit, the Scandinavian liqueur.

If you crush the seeds and simmer them in boiling water, you'll have an old home remedy for indigestion or intestinal gas. Chew the seeds as a breath sweetener.

Traditions: Archaeologists believe that caraway was part of meals in the Stone Age—5,000 years ago. It has been found in Egyptian tombs, and is mentioned in the Bible. Because it was believed to have the power to keep people from leaving, caraway was an ingredient in old love potions. In more recent times, a dish of seeds was often served with high tea in England, and in Scotland the custom was to dip the buttered side of bread in the seeds.

Catnip *Nepeta cataria*

PERENNIAL

SIZE: 1 to 3 feet

GARDEN: Sun or part shade; moist but well-drained soil

USED FOR: Tea, crafts

AVAILABLE COMMERCIALLY: No

Description: Catnip is first cousin to mint, and looks it: bright green, oval-shaped leaves with scalloped edges, set in pairs along a square stem, and small flowers tight against the stem at the end of the stalk.

Gardening: Start seeds in spring or fall or—which is far easier—start with a small plant, either from a nursery or from a friend. In either case, after it is established your plant will need to be divided regularly. It is an extremely tough plant, as those who consider it a weed will attest, and will withstand almost any kind of growing condition except waterlogged roots. Or cats.

If you have cats—and you probably wouldn't grow catnip if you didn't—they can roll around in the plant so energetically they completely crush it. Some gardeners compensate by growing catnip in a hanging container.

Uses: You either grow catnip to make toys for your cat, or tea for yourself, or simply for the curiosity of it.

The attraction for cats is well known; catnip oil has even been used by big-game hunters to attract lions and tigers. Dry the leaves and flowers, and sew them into a small sachet (see chapter 17) for your cat.

Less well known these days is its value as a pleasant, lemony tea. You might want to try it as a nighttime beverage, especially after a

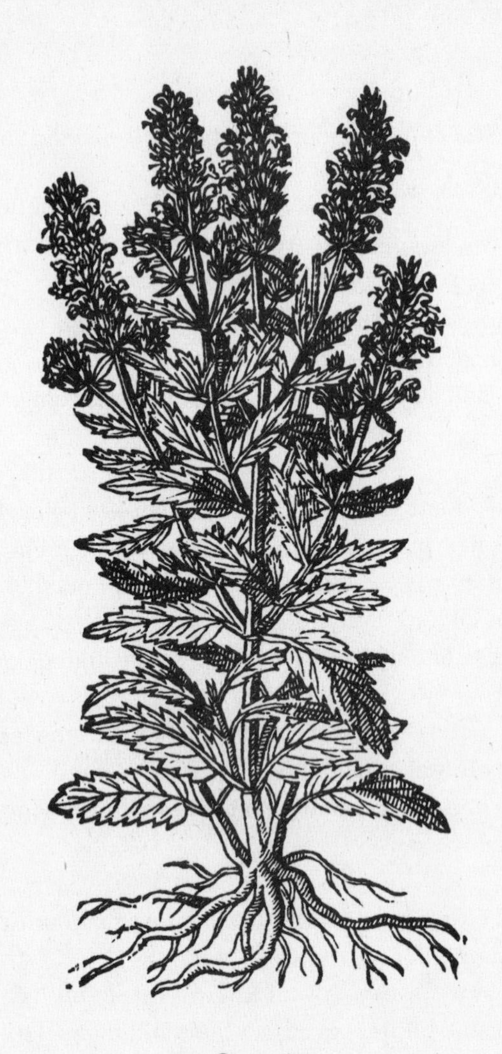

Catnip

hard day; it does appear that it helps people fall asleep. Dry the leaves (they're stronger than fresh) and steep them in a teapot, but do not boil or you will lose the essential oils.

Traditions: Catnip tea is not a new idea. It was prescribed hundreds of years ago, long before anyone had heard of vitamins, for sore throats and feverish colds (we now know catnip contains vitamin C). It also soothes upset stomach, and has long been given to colicky babies. In England it was the favorite tea beverage before black tea was imported from China.

Chamomile *Chamaemelum nobile (perennial)* *Matricaria recutita (annual)*

ANNUAL, PERENNIAL

SIZE: 2 feet (annual)
6 inches (perennial)

GARDEN: Full sun; tolerates most soils

USED FOR: Tea, cosmetics, medicinal

AVAILABLE COMMERCIALLY: Yes (packaged as a tea)

Description: There are two different plants called chamomile. The annual, which is usually called German chamomile, grows straight up; the perennial, known as Roman chamomile, is low-growing and spreading. To confuse matters further, Roman chamomile used to be named *Anthemis nobilis*, and you will still find that name in some references. The leaves of both plants are similar, light green and frilly, and both bear small white flowers that look like miniature daisies and smell like ripe apples.

Gardening: German chamomile must be started from seed the first year, but will reseed itself thereafter if you leave some of the flowers on the plant. Roman chamomile spreads by runners, making little baby plants in all directions. Roman chamomile is a good plant for putting between flagstones on a walk; it readily tolerates being walked on, and in fact is used in place of lawns in Europe. It's also a good plant for rock gardens or slopes.

In both cases it is the flowers that are used. When the flowers are fully open and the petals turn back, they are ready to harvest. Cut the flowers off very short, and spread on a screen or drying tray.

Uses: Chamomile is perhaps the most famous herb for making tea, and for very good reason: it is delicious and very soothing. It has

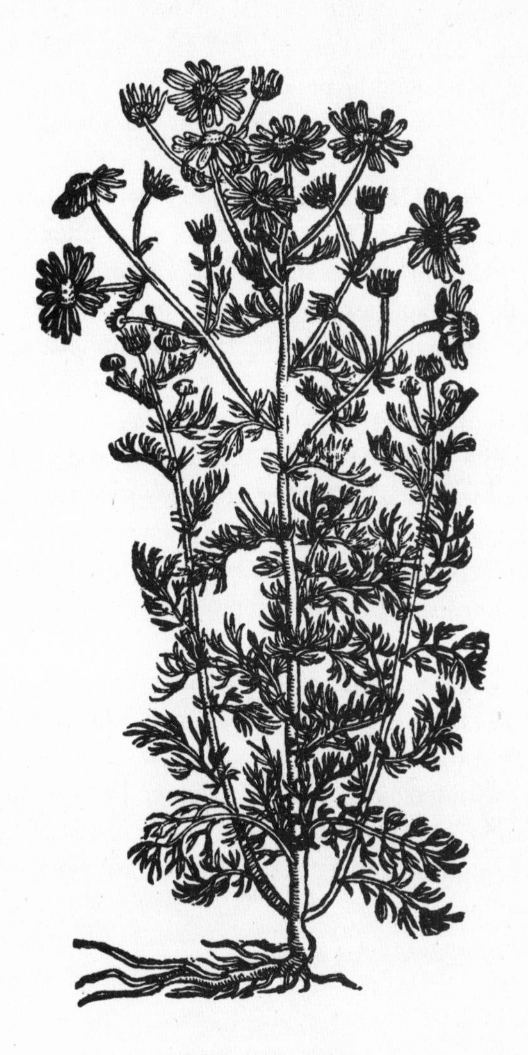

Chamomile

the reputation for helping people fall asleep, especially if they are restless, and it has been used for centuries to calm fretful children. It is widely available as a commercial product, or you can make your own tea from the dried flowers.

One word of caution: the pollen in the flower heads is the same as in ragweed, so if you already know you are allergic to ragweed, chamomile tea is not for you.

Dried flowers and leaves add bulk and a sweet undertone to potpourri and herb pillows. A strong herbal water added to the bath softens your skin and soothes irritated or sunburned skin conditions. Make a strong tea and use it to wash your face (makes skin soft); soak a washcloth in it and lay it over tired or irritated eyes. It makes an excellent hair rinse for blonds or light redheads; it brightens the color and conditions hair.

Chamomile has long been used medicinally, and modern science has confirmed beneficial ingredients; however, today there is some debate about whether those ingredients remain when the herb is brewed into tea. Chamomile oil, in any case, is used for stomach and menstrual cramps, and to treat skin problems.

Traditions: As far back as the ancient Egyptian civilizations, chamomile has been held in high esteem as a healing herb. In the Middle Ages, it was one of the most common strewing herbs, spread on floors as a disinfectant and room freshener. In monastery gardens, it was known as "the doctor for plants," for it appeared to invigorate sick plants and promote vigorous growth of whatever was planted nearby.

Chervil *Anthriscus cerefolium*

ANNUAL

SIZE: 1 foot

GARDEN: Partial shade; light, moist soil

USED FOR: Seasoning

AVAILABLE COMMERCIALLY: Yes

Description: The foliage of chervil looks very much like a fern, and the flower heads at the outer ends of the branches bear tiny white blossoms. Overall, a very light and airy look.

Gardening: Chervil seeds germinate quickly, and you'll have leaves ready for harvesting in two months or less. Sow seeds where you want the plants to be, for seedlings don't transplant well. In hot summer weather, the plant goes to seed too fast, which makes the foliage bitter tasting. So most gardeners sow seeds every few weeks, for a constant supply. One last sowing in the fall will usually produce an early crop the next spring. The plant is hardy and will survive light frosts, especially if you mulch around it. Heat is the enemy; plant under a tree or near large annuals that will provide shade in the middle of summer but let sunlight through in the spring and fall. Because it doesn't require constant sun, chervil also does well as an indoor herb.

Uses: Chervil is not as well known in American kitchens as it is in France, where it is considered one of the three herbs in the classic blend called fines herbes (the other two are parsley and chives). Chervil adds a very delicate anise flavor, and it also has the ability to enhance the flavor of other herbs. Perhaps best known in egg dishes, it is also used with chicken, fish, and veal; in cream soups and sauces; in chicken, egg, and potato salads; and to accent many vegetables, such as carrots, corn, and peas. For best flavor, always add

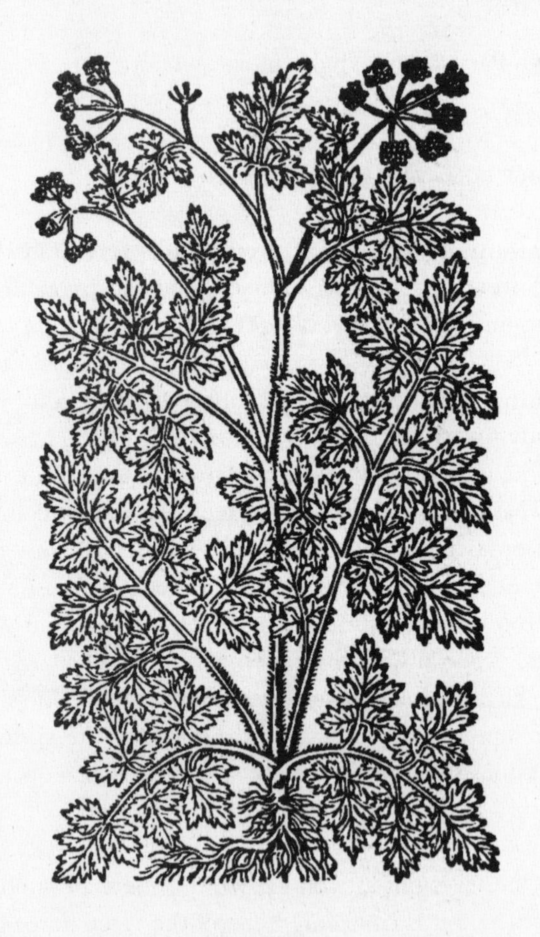

Chervil

chervil near the end of cooking. Chopped fresh leaves go well with cold tomato soup and green salads, and make a pretty garnish for almost any dish.

Chervil is disappointing as a home-dried herb; that's why people try to keep it growing from spring through fall, to use fresh. If you want to preserve it, try freezing ice cubes or herb butter (see chapter 6). Chervil butter is very tasty on broiled fish.

The very pretty leaves can be used in flower arrangements and tussy-mussies in place of ferns (see chapter 18).

Traditions: Pliny, the Roman historian of the first century A.D., said that vinegar in which chervil seeds had been soaked would cure hiccups. Throughout history, the leaves of chervil were eaten as a green vegetable, and for Christians chervil soup has been a traditional dish for Holy Thursday, after Lent.

Chives *Allium schoenoprasum*

PERENNIAL

SIZE: Up to 1 foot

GARDEN: Full sun; light but moist soil

USED FOR: Flavoring, ornamental

AVAILABLE COMMERCIALLY: Yes

Description: Almost everyone is familiar with the long, thin foliage—we can't really call them "leaves"—of a chive plant. But not everyone has seen the flower: a round pompom slightly smaller than a golf ball, mauve pink and fuzzy looking, that sits at the end of a stalk taller than the foliage.

Gardening: Chives belong to the onion family, along with garlic, leeks, shallots, scallions, and regular onions, and like them grow from an underground bulb, although it is quite small. What you see growing in the garden is a clump of bulbs, each of which puts out one or two green shoots. The bulb stores the plant's energy to carry it through the winter, foliage dies down in cold weather, and new stalks sprout in the spring. Bulbs multiply, so the clump keeps getting thicker, and about every four years it needs to be divided.

An interesting variety is garlic chives; it really does taste like garlic but has all the other chive virtues as well. The foliage is flat.

Harvest a chive plant by cutting a few green shoots on the outside of the clump. Always leave some leaves intact, otherwise the bulbs don't grow. For most flavorful leaves, keep clipping the flowers.

It is possible to start chives from seed, but it's much simpler to buy a small pot of plants already started. Potted chives are often found in supermarkets, and they will do reasonably well on your windowsill, although you won't get flowers or the garden's vigorous growth.

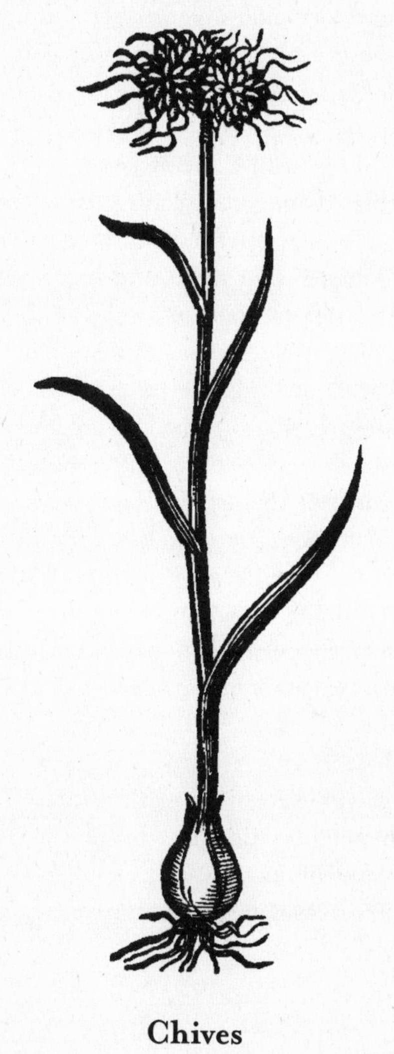

Chives

Home drying doesn't work well with chives; commercial products are freeze dried.

Uses: With their very mild onion flavor and pretty green color, chives may well be the most useful and versatile culinary herb in your garden. Sprinkle them on boiled potatoes, cream soups, scrambled eggs, and steamed carrots or cauliflower. Chop into bits and mix into cream cheese with a bit of lemon juice, and spread on crackers. Cut segments for green salads. Use entire stems as a garnish. For a special dinner, briefly steam long chive stems to make them more pliable, and wrap them like string around bundles of steamed julienne carrots or asparagus.

Chive flowers are edible and make a spectacular garnish. One other way to enjoy them, equally spectacular, is chive vinegar. It's also an easy way to preserve the goodness of chives for winter use. Fill a jar with chive flowers, pour in white vinegar to cover, and let sit for a couple of weeks, then strain. The vinegar turns a beautiful pink hue as it extracts both color and flavor from the blossoms.

As a garden plant, chives stay small and tidy and require almost no work (except dividing the clump every few years). Because of this, and because of the engaging flowers, they make a pretty ornamental for your flower bed or rock garden, and create very charming borders.

Traditions: Chives were used to flavor food in China in 3000 B.C. and were a popular cooking herb in ancient Greece and Rome. It is said that clumps of chives can be found today in the English countryside wherever Roman soldiers camped.

Comfrey *Symphytum officinale*

PERENNIAL

SIZE: 3 to 4 feet

GARDEN: Tolerates partial shade but full sun is preferred; rich, moist soil

USED FOR: Home remedies, ornamental

AVAILABLE COMMERCIALLY: No

Description: Comfrey is a *big* plant, with large, coarse, oval-shaped leaves as much as 12 inches long and a taproot that can reach as far as 10 feet down. The flowers, which are pink or purple, are small in comparison to the plant; they form in clusters at the top of the stem, and droop demurely downward.

Gardening: You can start comfrey from seed, or by taking a small offset plant from the root of your friend's plant. Or buy a small plant from a nursery. But whatever you do, think carefully about where to put it in your garden, because once it is established it's very hard to dig up. Most people grow comfrey as an ornamental, for the handsome leaves and pretty little flowers, but because of its size it does best as a background plant.

Uses: Primarily comfrey has value as a stunning backdrop for your flower garden. But if you happen to scrape your finger or twist your ankle while working in your garden, you can take advantage of its other safe quality: the leaves can be used as a healing poultice. Chop the leaves, mix with a little water, and apply to a sprain, scrape, or cut—any kind of small surface wound. And if after a day in the garden your muscles are sore or your skin sunburned, a soak in a comfrey bath will make you feel better.

Just don't drink it. In the past, many people made a tea of comfrey leaves or made a tincture from its roots, and used both of them

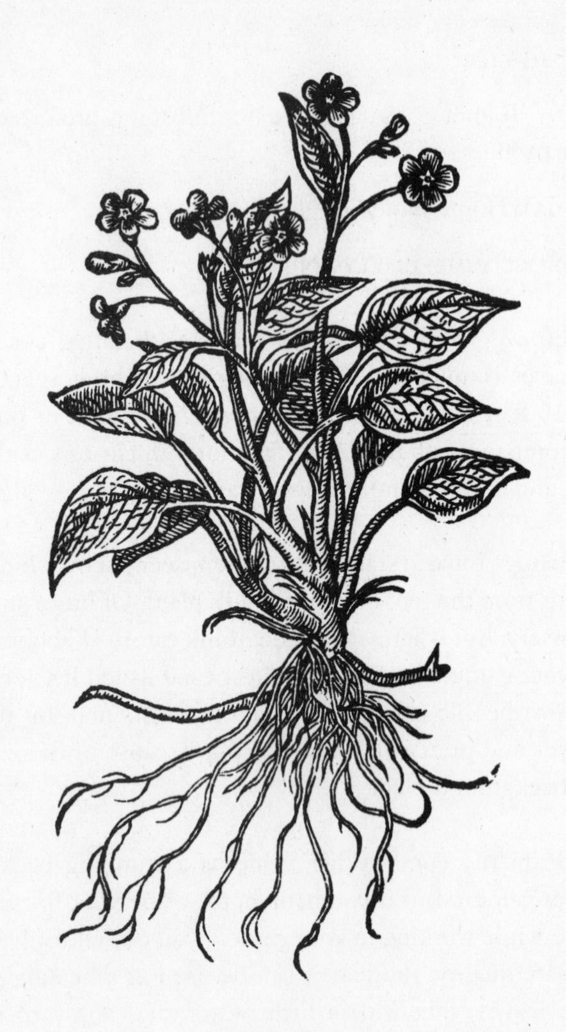

Comfrey

to treat a variety of illnesses. You will still find many books that recommend drinking comfrey tea for all sorts of medical problems. Don't do it. New research has opened the possibility that comfrey taken internally may be carcinogenic; until we know for sure, let's just enjoy it in the garden.

Traditions: Comfrey has a long tradition as a healing herb and has been used as a food for both humans (cooked like spinach) and animals (dried like hay). Old medical treatises prescribe it to stop bleeding, to set broken bones, and to heal wounds.

CAUTION: The safety of comfrey taken internally (as a tea) is now the subject of controversy.

Coriander/Cilantro *Coriandrum sativum*

ANNUAL

SIZE: 2 feet

GARDEN: Sun; rich, light, well-drained soil

USED FOR: Flavoring

AVAILABLE COMMERCIALLY: Yes, both dried seeds and fresh leaves

Description: Coriander and cilantro are the same plant; usually *coriander* is used when referring to the seeds, and *cilantro* the leaves. Actually, this plant has two kinds of leaves; the lower leaves are flat, roundish, and have scalloped edges (this is what we harvest as cilantro); the newer leaves, near the top of the stems, are very lacy and feathery. It produces masses of tiny white flowers in clusters at the top of the stem, which mature into tiny round seeds.

Gardening: If you intend to grow this herb for its production of seeds, plant seed in the ground as early in the spring as you can; you need a long growing season for the seeds to ripen. Green seeds do not have the characteristic coriander aroma. If you only want cilantro, sow small batches of seed throughout the spring for a continuous harvest. Seedlings don't transplant well; direct garden sowing is preferred.

When the foliage turns brown and the seeds are gray-brown, cut off the flower heads and dry them thoroughly indoors (hang upside down in a bag). If you leave a few mature plants in the garden, you may be rewarded with self-sown seedlings next spring.

Uses: Coriander seed is a common ingredient in many, many dishes, and it is widely available commercially if you don't want to grow your own. It is one of the ingredients in commercial curry powder and also the blend known as pickling spice. The hard-to-

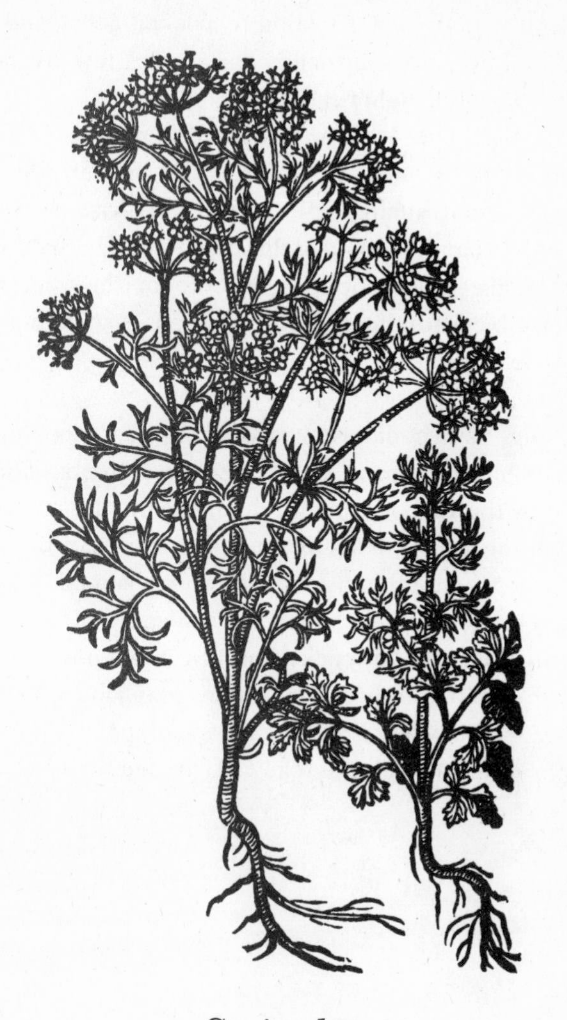

Coriander

describe flavor goes well in gingerbread, cakes, cookies, and sweet yeast breads; in baked apples and fruit salads. It also adds a rich note to poultry stuffing, spicy meat mixtures, meat loaf, stews, and sausage. It's the traditional flavoring for cooked beets, and its spicy tone goes well in many soups and casseroles. A few crushed seeds are delicious in coffee or hot chocolate.

Cilantro—the leaves—has an entirely different taste: spicy, peppery, tingly on the tongue. It has long been used in Mexican and Oriental cuisine but is fairly new to American cooks. As recently as 1967, a cookbook author wrote of this now-trendy herb: "I have met in my life exactly one American who uses them [the green leaves]—a well-known New York food editor." Perhaps that anonymous editor started the trend.

Traditions: Coriander has been used to flavor foods for at least 3,000 years; seeds have been found in Egyptian tombs. The plant is mentioned in the Old Testament, in an Egyptian medical treatise that was written when Moses was a young man, and in *Tales of the Arabian Nights*, where aphrodisiac qualities are claimed. It was one of the bitter herbs for the celebration of Passover. Writing around the time of Christ, Chinese physicians used it in potions they claimed would make one live forever. On a more mundane scale, Romans steeped the seed in vinegar and soaked meat in it as a preservative, and people of many cultures chewed the seed to sweeten the breath.

Costmary *Chrysanthemum balsamita*

PERENNIAL

SIZE: 3 feet

GARDEN: Sun (preferred) to light shade; almost any soil condition

USED FOR: Tea, crafts, cosmetics

AVAILABLE COMMERCIALLY: No

Description: Costmary leaves are long ovals, as much as 10 or 12 inches long, with serrated edges; the leaf stems are also long. The first leaves spring up directly from the roots, which grow at or near the surface of the soil, and spread to form new clumps. In full sun, the plant produces a tall flower stalk with tiny yellow flowers.

Gardening: Costmary is usually started with a piece of root from a friend's plant; it's an old-fashioned plant, one not easy to find in commercial nurseries. However, since it multiplies rapidly and needs to be divided every three years or so, your friend will be delighted to give you a start. After a few years a plant tends to die out in the middle; cut off some of the newer plants at the edges and start a new clump.

Uses: People generally grow costmary for nostalgia, or for the pleasant aroma of the leaves, which is something like spearmint. The dried leaves retain the scent and so are very good for making potpourri. It also makes a nice, gentle tea, and its minty flavor goes well in punch or iced tea.

A strong herbal water added to the bath is relaxing. Because it is astringent and mildly antiseptic, a costmary infusion is sometimes used as a skin lotion, especially for oily skin.

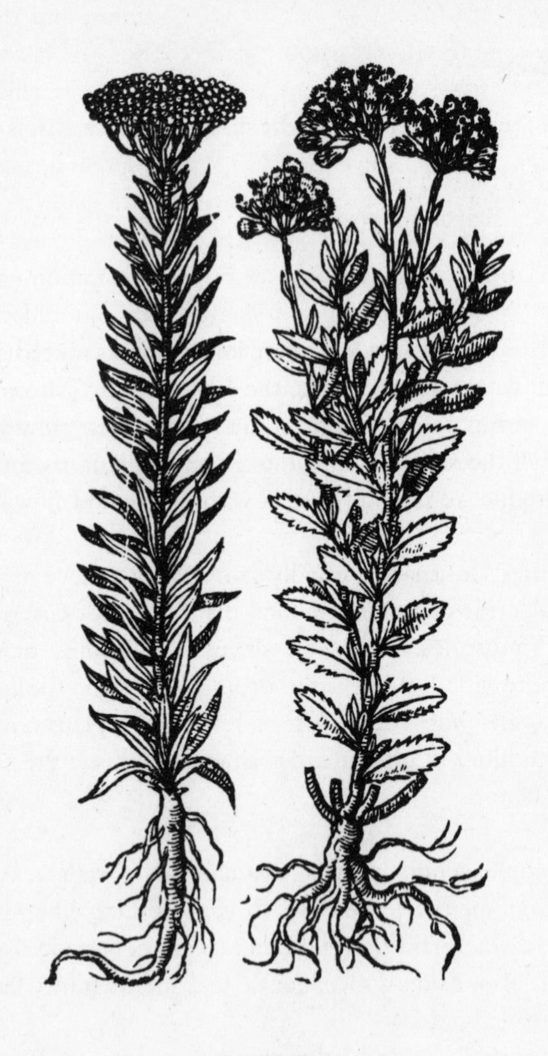

Costmary

Traditions: The name *costmary* means "Mary's herb"; some people believe that Mary used it medicinally during the birth of Jesus. The plant has two other common names, and they tell us much about the traditional uses of the herb. Before hops were introduced to the brewing industry, costmary was used in making beer and ale, for which purpose it was called alecost. In England, church parishes held fund-raising events known as church-ales, and alecost was often grown for this purpose in church gardens.

Having the herb so handy probably also led to its use as a bookmark in Bibles, from which derives the other common name: Bible leaf. Parishioners were handed a leaf as they entered the church doors; in those days of long sermons, parents encouraged children to nibble on the leaf to help them stay awake. In some areas today it is still used as a bookmark in both Bibles and secular volumes, and its scent is said to keep away the insects that could damage books.

Dill *Anethum graveolens*

ANNUAL

SIZE: 3 to 5 feet

GARDEN: Full sun; rich, moist soil

USED FOR: Seasoning, crafts, home remedies

AVAILABLE COMMERCIALLY: Yes

Description: Dill grows quite tall, with one main stem per plant and thread-thin, wispy leaves—in other words, big but very airy looking. At the top, the plant produces a flower head like an upside-down parasol, with tiny yellow-green flowers that ripen into the familiar seeds.

Gardening: Sow seeds early in the spring where the plant will stay, for they don't transplant well. Keep planting throughout the summer if you want a continuous supply; just before the ground freezes, plant one last time and you'll have dill early in the following spring. If you leave some seeds on the plant to fall to the ground, they'll self-sow for next year. The flower head is large and, when it is heavy with seed, the plant can be blown over by the wind. Either stake it up, or plant it in a spot that has some wind protection.

Clip the foliage any time. If you want to harvest the seeds, cut off the seed head when it turns brown, with a long stem section so you can hang it upside down; tie a paper bag around the flower head to catch the seeds.

Uses: The pickle industry could not survive without dill seeds. If you make your own pickles, you will discover that the flower head and the leaves can also be used, for visual appeal as well as taste. But dill has much more to offer than just pickles.

Dill is featured in many Scandinavian dishes. The seeds are used

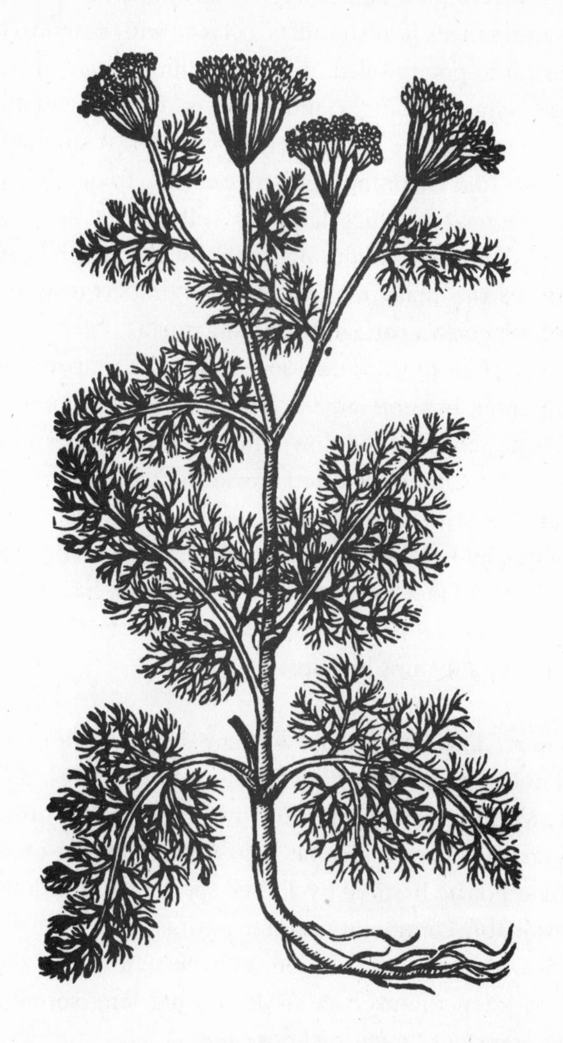

Dill

in breads, gravy and sauces, salad dressings, fish soup, and lamb or beef stew.

The leaves have, to a lighter degree, the same taste as the seeds. Snip them into sauces for fish (dill is a classic with salmon), into light cream soups, into potato salad. Add to cauliflower, green beans, carrots, squash, scrambled eggs and omelets. Combine with cottage cheese and cream cheese and spread on crackers. A summer salad of sliced tomatoes and cucumbers gets an extra zip from dill leaves.

The commercial product labeled "dill weed" is actually dill leaves, dried. You can dry your own, but they're much better fresh. This is one of the main reasons to grow dill: to enjoy the fresh leaves, for both cooking and a beautiful garnish.

Dill is so familiar to us as a seasoning that we may not think of it as an ornamental, but the large flower head is pretty enough to go into fresh bouquets. Cut the flower head before it goes to seed and hang it to dry, for a dramatic dried flower for wreaths.

For a very long time dill has been used as a mild sedative to calm colicky babies and help them fall asleep; simmer the seeds and strain the water. In fact the name comes from the Saxon word *dilla,* which means "to lull." From the time of ancient Egypt to now, people have believed it stops hiccups.

Traditions: The Greeks and Romans believed dill had special powers; Romans wove flower heads into a crown to recognize heroism. In the Middle Ages it was hung over doorways to protect those inside against witchcraft; anyone who carried a sprig of dill while outside could not be harmed by an evil spell. It is mentioned in the Bible as a valuable commodity used to pay taxes. Dill traveled to the New World with the English colonists, who so regularly chewed on the seeds to keep themselves awake during long sermons that it came to be known as "meeting house seed."

Fennel *Foeniculum vulgare*

PERENNIAL/ANNUAL

SIZE: 3 to 6 feet

GARDEN: Sun; very well drained soil

USED FOR: Cooking

AVAILABLE COMMERCIALLY: Yes, in the spice section (seeds) and the produce department (fresh bulb)

Description: Fennel has very feathery, lacy leaves and a broad, umbrella-shaped flower head at the top of the stem, which can reach as tall as a person. If you think that sounds like dill, you're right—they look a lot alike. If in doubt, cut off a stem section: if it's hollow, it's dill.

In botanical terms, *Foeniculum vulgare*, often called wild fennel, is a perennial; people grow it for the seeds, and it comes back every year. There is a variety called bronze fennel because of its very attractive bronze-colored foliage, grown mostly as an ornamental.

There is also a variety named *F. vulgare dulce*, known as Florence fennel. It sends up stems from a very thick, bulbous base that looks a lot like the base of celery, especially if the celery were pregnant. The bulb is sold as a vegetable in supermarkets, where it is sometimes labeled "finocchio." Because the plant is cut down in order to harvest the bulb, Florence fennel is for all practical purposes an annual.

Fennel nomenclature is confusing. The term *sweet fennel* is used for both the bulb type (which makes sense, for the *dulce* in its name means sweet) and the ordinary species. Here we will avoid the problem by avoiding the term "sweet" altogether; we'll call the one with the fat base Florence fennel and the other one wild fennel. The truth is, the licorice taste of the leaves makes them both sweet.

Gardening: Plant seeds where you want the plant to stay; transplanting doesn't work well. Keep soil moist, but good drainage is critical. If you are growing fennel for the leaves and/or seed, plant seed anytime from spring through summer. Gardeners who grow Florence fennel report more success with midsummer plantings. Harvest leaves any time, seeds when they turn brown (watch closely so you can get them before they fall). When the bulb of Florence fennel starts to thicken, pile soil around it (to keep it white) and cut off any flower heads that form. Cut off right at the soil line, and trim away all but the fattest portions of the stem.

Uses: Today fennel is mostly used in the kitchen—as a vegetable, a seasoning, or a tea. All parts of the plant are edible, and all have a soft licorice taste, similar to anise. Traditionally fennel is used with fish; make a sauce with seed or chopped leaves, or place whole leaves in fish cavity when baking or in water when poaching.

The leaves, in fresh form, are an especially pretty garnish for fish platters. They add a nice taste to tossed salads, soups, omelets, potato salad, and mild-flavored vegetables. Add to cooked dishes at the last minute, for the flavor is lost in long cooking. The seeds are used in sauerkraut, in meat stews, in breads, and to give a hint of sweetness to apple pie, cakes, and cookies. The bulb of Florence fennel is eaten raw, chopped into salads, or sliced crosswise and sauteed or steamed.

Traditions: If we are to believe the Greeks, fennel is a very powerful plant. Pliny, the historian and naturalist who is the source of much of what we know about everyday life in ancient Greece, says that when they shed their skin, snakes are temporarily blinded and eat fennel to restore their sight; for centuries afterward, humans drank fennel tea to improve their vision and used it as an eyewash.

Another ancient use, sure to pique interest today, concerned weight loss. Many people believed that fennel was an appetite suppressant; they would brew a strong tea from the seed while dieting, and also chew on the seed to quiet hunger pangs. In more modern times, pioneer mothers gave fennel tea to colicky babies, to calm them and settle their stomachs.

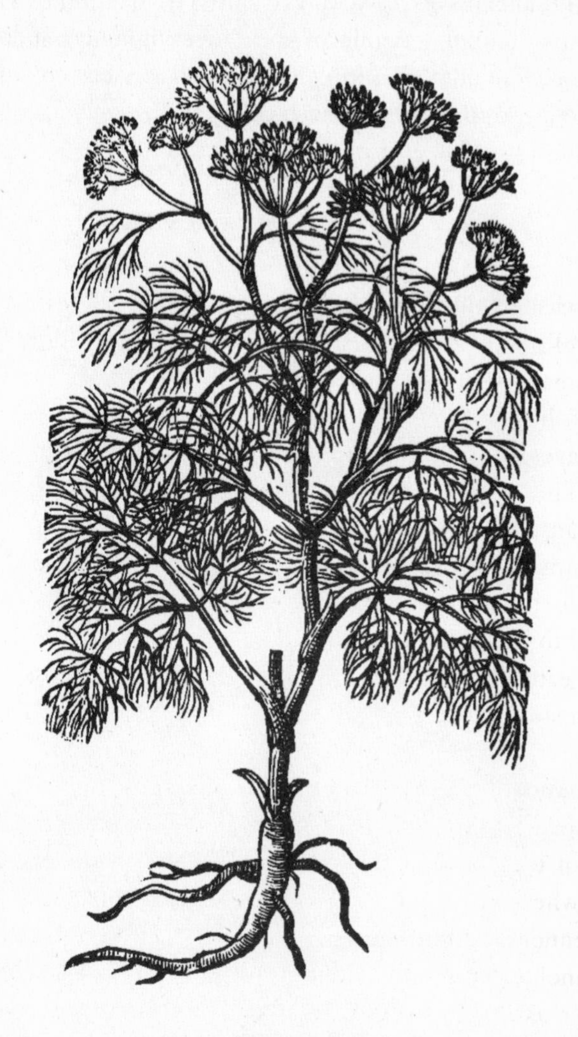

Fennel

In our country, the Puritans believed fennel had the power to protect people from Satan; they would stuff keyholes of bedroom doors with fennel leaves, to keep evil spirits from entering while the family slept. Fennel was one of the "meeting-house seeds": the sweet seeds were nibbled during long church services, to quiet restless children and rumbling stomachs.

Feverfew *Chrysanthemum parthenium*

PERENNIAL/BIENNIAL

SIZE: 2 feet

GARDEN: Sun or part shade; average soil

USED FOR: Ornamental, crafts, medical

AVAILABLE COMMERCIALLY: No

Description: Feverfew is in the same genus as garden chrysanthemums, and if you look at the leaves you will see the resemblance. The flowers, on the other hand, look like wild daisies, but in miniature.

Gardening: This plant grows easily in almost any garden space except deep shade, producing its dainty little flowers from spring till frost. It is either a biennial or perennial, depending on how you treat it. If you leave the flower heads on the plant to set seed, feverfew self-sows profusely, producing little plants that will flower the second year. Plant seed once, and you'll have an unending supply. If you remove the flowers, the foliage dies down in the winter but comes back the next spring.

Uses: Today we grow feverfew for its cute little flowers; they're not showy but very reliable and extremely easy, requiring no effort at all on the gardener's part. They go well in indoor bouquets, and dry very nicely for wreaths and dried arrangements. Cut an entire stem of flowers, then hang upside down until dry.

Feverfew was used in the Middle Ages and the Renaissance to treat a number of illnesses, some of which seem quaint today, but one aspect has current application. Medical researchers now believe that it may be an effective treatment for migraines.

Traditions: The name of this herb tells us its history: it has long been used to treat fevers. A famous herbalist of the seventeenth century suggested it for opium overdose.

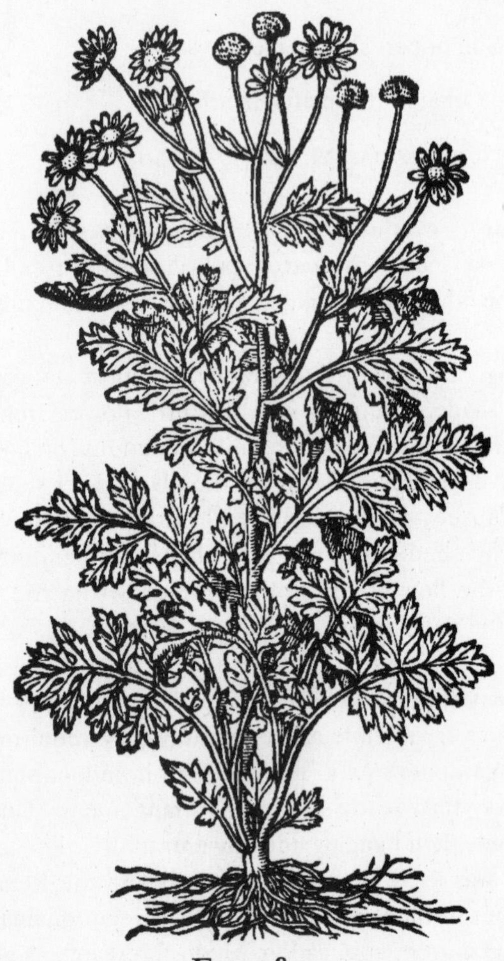

Feverfew

Garlic *Allium sativum*

PERENNIAL/ANNUAL

SIZE: 1 foot

GARDEN: Sun; moist, well-drained soil

USED FOR: Seasoning, crafts

AVAILABLE COMMERCIALLY: Yes

Description: Garlic is a member of the onion family, and while it is growing it looks like an oversized scallion: long, flat, grasslike leaves. The part we eat grows underground as a bulb; each bulb is composed of teardrop-shaped segments called cloves. There is a type called elephant garlic; the bulbs are gigantic but the flavor is much milder.

Gardening: Since garlic is available commercially in so many forms, why would anyone bother growing it? Because it's very easy and quite satisfying. Buy a bulb in the supermarket, break it apart into cloves, and plant each one; each individual clove will grow into a full bulb by fall, and then you'll feel virtuous and thrifty. Also, you can pull them from your garden with tops intact, make one of those garlic braids that costs a fortune in the market, and feel even more virtuous. One final reason: garlic produces a very interesting and very dramatic flower, and only those who grow it in their garden get to see it.

You can start garlic from seed, but it takes forever; much easier to start with cloves. Unless you have a very long growing season, you'll do best if you plant cloves in the fall, before the ground freezes, for the next year's crop. While the green tops are growing, keep the plants well watered. Keep flower heads cut so the bulb develops well. When the leaves look dead, the bulb is ready to be harvested.

Uses: You already know the many ways you and your family love garlic in cooking. A few ideas that may be new: Roast cloves in a

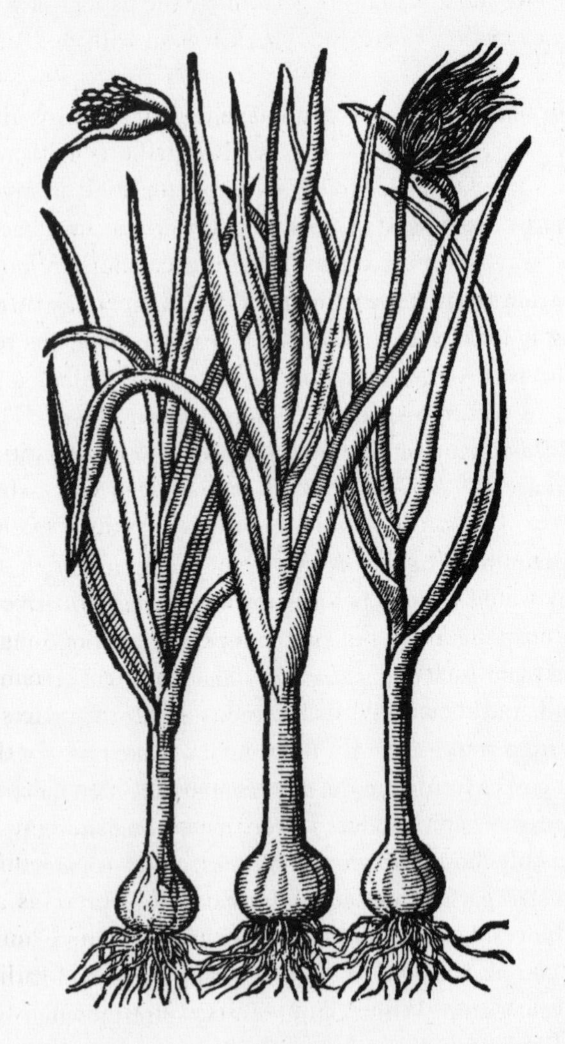

Garlic

325°F oven until they are soft, about 15 minutes, then spread on top of cream cheese and crackers. Cut a clove in half and rub on the inside of a wooden salad bowl. To remove the papery skin easily, lay a clove on a cutting board and whack it hard with the flat side of a large knife.

People who grow roses like to plant garlic nearby; they say it keeps aphids away. The flower head of garlic is a dramatic focal point in a mixed bouquet and dries nicely for dried arrangements.

Raw garlic contains an ingredient that works against bacteria very much the way penicillin does. Modern researchers are now finding evidence that supports other long-claimed properties: that it lowers high blood pressure, cures intestinal worms, and helps to prevent stomach cancer.

Traditions: Few herbs are so surrounded by superstition as garlic. Much of this folklore dates back thousands of years—but not all. As all lovers of old movies know, garlic is essential even now for keeping vampires at a safe distance.

Egyptian slaves who built the pyramids ate garlic every day as their main vegetable, as did Roman soldiers on their long marches across Europe; both cultures believed that it gave stamina. The Greek playwright Aristophanes has one of his characters feed his soldiers garlic cloves so they will have "greater mettle for the fight."

An early Christian legend says that when Satan departed the Garden of Eden, garlic sprang up wherever his right foot had stepped. Throughout the Middle Ages, garlic was prescribed for all manner of physical complaints. This belief in garlic as a cure-all persisted for centuries; in 1608, an Englishman wrote "our apothecary shop is our garden and our doctor a good clove of garlic."

In addition to medicine, garlic was used all those many centuries to flavor food. And Queen Victoria's chef, so the story goes, used to flavor dishes for the royal family by chewing raw garlic and breathing heavily over the food.

Scented Geraniums *Pelargonium species*

PERENNIAL (TENDER)

SIZE: 1 to 2 feet

GARDEN: Full sun; light soil, well drained, on the dry side

USED FOR: Crafts, cooking, ornamental

AVAILABLE COMMERCIALLY: No

Description: These are not the same as the familiar window-box geraniums that produce the cheerful red flowers, but they are related. Their full name is actually scented-leaf geranium, for the fragrance is in the leaves, not in the flowers.

This is a very large group, with literally hundreds of species and a very wide range of leaf shapes. The one thing they have in common is that the leaves are very fragrant—although the range of aromas is as different as leaf shape. Among the many scents are lemon, apple, cinnamon, nutmeg, pine, mint, coconut, and rose (there are more than 50 types of rose geranium). The leaves release their fragrance when they are rubbed or brushed against.

Scented geraniums do have flowers, although they are not nearly as showy as the garden geraniums. Each individual flower is an inch or less across, shaped rather like an orchid and often a delicate pink color. The flowers are pretty, but they are not the reason for growing these geraniums.

Gardening: You will probably buy a small plant from the nursery or a mail-order supplier. In the garden they need sun and rich soil. Botanically, they are perennials, but they are quite tender, so many people grow them as annuals, starting over with new plants each spring. They are often grown in containers so that they can be moved to a protected spot for the winter. It's possible to bring smallish plants indoors—not guaranteed, but worth trying. Many garden-

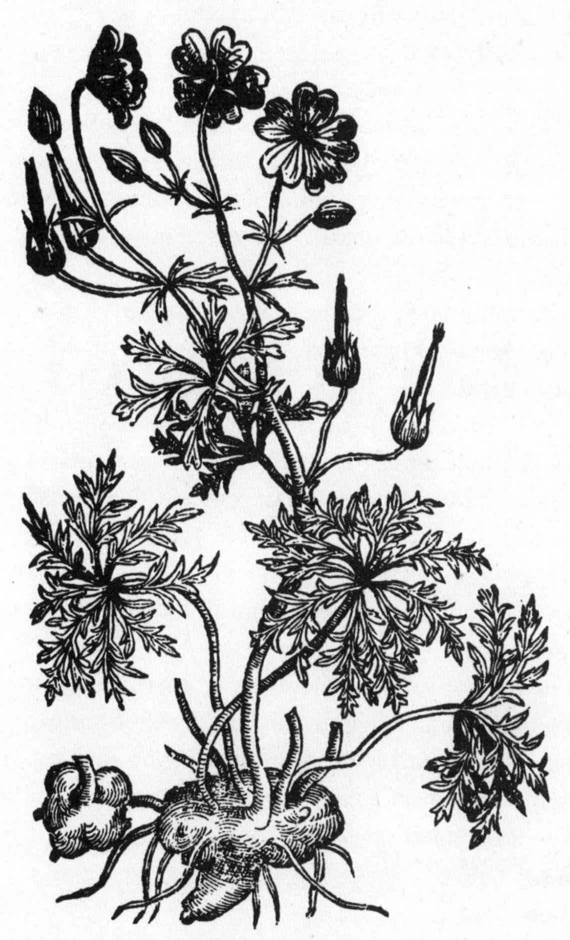

Geraniums

ers take cuttings in late summer, root them on the windowsill during the winter, and have new plants for the following spring.

There are so many varieties, with so many intriguing scents, that anyone who buys one scented geranium soon adds others; trading cuttings with a friend who has other varieties is a favorite pastime for geranium collectors.

Uses: With their intriguing scents, these geraniums are mainly used for potpourri and sachets. The dried leaves lose some of their color and so are particularly appropriate for sachets (where the mixture isn't seen) or as the "extra" fragrance in mixtures with lots of flower petals.

A kitchen tradition that comes to us from the Victorian days is to use geranium leaves to flavor cakes; lay lemon- or rose-scented leaves on the bottom of the cake pan before pouring in the batter. Then, for a really special occasion, make frosting from rose-scented sugar: put alternate layers of leaves and sugar in a jar, cover tightly, and let sit in the cupboard for 2 to 3 weeks; the fragrance will be transferred to the sugar. You can use the same idea with homemade jelly, especially mild-flavored types like apple: put a leaf with a compatible fragrance (cinnamon, lemon, rose) in the bottom of the jar before you pour in the hot jelly.

Dried leaves are used to make tea or, more likely, added to tea blends for their hint of fragrance. The perfume industry uses oils distilled from geranium leaves—especially the rose types. In your garden or parlor, you can enjoy the natural perfume in a far simpler way: position the plants where people will brush against them as they walk by.

Traditions: The pelargonium genus is native to southern Africa, and the plants were brought back to England in the seventeenth century by crewmen sailing around the Cape of Good Hope. When French perfume makers discovered their oils, scented geraniums became an important commercial crop.

Germander *Teucrium chamaedrys*

PERENNIAL

SIZE: 1 to 2 feet

GARDEN: Sun or light shade; average soil

USED FOR: Ornamental

AVAILABLE COMMERCIALLY: No

Description: A small shrubby plant with rich green leaves; the leaves are oval shaped, about an inch long, and have jagged edges. In the summer, flower stalks appear, with pretty pink blossoms tight against the stem. There is a variety that grows low to the ground, used for ground covers or rock gardens.

Gardening: Germander will live in some shade but prefers full sun; any well-drained, light soil is acceptable. Most people who grow germander start with small plants, for seeds take a very long time to germinate. Germander keeps its leaves all year long, but in very cold winter it needs a protective mulch.

Uses: Today we have germander only for its looks: the rich, dark green foliage that can be pruned into a hedge. It is often planted as a border, for it makes a neat little wall that sets off the more boldly colored herbs and flowers. It is especially important to those traditionalists who maintain a knot garden; the classic knot garden design interweaves gray and green-colored plants—and germander is almost always the green.

Traditions: Germander's use in intricate knot gardens goes back centuries. Even earlier than that, it was used as a medicine, principally for gout. As we don't see too much gout these days, there is no modern evidence about this cure. In ancient Greece, it was part of an elaborate formula for a general tonic that was said to

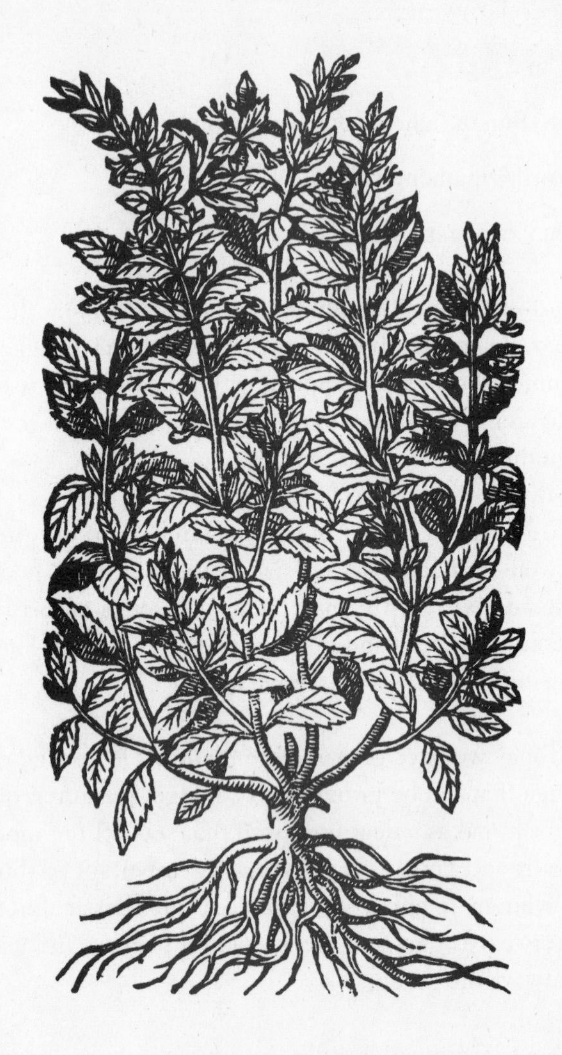

Germander

cure just about everything, including snakebite. Germander and several other herbs were mixed with wine and honey and one other amazing ingredient: ash of viper, which is obtained by burning the skin of a snake. Mix it all up, and eat with a spoon.

Hop *Humulus lupulus*

PERENNIAL

SIZE: 20 to 30 feet (vine)

GARDEN: Full sun; rich, well-drained soil

USED FOR: Ornamental, crafts, medicinal

AVAILABLE COMMERCIALLY: No

Description: This plant grows as a vine; each fall it dies back to the ground, and it sprouts again the following spring. The leaves are shaped somewhat like a grape leaf, but smaller, with each leaf divided into three segments. On the female plant, the flower, which is quite small, produces something that looks like a small cone and contains the true fruit and its seed; most people call that pretty little cone the flower, and so shall we.

Garden: Try to get a rooted cutting of a hop plant; otherwise, you can grow hops from seeds, planted early in spring. The first year, your plant will be small; after the second year, it's a vigorous grower. Plan some sort of support like a trellis, for this vine needs something to grow onto. Cut off the flower cones in late summer, and then cut the vine back at ground level in late fall.

Uses: Hops are used commercially to make beer, and if you are interested in making beer at home, you'll need to grow hops. However, most people use this as a pretty garden plant to create a screen. It grows amazingly fast—some say as much as a foot a day. So if you plant a few vines to grow up a trellis on your porch or patio, you can have almost instant shade in the summer. Then the plants die back in the winter, letting sunlight through when you want the warmth.

We know that hops are a mild sedative, and so the old custom of using them in a sleep pillow has a scientific basis. A tea made from the flowers has the same properties and is good to help you fall

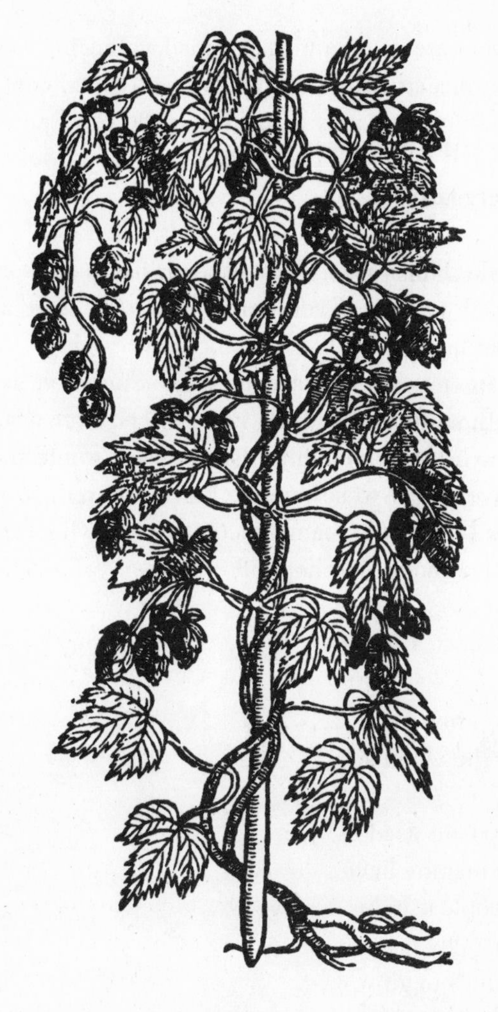

Hop

asleep. The plant is somewhat antiseptic, and a poultice made from the flowers will help reduce inflammations and ease skin infections. In northern Europe, some people cook the young stems like asparagus.

The flowers are quite unusual: small green bracts, like petals, overlap to form a structure that looks like a green cone. With their unique look, they are very attractive in flower arrangements and dried wreaths. If you are a basket maker, you can weave the stems, which are very flexible.

Traditions: Hops have been used to flavor and preserve beer since the ninth century. Even before that, they were an important medicinal herb, prescribed for just about everything. The most classic application takes advantage of their reputation as a sedative. Sleep pillows, stuffed with dried hop flowers, were a standard item for those who had trouble falling asleep; users would sprinkle water or alcohol over them to soften the herbs and reduce scratchiness. King George III and Abraham Lincoln are two who were said never to have been without their hop pillows.

Horehound *Marrubium vulgare*

PERENNIAL

SIZE: 1 to 2 feet

GARDEN: Sun; average to poor soil, well drained

USED FOR: Medicine, ornamental

AVAILABLE COMMERCIALLY: Occasionally, in the drugstore: lozenges and cough syrup

Description: Horehound belongs to the same family as mints, as its square stems show. It tends to grow in upright clumps, and the leaves and flowers grow tight against the stem. Stems and leaves are covered with fuzz; each individual stem has a dense, furry look. The leaves are gray-green and crinkled on top, like seersucker, and the tiny white flowers grow in a dense circle completely around the stem.

Gardening: Seeds are somewhat slow to germinate, but once they are started you will have horehound for life. The plant produces flowers the second year and self-sows enthusiastically thereafter; be watchful, or you'll have it everywhere. The seeds stick easily to animal fur or people's socks, and in that fashion they are carried miles from the original plant. Dioscorides, writing in the first century A.D., said it was a common roadside weed in Greece. Horehound, like its mint cousins, will also spread by rooting wherever a node touches the ground. It grows on any kind of soil and will survive periods of drought better than most plants.

Uses: Horehound—in the form of candy, throat lozenges, and cough syrup—has been used to treat coughs and sore throat for many centuries. Thanks to modern science, we now know that it contains vitamin C, and it also has a high content of mucilage, which is slippery and therefore coats throats made raw from coughing. Even today, commercial cough syrup often contains horehound, and

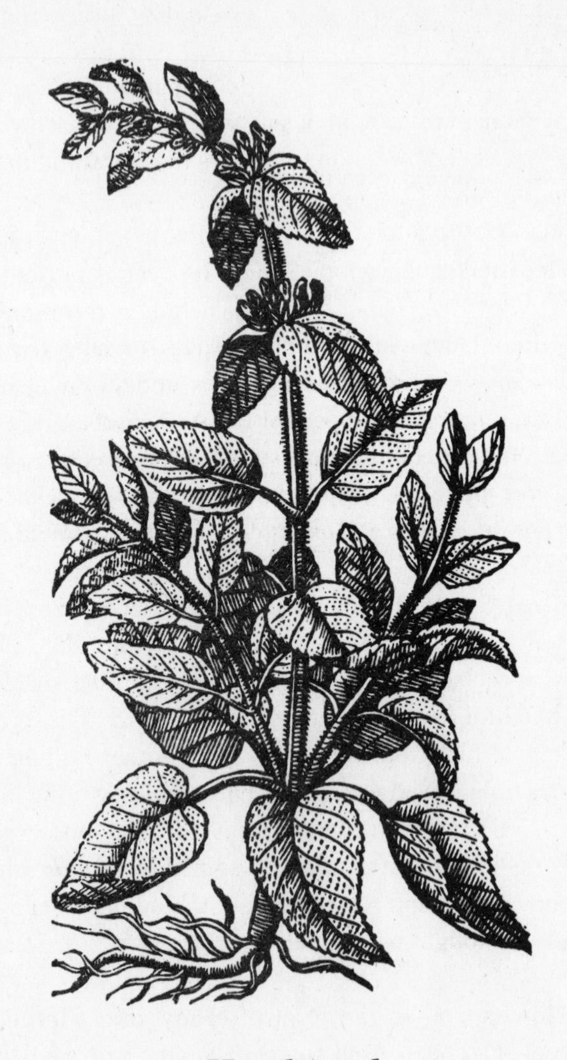

Horehound

up until very recently cough drops made of horehound were sold in every neighborhood pharmacy. Earlier in the twentieth century the Girl Scouts sold horehound candy door to door, just as they now do those sinfully good cookies.

Horehound also has value as a garden ornamental. Its gray foliage provides a good contrast with dark green plants. Bees love its flowers, and every vegetable gardener knows that anything that attracts bees to your garden is a good thing.

Traditions: The Greek physician Hippocrates prescribed horehound for many diseases of the day, including the bronchial and throat conditions for which it is still used. It was also considered effective for snakebite and scorpion stings, and was given as an antidote to anyone who had drunk poison. And it was a good plant to have around if someone had cast an evil spell on you, for it had the power to break the spell.

Hyssop *Hyssopus officinalis*

PERENNIAL

SIZE: 1 to 2 feet

GARDEN: Sun or light shade; any well-drained soil

USED FOR: Ornamental, medicinal, seasoning, tea

AVAILABLE COMMERCIALLY: Yes, in natural food stores, as a tea

Description: Hyssop belongs to the same botanical family as all the mints and in some ways resembles them; most of all, it looks like a cross between tarragon (narrow leaves) and lemon balm (upright growth). The leaves are small and thin but a rich green in color, and the plants are green almost all year long. The tiny flowers are a soft purple-blue (sometimes pink, sometimes white) and clustered in tall spikes that sit up above the foliage like beautiful plumes.

Gardening: You can start hyssop seeds, order a small plant, or take cuttings from a friend's plant. By the second year, you'll have a tidy, compact little shrub. One of the easiest of herbs to grow, hyssop will tolerate almost any soil and will grow in shade as well as sun, although in shade it will get lankier. Cut the flower heads off to maintain a green border plant, or leave them for your family and the bees to enjoy.

Uses: Hyssop should be included in all flower gardens, for—with almost no effort on the gardener's part—it produces its delicate flowers from early summer all the way through to fall. The flowers are favorites of both bees and hummingbirds, and hyssop honey is considered a gourmet treat. This plant is also used quite often as a small border shrub, because it can be regularly pruned and shaped without damaging the plant; to do so, however, means that you must sacrifice the flowers.

Hyssop is less well known in the kitchen, because the flavor is

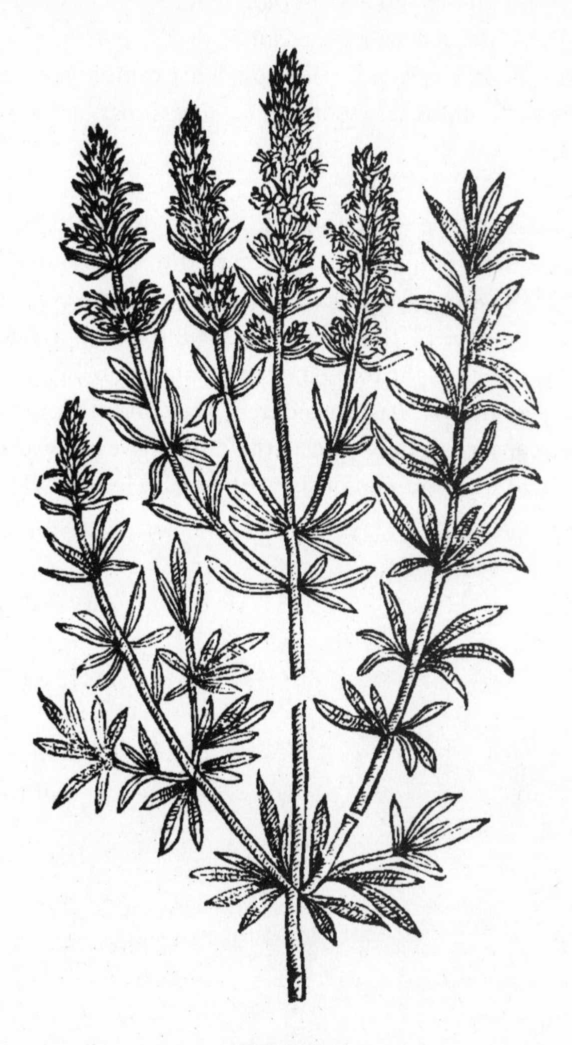

Hyssop

rather strong and medicinal and it's not to everyone's taste. The leaves are most often used in meat dishes such as stews and pâtés. The flowers are edible and add a bright color spot to tossed salads.

When dried, the leaves have a smell that is part mint and part camphor (think of Vicks and you know what camphor smells like), and a tea made from them is soothing for sore throats and respiratory congestion.

Traditions: Hyssop is mentioned often in the Bible, but no one is certain whether the plant that is referred to is the same one we know today as hyssop. We do know, though, that it was used in the Middle Ages as one of the primary strewing herbs, especially in sickrooms; it was thought to be a disinfectant, probably because of its camphor aroma. It was considered a sacrificial herb, used to cleanse and consecrate holy places; the altar at Westminster Cathedral in England was ceremoniously washed with hyssop when it was first built.

Lady's Bedstraw *Galium verum*

PERENNIAL

SIZE: 1 to 3 feet

GARDEN: Sun or part shade; rich, moist soil

USED FOR: Ornamental

AVAILABLE COMMERCIALLY: No

Description: Lady's bedstraw is a delicate plant, with a soft, wispy look and airy puffs of golden flowers. The leaves are small (less than an inch long) and quite narrow, set in circles all around the stem at regular intervals.

Gardening: Bedstraw grows along streams and other naturally damp areas, and in our garden wants the same kind of condition: moist but well-drained soil, rich in compost or natural fertilizer; full sun is fine, and so is a mixture of sun and shade. The best way to start is with rooted cuttings from a friend's garden or a mail-order supplier. The plants soon spread on their own, and by the third year they will probably need to be divided.

Uses: Lady's bedstraw, with its lacy foliage and honey-colored flowers, is a beautiful garden plant, especially in areas where there are also heavy-looking plants with large leaves and flowers. Bedstraw has a tendency to sprawl and spread, and so works very nicely in rock gardens. It adds lightness and softness to mixed-flower bouquets.

Traditions: Along with its delicate look, the main charm of this plant is the wonderful romantic traditions that are associated with it. An early Christian legend tells that Mary used stems of this plant to prepare the bed for the baby Jesus, and that the original white flowers turned to gold when he was laid upon it. From this, the herb was long called Our Lady's bedstraw.

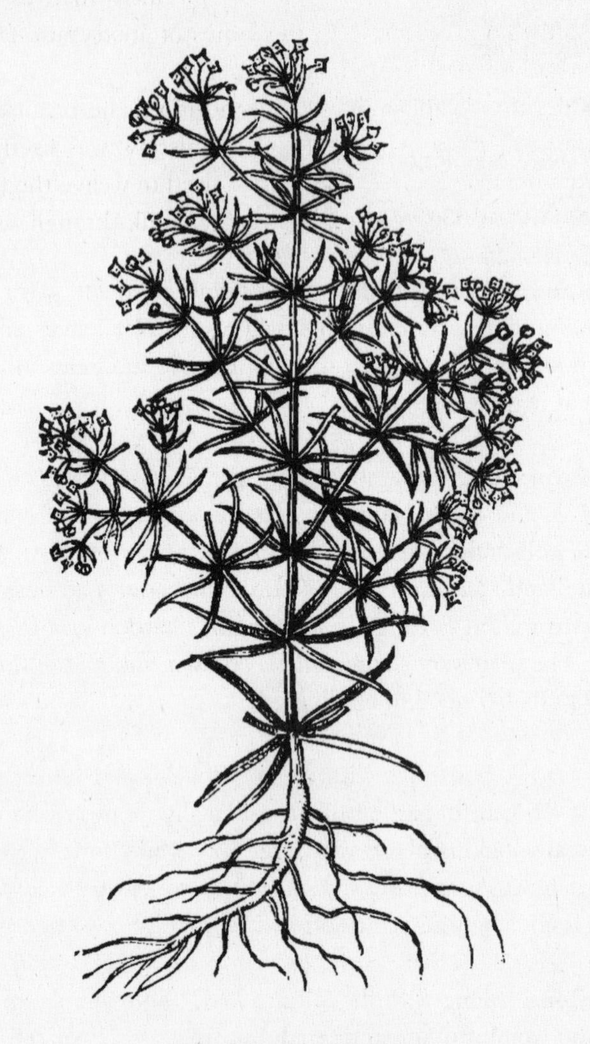

Lady's Bedstraw

Throughout the Middle Ages and Renaissance, it was indeed used as its name would imply: as mattress stuffing. Because it remains springy when it is dry, bedstraw produces mattresses that are very soft; they were used by the ladies of aristocratic families, while men had rougher bedding.

One of the chemical components found in this herb causes milk to curdle, and as early as A.D. 50 lady's bedstraw was used in the manufacture of cheese. Greek shepherds used to weave the flexible stems into a tight basket and pour the goat's milk through, as a first step in cheese making.

Lavender *Lavandula angustifolia*

PERENNIAL

SIZE: 1 to 3 feet

GARDEN: Full sun; light, well-drained soil

USED FOR: Cosmetics, crafts, ornamental

AVAILABLE COMMERCIALLY: Occasionally in craft shops (dried flowers)

Description: The basic lavender plant is a low shrub with many branches, gray-green leaves that are comparatively long and quite narrow, and a tight cluster of tiny purple flowers at the end of a long stalk. More precise descriptions are impossible, for there are literally hundreds of varieties and subspecies: those with pink, soft blue, and even white flowers; compact types that remain quite small; and a wide range of leaf shapes and sizes.

Gardening: The naming of all these varieties has become muddled, and that makes buying a lavender plant tricky. Several scientific names are used interchangeably, and common names—such as English lavender, French lavender, Dutch lavender, spike lavender—are broadly applied to many different plants.

The very best thing to do, if possible, is to buy lavender plants from a nursery that has many varieties, and to visit the nursery when the plants are in bloom, so you can see what you're getting. Next best is to take a cutting from a friend's plant; it will take a while to root, but you can enjoy it on your windowsill in the meantime.

In the garden, lavender likes soil on the alkaline side of the pH scale; if you already know you have acid soil, work in some lime. Early each fall, cut the stems back until they are about one-third the original length; if you don't, next year's growth will be out at the ends and the center of the plant will be bare. Some people find

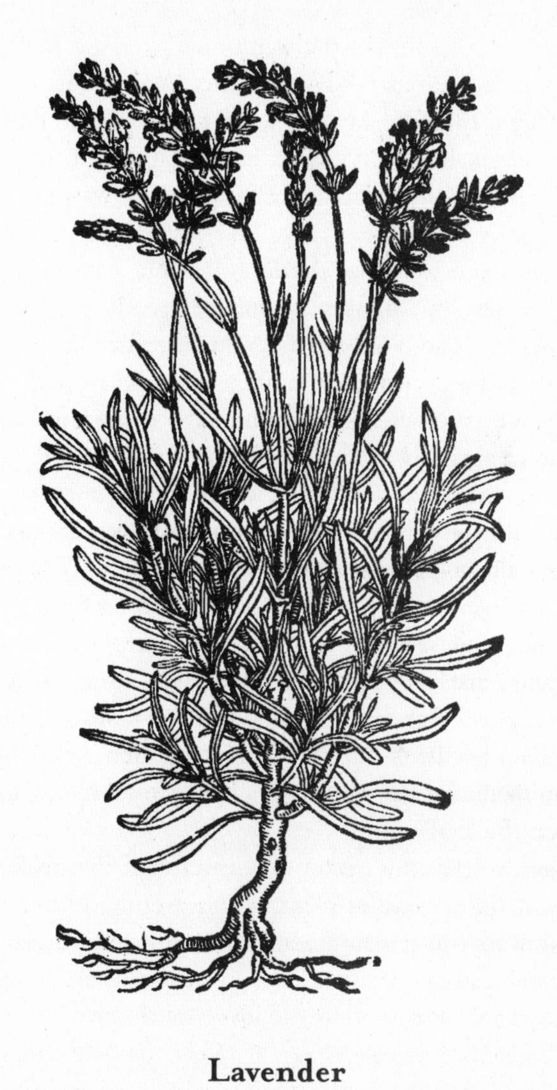

Lavender

that their lavender plants lose vigor after five years, and so they constantly rotate in new plants. Lavender also does well in containers.

The leaves have some of the traditional lavender fragrance, but the flowers have the most; they are at their most aromatic when the first buds begin to open. At that point, cut off entire flower stalks and bring them inside to dry; either hang a bundle upside down, lay flat on screens, or stand upright in a vase with no water.

Uses: I've been told that there are people who don't like the smell of lavender, but frankly I don't believe it. Surely everyone finds the sweet, clean, nostalgic fragrance irresistible. And that fragrance is lavender's raison d'être; it is captured in perfume, soap, and other toiletry products by commercial companies, and in all kinds of sweet-smelling homemade items.

Lavender vinegar is delightful when added to your bath and makes a beautiful rinse for dark hair. Lavender water (made from a base of grain alcohol) can be used as a light cologne. The most common form of lavender is the dried flower buds, which retain their scent for a very long time; in this form it is found in many potpourri mixtures, and pure lavender makes the classic closet sachet, to protect clothes and linens from insects. For those who would like to make lavender products but don't have a garden, essential oil distilled from lavender is widely available from many mail-order sources and local craft shops.

In the garden, lavender is an easy-care plant that makes a good small-sized hedge or border plant, with a wonderful bonus—those heavenly flowers—in the summer. Plant a row of lavender close by your front walk, so that visitors brush against it when they approach your door and are welcomed by the lovely perfume.

Traditions: Lavender was known and used by the ancient Greeks and Romans, who valued it highly and wove it into crowns to recognize outstanding achievement. They believed that the asp (a snake for whose venom there was no known antidote) made a nest under lavender plants; only a few brave souls dared to harvest the flowers, which made them all the more precious.

In the Middle Ages lavender was considered a luxury for aristocracy; satin cushions were stuffed with dried lavender for members of Europe's royal families. As it became evident that the plant was hardy and easy to grow (and not infested with snake nests), lavender became more common, and its use spread to the common folk.

Lavender (the plant) is not named for the color, but rather the other way around. The name derives from the Latin word *lavare,* which means "to wash," and that gives us a clue to its historic use. With its clean fragrance and antiseptic properties, lavender was used to clean the musty rooms of medieval dwellings, especially sickrooms. For the same reasons, it was one of the most important strewing herbs. Through the centuries, homemakers have included lavender in the rinse water to impart a freshness to laundry.

Lavender had medicinal applications too. It was part of the formula for smelling salts, and in Elizabethan times the long stems of the flower stalks were woven into a cap that was worn as a cure for headache. Even today, practitioners of herbal medicine treat headaches with lavender: either a cold cloth dipped in lavender water, or massage oil rubbed on the temples. Until the beginning of the twentieth century, fresh lavender was used to dress battlefield wounds.

Lemon Balm *Melissa officinalis*

PERENNIAL

SIZE: Up to 2 feet

GARDEN: Sun or shade, but partial shade is ideal; moist but well-drained soil

USED FOR: Tea, seasoning, fragrance, home remedy

AVAILABLE COMMERCIALLY: In some natural food stores, as a tea

Description: Lemon balm—also known as balm, sweet balm, and bee balm—is closely related to the mints, and the family resemblance is very apparent. The plant has square stems and leaves about 2 inches long, with a crinkled surface and scalloped edges. In summer, very small white flowers develop near the tops. There is a variegated type known as golden balm, with yellow-splotched leaves.

Gardening: This sturdy plant will grow just about anywhere, but is happiest in areas that get shade part of the day; like all mints, it thrives in moist spots. It grows in a rather haphazard way, sending up stems from a clump at the ground, and like its mint cousins will spread to China if you let it. In winter it dies back to the ground, but the roots are indestructible and will send up new shoots next spring, whether you want them or not.

It is possible to start lemon balm from seeds (although germination is slow), but it's much easier to buy a small plant or get a start from a friend. Once planted in your garden, it's there forever, unless you deliberately dig it all out. Also, if allowed to go to seed, plants in moist areas will self-sow, and you'll have a brood of baby plants next spring.

Harvest leaves for drying by cutting stems anytime; cutting only encourages more growth. Tie in bundles and hang to dry.

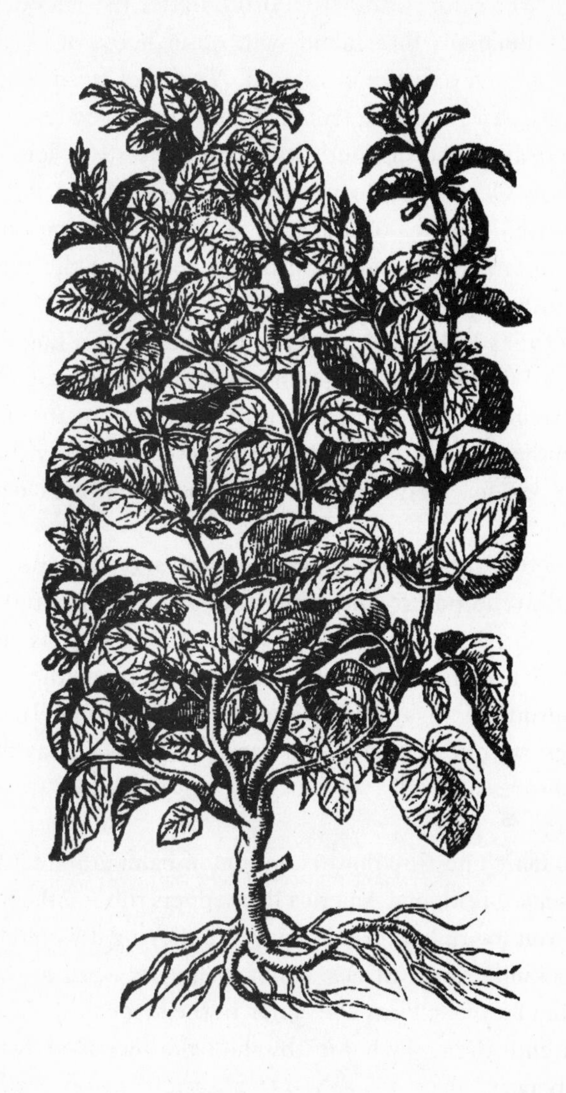

Lemon Balm

Uses: Lemon balm makes a wonderful minty/lemony tea that is delicious hot or cold; fresh leaves make better tea than dried. It is particularly delicious in a blend with other herbs or as a lemony addition to punch or other beverages. A sprig of fresh lemon balm leaves is nice as a garnish in lemonade or regular iced tea.

When cooking, use this herb wherever the taste of lemon would be appealing. Chop a few leaves and sprinkle in fish dishes. Add to stuffings for chicken, to fruit salads, to rice. Old recipe books suggest putting one lemon balm leaf in the bottom of the canning jar when putting up pear butter.

For centuries lemon balm tea has been used as a home remedy for colds and flu. A French liqueur known as *eau de melisse* is made from lemon balm; the original patent for this fragrant drink was granted to the Carmelite friars by Louis XIV. Originally the cordial was produced for medicinal purposes, particularly as a cure for headache.

The dried leaves retain their fragrance and so are a common ingredient in potpourri and other items using scented blends. Added to the bathwater, it soothes the skin as well as the spirit. Another old use that still makes sense today: rub the leaves on wooden furniture for a natural lemony furniture oil. Try rubbing fresh sprigs on your picnic table to keep mosquitoes away from your summertime feasts.

Traditions: The tiny flowers on lemon balm are great favorites of honeybees. In colonial America beekeepers rubbed the insides of the hive covers with lemon balm leaves, believing it would keep the bees from flying away. In fact lemon balm has been grown for its nectar for 2,000 years; Pliny the Elder, in the first century A.D., wrote that bees "find their way home" by the balm fragrance "when they are strayed away."

The medicinal value of lemon balm was well respected. Crushed leaves were mixed into a poultice for insect bites and skin injuries. An herbalist in the seventeenth century wrote that if taken every morning (as a tea, presumably), it would "renew youth, strengthen the brain, and prevent baldness." It was widely believed that balm tea would cure depression and melancholy and raise the spirits; an old Arab saying claims that it "makes the heart merry." Balm is known as the herb of sympathy. The oil distilled from the plant, still an ingredient in many perfumes, was often used ceremonially; Shakespeare's characters speak of being "anointed with balm."

It was the custom in ancient Rome to rub a guest's chair with sweet-smelling herbs just before the guest arrived, to drive away evil spirits (not incidentally, the aromas also helped disguise body odors). Lemon balm was a favorite for this use, which continued into the eighteenth century; and for the same reasons balm was one of the favorite strewing herbs.

Lemon Verbena *Aloysia triphylla*

PERENNIAL

SIZE: 2 to 10 feet, depending on climate

GARDEN: Full sun; rich, well-fertilized soil, kept moist

USED FOR: Tea, seasoning, crafts, cosmetics

AVAILABLE COMMERCIALLY: Tea, in natural food stores

Description: In South America, its native home, lemon verbena grows as a large shrub or small tree. In southern California, it is grown as an outdoor hedge; in the rest of the country, it is generally a container plant, so it can be moved indoors for winter protection, and in containers it stays much smaller. The leaves are long and narrow, dark green, and attached to the stem in sets of three (*triphylla* means "three leaf"). There is a stretch of bare stem between the leaf sets, giving a rather sparse look to the plant overall. The flowers are very tiny, set on airy branches at the ends of the stems.

Gardening: Everywhere but extremely mild climates, lemon verbena is generally grown in a large pot or tub, so that it can be more easily moved indoors in winter. Some people, in fact, grow it as a houseplant year-round. Outdoors in the summer, it grows rapidly during the hot weather, especially if you can keep it against a south wall.

When the weather starts to turn cold, move the plant inside; an enclosed porch or garden room would be fine. The leaves may very well drop off—but don't panic. Lemon verbena is deciduous, which means it loses its leaves every fall, just like oak trees. But never fear, new leaves will sprout in the spring. During the dormant period in winter cut way back on the watering, but don't let the root system go completely dry.

In February or March, cut the stems back to about 6 inches high, so you'll have a bushy plant when it begins to leaf out. While it's

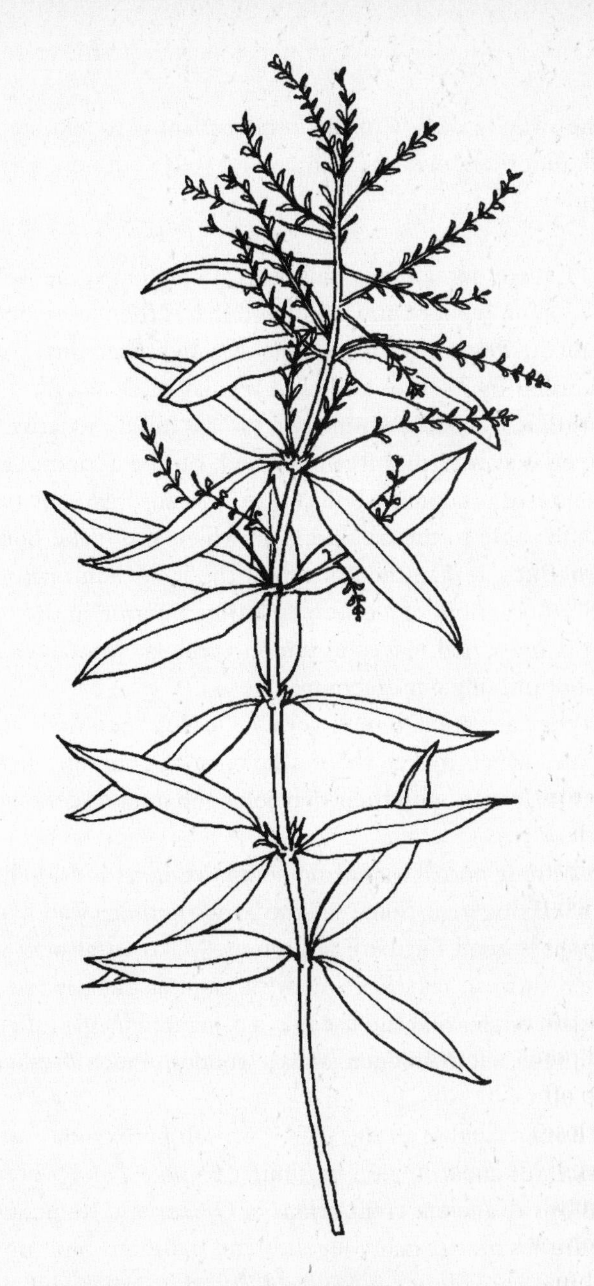

Lemon Verbena

actively growing, lemon verbena needs organic fertilizer and moist soil.

Another way to deal with this tender plant is to take cuttings in early fall, root them over the winter, and start with new baby plants in the spring.

Uses: Except for lemons themselves, lemon verbena has the strongest lemon scent of any plant, and that is the reason people are so fond of it. The dried leaves make a light, lemony tea, to be enjoyed either by itself or added to regular black tea for a layer of lemon taste. It's a good bedtime tea, for it is mildly sedative.

Chopped leaves, either fresh or dried, can be added to any dish where the taste of lemon would fit: fruit salads, fish, chicken, fruit punch. Add some to the custard from which you make homemade ice cream. Put a leaf in the bottom of the jars when making apple jelly, or in the bottom of a cake pan before pouring in the batter. If you have a few dried leaves of lemon verbena, you never need to worry about running out of lemons.

When they are dried, lemon verbena leaves keep their aroma for a long time, which makes them a favorite of potpourri and sachet makers. The leaves, with their rich color and lemon scent, go nicely in tussy-mussies.

Make a strong herbal water from lemon verbena and add it to your bath for a relaxing soak. Some say the lemon verbena water, used as a mouthwash, is good for teeth and gums. Make an alcohol infusion (fill a jar with fresh leaves, cover with grain alcohol, let sit for two weeks, strain out leaves) and use it as a cologne. Vinegar infused with lemon verbena, set in an open jar, is a wonderful room freshener.

Traditions: Almost all the plants we call herbs today are native to the Mediterranean region or similar climates, and were known and used by the ancient civilizations of Greece and Rome. Over the many centuries of use, many legends and traditions built up around them. Later, as explorers discovered and then colonized the New World, the plants and their history were transported to America.

But not lemon verbena—it was already here. This plant, which is native to South America, was discovered by Spanish explorers and taken back to Europe in the seventeenth century. In the history of herbs, three hundred years is a short time, not long enough for folklore to develop.

Lovage *Levisticum officinale*

PERENNIAL

SIZE: To 6 feet

GARDEN: Sun or part shade; moist, rich soil

USED FOR: Cooking, medicinal

AVAILABLE COMMERCIALLY: No

Description: Lovage sends up tall stalks from its roots each spring; by late summer, there are dusty yellow flower clusters, shaped like parasols, which develop into seed heads. In winter the plant dies to the ground, only to return the following spring. The leaves look very much like the leaves of celery, except larger and darker green.

Gardening: One small piece of root will grow into a tall, bushy clump, and one clump produces all the lovage that most families need. Therefore, the best thing is to buy a small plant at a nursery, or get a friend to give you a root cutting in the spring just as the new shoots are starting (make sure it has at least one green bud). Plant it in rich soil to which you have added compost or organic fertilizer, and keep it watered.

Harvest the leaves anytime, but wait for the second year to cut stalks or harvest pieces of root. The seeds dry on the plant and will self-sow unless you clip off the seed head, which you will want to do anyway since the seeds are so useful in the kitchen.

Uses: Every part of the plant is used—leaves, stems, seeds, and root—and every part has the same taste: like celery with spicy-sweet undertones. We could say it's a substitute for celery, but actually it's better, because it's much easier to grow and stays in the garden for a long season; if you've ever uncovered a yucky brown mass of old celery in your refrigerator, you'll be glad you have lovage growing outside in the garden.

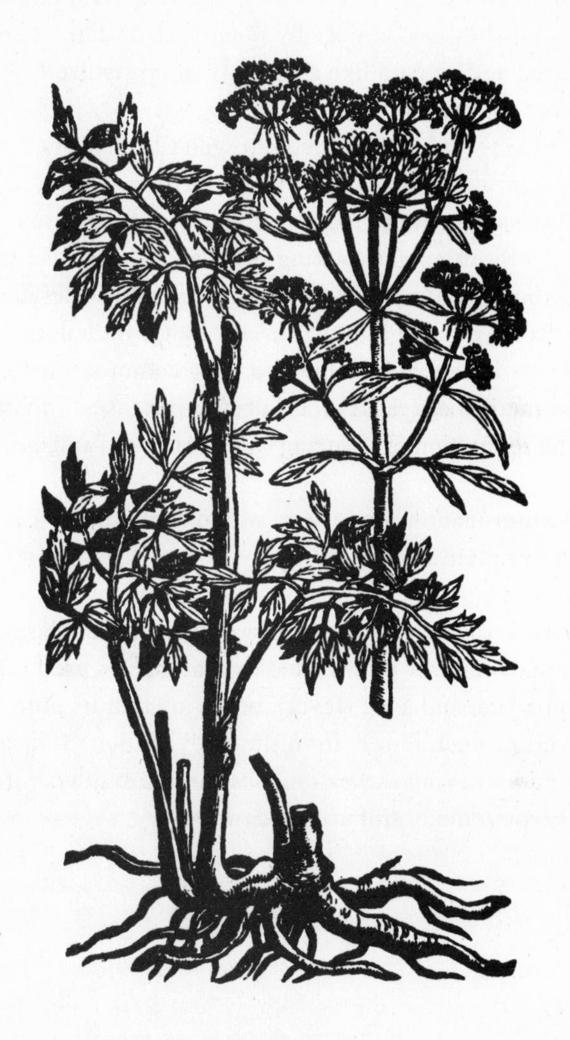

Lovage

The leaves are good fresh in green salads; some people steam the larger leaves as a vegetable, like spinach. Both leaves and stalks, chopped fine, go well in soups, stews, chicken salad, poultry stuffing, seafood dishes, and especially potato salad. The young stems can be peeled and cooked like asparagus, or crystallized for a sweet snack or cake decoration.

Seeds, either whole or crushed, are good in biscuits and homemade bread, in soups, stews, and vegetable dishes. They are a main ingredient in salt-free herb blends, and can be used to make a tasty vegetable broth either for cooking or drinking. Because the seeds dry easily, you can have a year-round source of this celerylike flavor.

An old cookbook suggests that lovage root, candied, can be used instead of crystallized ginger, but the more common use of the root is to make medicinal tea. It is a diuretic (increases urination) and thus has the reputation of reducing water retention and easing flatulence.

Herbal water made from lovage, added to the bath, is said to be soothing for irritated skin.

Traditions: In the past, lovage was more often thought of in medicinal than culinary terms. Medieval herbalists used it for jaundice, rheumatism, and ague (fever), believing that its diuretic properties served to flush illness from the body. Serious skin problems were treated by having the patient soak in a tub filled with lovage water—a home remedy still used today.

Marjoram *Origanum majorana*

PERENNIAL/ANNUAL

SIZE: 1 to 2 feet

GARDEN: Sun; rich soil

USED FOR: Seasoning, home remedies

AVAILABLE COMMERCIALLY: Yes

Description: Marjoram is a small bushy plant with sweetly pungent small leaves and tiny white flowers. The *origanum* genus is important to herb lovers, for it contains both oregano and several kinds of marjoram.

This is another case of confusing nomenclature. The herb that is most used for cooking is *O. majorana,* known as sweet marjoram or knotted marjoram; the common name "marjoram" is derived from the species name, probably the result of the medieval equivalent of a typographical error. It is called "sweet" because the aroma does have a kind of sweetness, and "knotted" because the flowers look like little green embroidery knots.

Two other members of the genus are *O. onites,* called pot marjoram, which is often grown in a hanging basket on patios or even indoors; and *O. vulgare,* known as wild oregano. And that's where the confusion comes in. If you buy a jar labeled "oregano" it might be *Origanum vulgare,* or any one of several subspecies, or possibly even a different genus altogether (see separate entry on oregano). Marjoram is a lot like oregano, but milder and sweeter.

Gardening: Although it is technically a perennial, sweet marjoram is a tender plant that will live through only the mildest winters; in most of the country, it is grown as an annual. Start seeds in the spring; they are very tiny and slow to germinate, so you may prefer to start with a small plant. It grows best in full sun and well-drained soil, on the dry side. Cut stems from the plant throughout the sum-

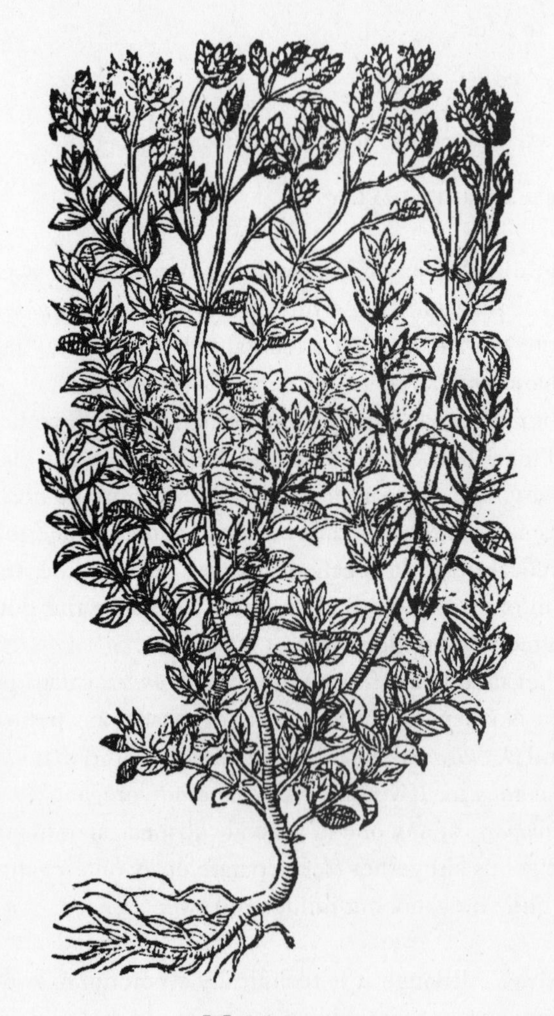

Marjoram

mer, to maintain a bushy shape. The leaves dry wonderfully, retaining the characteristic fragrance.

Uses: Although it still has its place as a home remedy, mainly for colds and sinus congestion (taken as a tea), sweet marjoram is found primarily in the kitchen these days. Its sweet/spicy flavor goes well with many, many foods: hamburgers, meat loaf, stews, chicken pot pie, fish dishes, cottage cheese, scrambled eggs, and many vegetables, including cabbage, peas, carrots, and beans. Add to tomato juice, to clam chowder, and almost any kind of soup. It is a common flavoring for sausage, especially in Germany, where it is known as *Wurstkraut*, or "sausage herb."

Marjoram vinegar (steep leaves in vinegar for two weeks, then strain) is delicious on salads. The classic herb mixture known as bouquet garni usually has marjoram, parsley, thyme, and bay leaf. In fact marjoram is so versatile, and so delicious, it's hard to imagine cooking without it.

Traditions: Marjoram and wild oregano grow along the rocky slopes of Greece and southern Italy, and so these herbs appear in Greek and Roman writings dating back several thousand years, sometimes as medical prescriptions and sometimes as pure legends.

Two myths have grown up to explain how marjoram was created. One concerns the goddess of love. One day Venus (or Aphrodite, as she was known in Greek mythology) was accidentally shot in the arm by one of Cupid's arrows. She could not find at hand any of the healing herbs to stop the bleeding, so she commanded another to spring up, and that was marjoram. Unfortunately, in her anxious state she gave the new plant the wrong power, and her wound, instead of healing, became more inflamed with Cupid's poison; Venus fell in love with the next man she saw. From this came the tradition of marjoram as a love herb; it was believed to have the power to attract the attention of one's beloved, and garlands woven from it were used in wedding ceremonies.

The other myth has a darker side. It seems that a young page in the court of the king of Cyprus stumbled one day while carrying a jar of precious perfume. The jar shattered, and the terrified young man, fearing that he would be killed instantly, fainted and fell to the ground. A sympathetic god, observing his plight, saved the doomed young man by changing him to a fragrant plant—sweet marjoram. From that day, marjoram was planted on grave sites, to comfort and soothe the dead.

In medieval times, sweet marjoram was one of the most common strewing herbs used to freshen rooms, and was added to potpourri (it still is, in fact). Sprigs of the herb were stored with clothes and linens, to keep them smelling sweet and deter moths. But mostly it was used medicinally, to treat a whole catalog of illnesses, from toothache to melancholy. A medical book published in 1597 suggests marjoram tea for those who are "given to overmuch sighing."

Marsh Mallow *Althaea officinalis*

PERENNIAL

SIZE: 4 to 6 feet

GARDEN: Sun; damp soil

USED FOR: Medicinal

AVAILABLE COMMERCIALLY: No

Description: Marsh mallow is a tall plant with a very long root; leaves are triangular shaped and covered with fine hairs that make the leaves feel like velvet. Flowers are pale pink or white, about an inch across, and set tight in against the leaves near the top of the stalks. This plant is related to cotton and to garden hollyhocks, which it somewhat resembles.

Gardening: Marsh mallow grows in marshes, as its name suggests, and salt marshes at that. This tells us that in the garden it prefers soil that is damp, and it likes sun. Given those conditions, the plant will thrive; after all, any plant that lives in salty soil must be very hardy. A piece of root from an established plant is enough to start a new plant; the best time to make a root cutting is in the fall, after the stalks have died back.

Uses: All parts of the marsh mallow plant contain a thick substance called mucilage, which is both sticky and slippery, somewhat like the glue you used in grade school. It is very soothing to irritated tissues, especially mucous membranes. Marsh mallow preparations are used both externally and internally. Leaves and flowers are made into a poultice for skin injuries or a healing tea for sore throats and chest congestion; mostly, though, the roots are used, for they have the highest mucilage content. Many home remedies start by boiling the peeled roots to release the mucilage; the roots also have a high content of starch, which rises to the surface and is easily skimmed

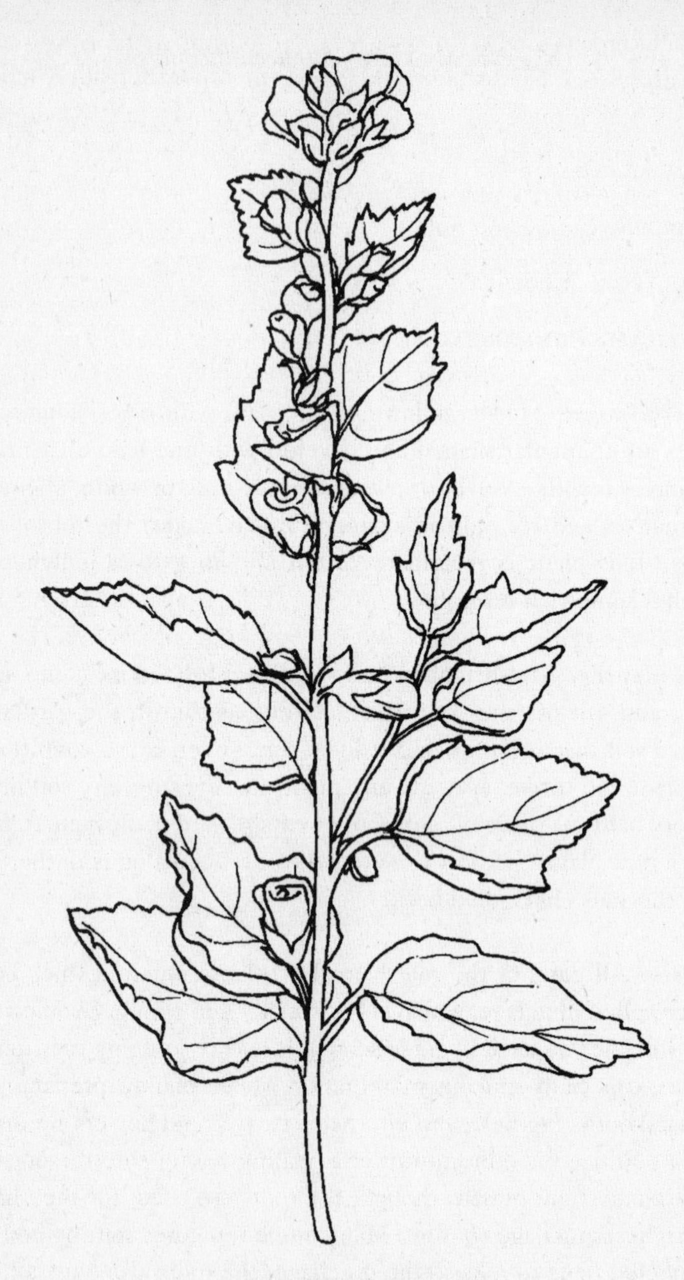

Marsh Mallow

away. The mucilaginous liquid can be turned into a lotion for sunburn, a face pack for dry skin, and even a treatment for skin conditions such as psoriasis. In some countries mothers rub the liquid onto the gums of teething children.

The inner part of the root is rather sweet, and in earlier times children chewed on a piece of root (after it had been peeled) the way some now enjoy sugarcane. That sweetness, plus the gluelike qualities of mucilage, led commercial confectioners to use marsh mallow root in candy manufacture. And that is the origin of the puffy white gooey treat we call marshmallow, although today's product contains nothing from the marsh mallow plant except its name.

Traditions: Marsh mallow has always been used as a medicinal herb, and nothing else, but that use extends several thousand years, back to the ancient Egyptians and Syrians. They used it to treat insect bites and toothaches, to dress wounds, and to ease urinary infections. Herbal physicians—then and now—use it as a mild laxative.

Mint *Mentha species*

PERENNIAL

SIZE: 2 inches to 2 feet, depending on species

GARDEN: Sun or shade; damp soil

USED FOR: Tea, seasoning, crafts, medicinal, ornamental

AVAILABLE COMMERCIALLY: Yes, dried (tea) and fresh

Description: There are more than 400 varieties of mint; all have square stems, aromatic leaves, and dainty flowers. Most grow upright, although some are low mats, and all have an invasive root system by which they will spread to the next county. Some of the major varieties are:

spearmint	the one used to flavor candy, chewing gum, medicine, and so on
peppermint	the source of menthol
Corsican mint	unbelievably tiny leaves; used as a ground cover
pennyroyal	a low-growing plant used to keep fleas away

Among the many unusual varieties are orange mint, apple mint, pineapple mint, chocolate mint, and candy mint; each one really does taste like its name.

Gardening: The biggest trick to growing mint is to decide whether you want to contain it or let it have its way. Mint will quickly take over, for it roots wherever a node touches the ground and also spreads by underground runners; with no trouble at all it will grow under a driveway and come out the other side. If you want to keep it in one limited spot, you have two choices: build some kind of barrier, or keep digging out the parts you don't want. Build a

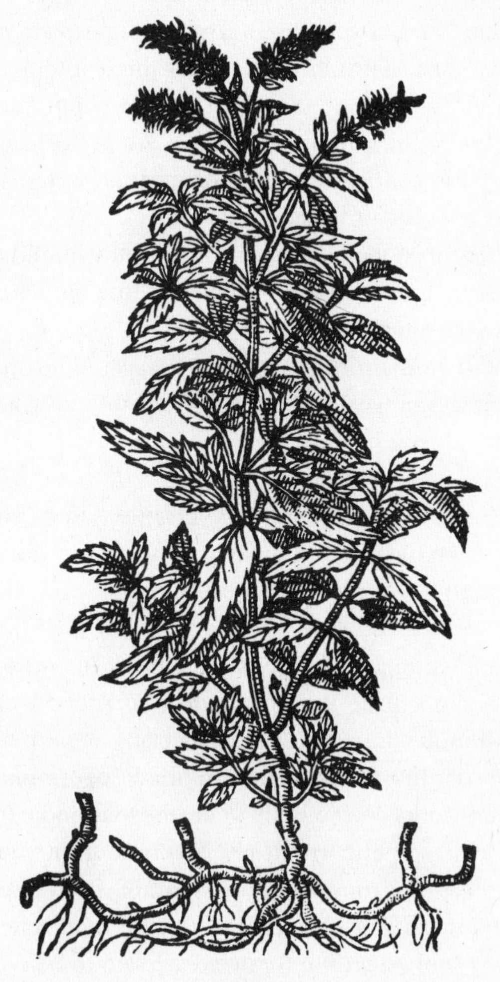

Mint

border of lumber or sheet metal sunk endwise in the ground; be sure to seal the corners, because mint can sneak through an opening the thickness of a fingernail. Or cut the bottom out of a restaurant-size tin can and bury all but the top 2 inches. Even so, be vigilant.

On the other hand, if you have a large enough space, give over an entire area to mint and just let it go. Every three or four years, divide each patch and discard the oldest parts; move peppermint to a new location entirely. A third alternative: mints are perfect candidates for growing in a patio container, even indoors as a houseplant; you can root a cutting in a glass of water.

Mints prefer moist locations; very often you will find them growing as volunteers around dripping faucets. But they are incredibly tough, and will tolerate drought.

You can start mint from seeds, but any gardener in the world, even a complete stranger, will be delighted to give you a root cutting, and that's all you need.

Uses: It's hard to imagine a more versatile, safer group of herbs than the mints. Home remedies, flavoring for home and commercial use, and wonderful teas are just the beginning.

Medicinal: Mint leaves, rubbed on itchy skin, are cool and have a slight numbing effect; thus they are also rubbed on gums for toothache. All mints help digestion, especially spearmint; the after-dinner mint is not just for your sweet tooth. Peppermint contains an ingredient that works on the body as an antispasmodic (reducing all kinds of spasms), so peppermint tea is very soothing for menstrual cramps, diarrhea, and tummyaches. Menthol, from peppermint, is used to treat sprains and bruises, and to ease toothache pain. Peppermint leaves rubbed on the forehead are said to be effective for a headache. Pennyroyal was used in A.D. 1000, and still is used in the twentieth century, to prevent seasickness.

Flavoring: Essential oil of mint is used commercially to flavor cough syrup, mouthwashes, and breath mints; peppermint oil is the key ingredient in creme de menthe. At home, we use mint leaves to add both flavor and a pretty garnish to all sorts of beverages; for party punch, freeze individual leaves in ice cubes. Theodore Roosevelt planted a bed of spearmint on the White House lawn, to be added to drinks for his cabinet meetings. Mint sauce is the classic accompaniment to roast lamb, and chopped mint leaves (either dried or fresh) perk up fruit salads, cream soups, and vegetables such as beans, peas, carrots, and potatoes. Mint vinegar, made from any mint you happen to have, makes a delicious dressing for tossed salad or fruit salads. For a party sandwich, mix cream cheese with chopped mint, spread on date nut bread.

Household: With its fresh, clean scent, you won't be surprised to learn that mint was just about the favorite strewing herb (strewn on floors as a room deodorizer), and it's still useful today. Fresh mint leaves in your pantry will keep mice away. Pennyroyal grows well in pots indoors, where it helps keep the mosquito population down; dry some leaves and add them to your dog's bed as a flea repellent. Make a mint infusion (steep leaves in boiling water, strain) and wash your face with it; it is both cooling and stimulating. Mint water added to your bath is cooling and very refreshing, especially in hot weather.

Traditions: The Greek god Pluto was already married when he fell in love with a beautiful nymph named Minthe, and his jealous wife changed the maiden into a plant. Pluto was unable to save her, but he did give Minthe an everlasting sweetness that could not be destroyed even when crushed underfoot.

Ever since, mint has been cherished for its healing powers and its delicious taste. Romans rubbed their banquet tables with mint leaves; the oil was good for the wood, and the smell stimulated the appetite. For a time in ancient Rome, women were prohibited by law from drinking alcohol, and the punishment was death. Adventurous women drank wine anyway and used mint to disguise their breath.

Pliny, the Greek historian and naturalist, recommended that students wear a crown woven of mint while they were studying; he said it would exhilarate the mind and stimulate the brain. He also described a mint poultice for mad-dog bites, and suggested mint as a cure for diseases of the spleen, but only if taken in a certain way: for nine days in a row, the patient had to take a mint leaf (being careful not to pull up the plant) and nibble it while standing in the garden, simultaneously saying out loud that he was doing this specifically for the purpose of benefiting the spleen. Whether you accept those prescriptions, we do know that Pliny's pronouncement that mint is "marvellous wholesome for the stomacke" is indeed accurate.

A fourteenth-century monk developed this prescription for infected sores: "Take eggis that be rotyne [rotten] and breke them and ley them on the sore and it shall sleye [slay] the worme; and whoso hath none eggis take thereof the Ius [juice] of mynte and it will do the same." By the fifteenth and sixteenth centuries rotten eggs had fallen out of favor, but physicians still recommended mint to promote digestion, to ease fevers and influenza, and to cure toothaches—all uses that continue to this day.

Nasturtium *Tropaeolum majus*

ANNUAL

SIZE: 2 to 10 feet

GARDEN: Full sun; average soil

USED FOR: Ornamental, cooking

AVAILABLE COMMERCIALLY: No

Description: Nasturtiums have very flat, round leaves that somewhat resemble lily pads but are much smaller, and the familiar and spectacular flowers in brilliant orange, yellow, and red. There are two types: vines, which creep and sprawl until they find something to climb on, and dwarf shrubs that stay small and compact; the dwarf type is *T. minus.*

Gardening: Start seeds directly in the garden in spring; they germinate in about a week. If you have the more common vining type and can give it something to climb on, it will reach as high as 10 feet. Both it and the bush type keep up their blazing display of color right up until frost. If you are more interested in flowers, keep the soil rather dry and fertilize only lightly; moist soil with lots of compost produces rich leaf growth. Both kinds are very popular with aphids, so if you plan to eat leaves or flowers, wash them well first. Some vegetable gardeners plant nasturtium as a trap plant, to lure aphids away from other plants; maybe it works, maybe not, but they do get to enjoy the wonderful flowers. Nasturtiums are a good choice for window boxes and large patio containers, especially those with several different kinds of plants; they'll cascade down the side, and provide a bright color accent.

Uses: Both leaves and flowers of nasturtiums have a tangy, peppery bite that will remind you of watercress, a fact that is reflected in its name: "nasturtium" is the Latin name of watercress. They are in

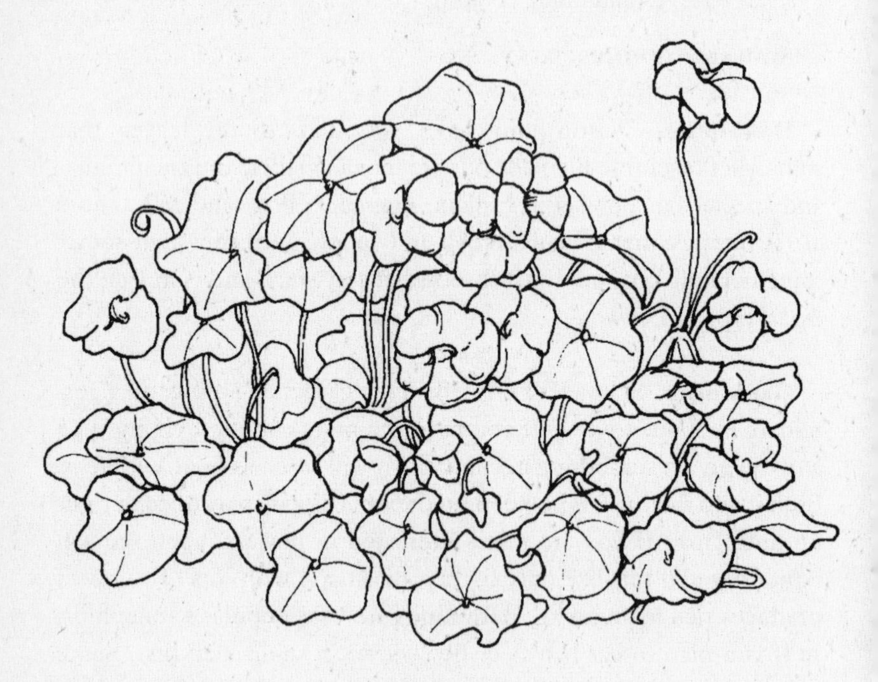

Nasturtium

herb gardens for two reasons: to delight the eye and to serve as a salad herb. Both leaves and flowers are edible; the leaves can be added to a green salad, although the taste is so strong you probably wouldn't want a whole salad of them. The flowers are a knockout garnish for salads, fruit platters, or the punch bowl.

Traditions: Nasturtiums are native to the Andes Mountains in South America. They were discovered by Spanish explorers and brought back to Europe in the early part of the seventeenth century, to be planted in the garden of King Louis XIV of France.

Oregano *Origanum vulgare*

PERENNIAL

SIZE: 2 feet

GARDEN: Sun or partial shade; average soil, well drained

USED FOR: Seasoning

AVAILABLE COMMERCIALLY: Yes

Description: *Origanum* is the name of a genus that contains both marjoram and oregano, and several subspecies of each. They all look a lot alike: small (1-inch), pointy leaves, small flowers at the top of the stem, and a rather sprawly way of growing. Dip into that genus for one specific plant, and you find confusion. *Origanum vulgare,* which is known as wild marjoram, is the "basic" oregano, and there are a number of varieties, many of which have pretty flowers but not much taste. The one that most people agree has the best flavor is *O. heracleoticum,* known as Greek oregano. The product we buy in the supermarket is actually a blend of several different types.

Uses: Oregano is primarily a cooking herb, and its flavor is very close to its first cousin, marjoram, although quite a bit stronger. It is an important seasoning in Italian, Spanish, and Mexican cuisines (and it grows vigorously in all those warm-weather climates). World War II soldiers who served in Italy returned home with a taste for Italian cooking, and sales of oregano and other Mediterranean herbs in American markets increased dramatically.

Oregano is a familiar taste to every person who has ever eaten spaghetti or pizza, but we don't have to limit it to spaghetti sauce. It goes well in bean or lentil soup, poultry stuffings, chili, hamburgers, meat loaf, squash, eggplant, and beans.

Fresh oregano, especially when it is flowering, is pretty in small flower bouquets and tussy-mussies.

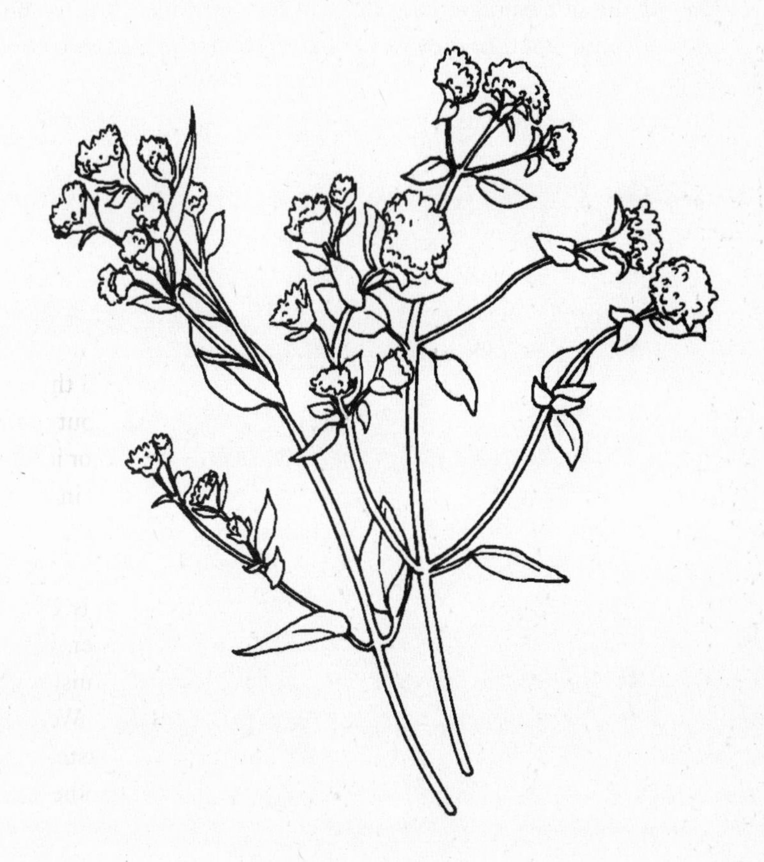

Oregano

Traditions: Oregano was known to ancient Greeks as the herb of happiness, and wedding ceremonies concluded with the bride and groom being crowned with a wreath of marjoram. For much the same reason, it was planted over the tops of graves, to make the journey into the next life more peaceful.

Many of the old medical formulas call for "origano," but we do not know for sure whether they were talking about the plant we now call oregano.

Parsley *Petroselinum crispum*

BIENNIAL

SIZE: 18 inches

GARDEN: Sun or part shade; rich, moist soil

USED FOR: Cooking, home remedies

AVAILABLE COMMERCIALLY: Yes, fresh and dried

Description: The parsley we know best, with the familiar, tightly curled green leaf, is called curly parsley. A less common variety is Italian parsley; the leaves are flat with scalloped edges and appear in bunches of three leaflets. It somewhat resembles cilantro, but it is not the same, even though cilantro is sometimes called Chinese parsley.

Garden: Parsley is a biennial, a plant that lives two years. In the garden, sow seeds one spring and you'll get leafy growth that summer. In some cold areas the foliage may die down in the winter, but often you can harvest parsley right through the year; in any case, the roots are alive, and in the second spring new leaves will sprout. Early that second summer, the plant produces a flower stalk and seed, then dies completely. The leaves get coarse and less flavorful when the plant flowers, and so many gardeners grow parsley as an annual, starting over with new plants (or seeds) every year. In mild climates, some are able to keep it as a perennial by nipping off all flower stalks.

There is an old bit of folklore that parsley seed has to go to the devil and back seven times before Satan permits it to break through the ground; in other words, parsley is extremely slow to germinate. If you want to start seed, you can speed the process along by soaking the seeds overnight before you plant them, or pouring boiling water over them once in the ground. Parsley also grows well in window boxes and in pots on the windowsill indoors.

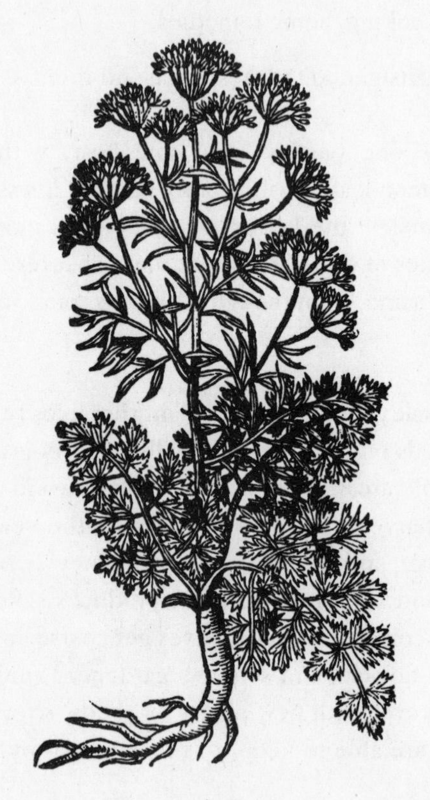

Parsley

Because parsley grows year-round or nearly so, you can enjoy it fresh for many months, but if you have a large crop you may want to preserve some. Parsley lends itself especially well to microwave drying (good taste and excellent color), and it also freezes very well: the leaves will be limp when defrosted, but the color and taste are just like fresh.

Uses: If you think of parsley only as a garnish, you are missing out on an excellent all-around kitchen herb. Parsley has a mild flavor that combines well with many dishes, adding its bright color and fresh taste to soups, stews, sauces for pasta and vegetables, herb butter for bread, fish, and poultry, and green salads. And there's a bonus: parsley is rich in iron, calcium, and vitamins A, B, and C—in fact, it has more vitamin C than an equivalent amount of oranges.

Italian parsley has a richer, spicier taste than curly-leaf parsley; and in both cases, the stems are more flavorful than the leaves. If you chop the leaves fine for parsley butter or sauces, save the stems for the soup pot.

European cooks dip parsley clusters in batter and deep-fry them, and parsley jelly is popular in England as an accompaniment to roast meat and chicken. Parsley is one of the herbs in the classic French herb blend known as fines herbes, and it is often included in a bouquet garni mixture.

Parsley tea has mild diuretic properties (stimulates urination), and it also has an effect on the digestive system, so it is sometimes used as a home remedy for stomachaches. Fresh leaves sweeten the breath, so be sure to eat that garnish when you're out at a restaurant.

Traditions: The Greeks considered parsley a symbol of honor, for it was said to sprout wherever a hero's blood was shed upon the ground. Greek soldiers and athletes ate large amounts of parsley because they believed it provided strength and stamina, and victorious athletes were crowned with a wreath of parsley. The Romans fed it to the horses before a chariot race, to give them stamina. They also used it liberally on the banquet table, in the belief that the herb would absorb the fumes from the wine goblets, so that the imbibers would not get too drunk.

In more modern times, parsley was primarily considered a kitchen herb, although tea made from it was used for rheumatism. It was so common in Europe that almost every home had a parsley patch outside the kitchen door, which probably is the source of the old story that mothers told inquisitive youngsters when they asked where babies came from: we found them in the parsley patch. A book of home remedies published in 1775 suggested a surefire way to prevent baldness: "Three nights a year, powder your hair with parsley seed [ground into a powder] and the hair will never fall off."

Rosemary *Rosmarinus officinalis*

PERENNIAL

SIZE: To 6 feet

GARDEN: Sun; alkaline soil, well drained

USED FOR: Seasoning, cosmetics, crafts, ornamental

AVAILABLE COMMERCIALLY: Yes

Description: Rosemary grows as a medium-sized shrub, with stems that become tough and woody after the first year, and foliage that looks like the needles on a fir tree: about an inch long, extremely narrow, dark green on top and gray on the bottom. In warm climates, it develops tiny pink or lavender flowers like a fairy's orchid; the flowers are very attractive to bees. There are creeping types that are pretty in rock gardens and hanging containers. The fragrance of the plant is very strong; it is said that off the coast of Spain and Portugal, where it grows wild, you can smell it twenty miles out to sea.

Gardening: The Latin name is a combination of *ros* meaning dew, and *marinus*, meaning sea; *rosmarinus*, "dew of the sea," grows wild on the coast of warm Mediterranean countries. Think about that, and you will know what kind of growing conditions it needs: moist but very well drained soil (like the sandy soil of the coast), mild climate, and humidity.

Rosemary is a very tender plant; freezing temperatures will kill it. Therefore, in much of the country it is grown in a container so it can be moved indoors in winter without having to dig it up, which could damage the rather fragile roots. It also does reasonably well as an indoor plant year-round. Outdoors, it prefers sun but will grow in some shade; soil drainage is very important, for the roots are susceptible to rot. Rosemary does best in alkaline soil; add lime or crushed eggshells if your soil is acid.

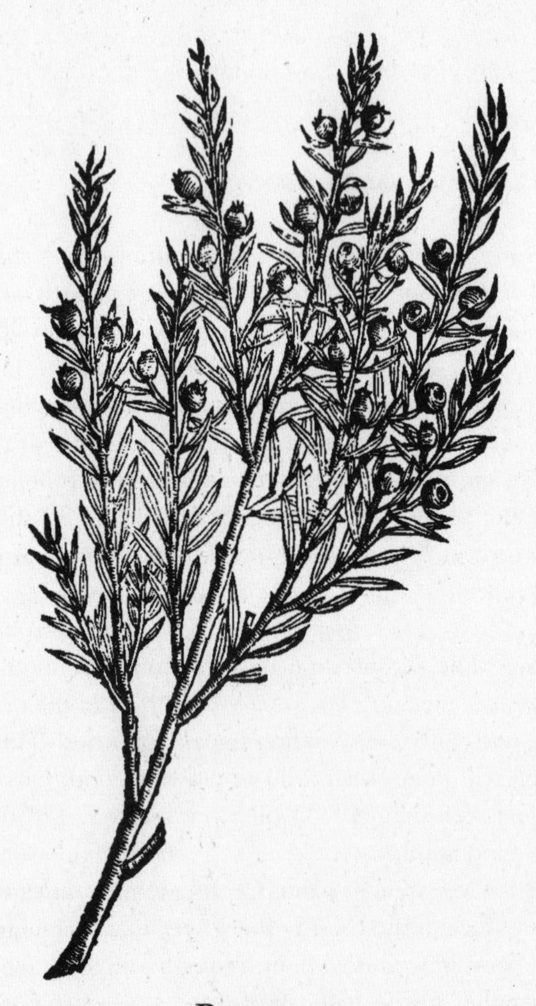

Rosemary

Uses: It's a fair bet that no herb known to humankind has a longer history of multiple uses and more legends than rosemary. It has been used as a flavoring herb since the time of the Greeks and Romans. Rosemary has a rather strong taste that will make you think of pine trees; add to roast meats, pea soup, minestrone, beef stew, chicken dishes, breads, yogurt dips, and mild-flavored veggies like cauliflower, potatoes, and beans. If you dry leaves from your plant, store them in whole form to preserve the most flavor, but crush them before cooking (or use a cheesecloth bag), because when dry they are very hard and could cause choking.

The pungent aroma of rosemary makes it popular as a potpourri ingredient, and it is excellent in moth-repellent sachets. Even a sprig of rosemary all by itself, laid among your clothes and linens, helps keep insects away.

Rosemary has many cosmetic applications. It makes a marvelous rinse for dark hair: it enriches the color, adds body, stimulates the scalp, and helps prevent dandruff. Herbal water (make a tea, strain out leaves) makes a good face wash, especially for dry skin, and is said—but not proved—to fade freckles. The same rosemary water can be used as a mouthwash: it kills bacteria and leaves the mouth very fresh. A lotion made by steeping leaves in rubbing alcohol is very soothing.

Rosemary contains an oil that stimulates the flow of blood to the skin and is used in several commercial products for sore muscles; rosemary water added to the bath is both invigorating and soothing for tired bodies.

Traditions: Several Christian legends attach to rosemary. When Joseph and Mary fled into Egypt with the baby Jesus, Mary washed out the infant's clothes and spread them over a rosemary bush to dry, and the plant immediately burst into bloom. On the same trip, she laid her own robe over a rosemary bush while she sat down to rest, and the flowers turned from white to blue. For years people believed that a rosemary bush would not grow taller than 6 feet (Christ's height when he was on earth) or live longer than his thirty-three years.

Rosemary is known as the herb of remembrance and thus of friendship. Students sniffed it while studying for their exams, to help them remember their lessons, and sprigs of the herb were sent to special friends as a New Year's greeting. At burials, rosemary branches were thrown into the grave, a symbol that the departed friend would not be forgotten. This custom probably originated for a very practical reason: rosemary was considered an antiseptic that would prevent spread of the terrible plagues that killed so many. For that same reason, people carried it in their hand when they went outside and held it close to their mouth when greeting another person. Later, it was one of the herbs carried in a pomander, the small filigree ball worn around the waist to mask body odors.

Somewhere along the way, it came to be an important symbol of married love and was often carried in the bride's bouquet. At her wedding to Henry VIII, Anne of Cleves, the king's fourth wife, wore a crown woven of rosemary and set with precious jewels.

Rosemary was believed to have very strong powers against evil, and so people put a piece of it under their pillow at night to protect against nightmares and evil spirits. So great was this power that in churches rosemary was hung on the walls and strewn on the floors, and it was burned at the altar like incense. In fact, rosemary was so important in religious life that it was said that it would not grow in the garden of "one who is not just and righteous."

Women of today might be inclined to adopt it as their special symbol, to honor the long tradition that rosemary grows vigorously in gardens where the wife rules the household and poorly where the husband is the dominant partner.

Rosemary has been used medicinally since before the time of Christ, to treat disease, injuries, and poisonous bites. Indeed, one old medical book, probably reflecting ideas that date back to the sixth century, says: "It is good for every disorder which can exist in the human body." And in the early sixteenth century, this all-purpose formula is described: "seethe [steep] much rosemary, and bathe terin [therein] to make thee lusty, lively, joyfull, and youngly."

Rue *Ruta graveolens*

PERENNIAL

SIZE: 2 to 3 feet

GARDEN: Sun or light shade; average soil, well drained

USED FOR: Ornamental

AVAILABLE COMMERCIALLY: No

Description: Rue grows into a small shrub, with an overall rounded shape that manages to look dense and frothy at the same time. The leaves have a blue cast that is very distinctive, and each leaflet has a rounded end that contributes to the plant's soft look. Small yellow flowers in clusters.

Gardening: Rue is a native of dry, rocky landscapes of the Mediterranean and requires soil that has very good drainage; in fact, it will do very nicely in sandy, unfertile soil that little else could live in. Although it will live in some shade, it prefers full sun.

The oil present in rue causes a skin rash in some people; it is somewhat like poison ivy, and seems to occur most often on sunny, warm days (when the oils are most volatile). Gardeners are advised to wear long sleeves and gloves when working around rue in the summertime.

Uses: In centuries past, rue was a potherb (eaten as a green), and in older cookbooks you will still find occasional suggestions that call for rue. Today, eating rue or drinking tea made from it is not recommended; the same oils that cause skin rash externally can create internal problems. And if you're pregnant, **absolutely** do not use it internally.

In the garden, however, it is a visual delight. The soft blue-tinted foliage makes a pretty contrast to both dark green and gray-green leaves of other plants, and a hedge border of rue is striking. The same pretty foliage goes well in flower arrangements and makes an attractive base layer in tussy-mussies.

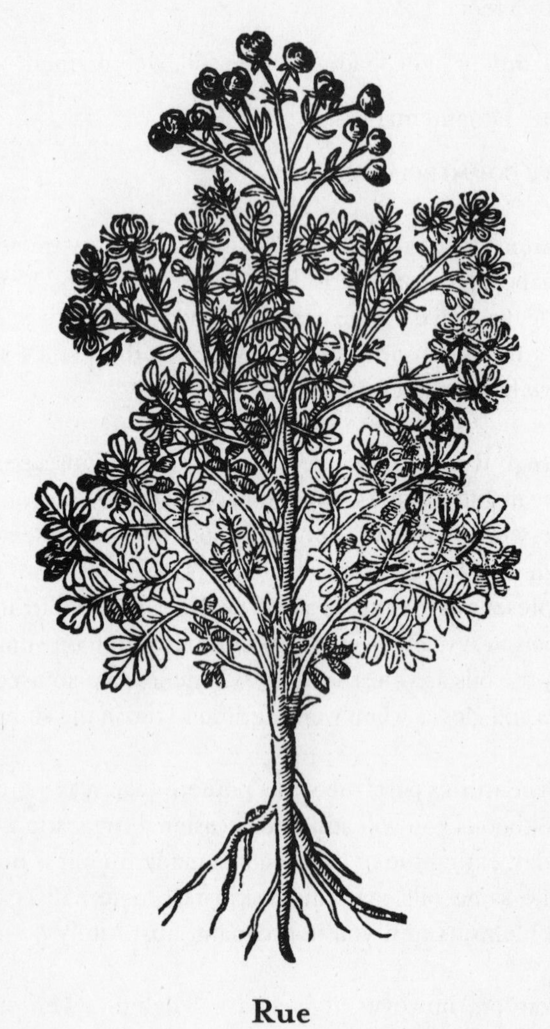

Rue

Traditions: Rue has a very unusual smell that most people describe as bitter. That smell probably accounts for its use in the Middle Ages as protection against disease, witches, and evil spirits; surely anything so pungent would drive away danger. It was a strewing herb in churches, hung from doorways in houses, and carried in hand during times of plague. In England judges kept rue in a vase in court so they would not catch "gaol fever" from the prisoners brought before the bench. That practice continued up through the nineteenth century, although by then it was done more for tradition than for protection.

Rue has an important place in the lore of the Catholic church. Priests dipped a sprig of rue in the holy water and sprinkled it on worshippers, symbolically washing away their sins. From this practice, rue came to be known as the herb of grace; into the middle of the twentieth century, it was called "herbygrass" in some parts of England.

In medieval times rue was used medicinally, to treat everything from boils and snakebite to tuberculosis. It was especially renowned for treatment of fading eyesight, although from what we now know of its potent oils it's hard to imagine putting it in your eyes. In the days when so many died from the plague, a band of looters known as the Four Thieves concocted a very strong herb vinegar, made from rue and other herbs, and rubbed it into their skin to keep them from catching the Black Death while they were pillaging the homes of recent victims. A less gruesome note is this thirteen-century prescription for a tonic intended to keep people from talking in their sleep: "Take leaves of rue and pound with vinegar till it becomes a mass, then mix it well in old ale, strain, and let the patient drink it." More likely the ale, not the rue, produced sound sleep.

CAUTION: Rue is considered unsafe for internal consumption.

Sage *Salvia officinalis*

PERENNIAL

SIZE: 1 to 2 feet

GARDEN: Sun; light, well-drained soil

USED FOR: Flavoring, tea, cosmetics, crafts, ornamental

AVAILABLE COMMERCIALLY: Yes

Description: Sage grows as a thick mass, with many short branches sprouting from the main stem. The leaves are long, oval-shaped, and have a rough, pebbly surface texture; small flowers sit on stalks up above the leaves. Garden sage has rich blue flowers, and other varieties have pink and lavender blossoms; all the flowers are richly attractive to bees.

Common garden sage has light green leaves with a grayish cast. There are several varieties, interesting for their colorful leaves: variegated sage is yellow and green; tricolor sage is pink, white, and gray-green; purple sage is reddish purple with an overlay of gray. Pineapple sage has pointy leaves that smell remarkably like fresh pineapple.

Gardening: To keep your plants bushy and trim, cut them often. Even so, after three or four years, the center tends to get bare, with all the new leaves out at the ends of woody stems. Replace with new plants, which you can start from cuttings taken from the original plant; they root easily.

Pineapple sage is not hardy in cold winters (it makes a nice houseplant), but most other sages will do fine all year round in moderate temperatures. This means you can harvest leaves anytime, which you will want to do, for the fresh leaves are milder than dried and have a lemony undertaste that is lost in the drying process.

Uses: We tend to think of sage in connection with Thanksgiving turkeys and not much else, which is too bad, for its rich flavor complements many dishes: fish chowder, beef stew, hamburgers, cornbread and other breads, stewed tomatoes, cheese spreads, and many vegetables. It is the main flavoring in classic welsh rarebit (cheese, beer, and sage), and it has a natural affinity for pork (and appears to help with its digestion). Fresh leaves, with the light taste of lemon, can be crystallized and served like after-dinner mints: paint both sides with beaten egg white, roll in sugar, dry in a very low oven.

Sage tea is surprisingly good (especially with a little lemon added); it is an old home remedy for fever, since it reduces perspiration. Purely as a beverage, it was a favorite tea in England before black tea was introduced from China. Then, interestingly enough, the Chinese developed a taste for it, and European merchants traded sage in China for black tea to bring back to England.

Sage vinegar is delicious, especially that made from fresh flowers; if you use white vinegar and sage's blue flowers, you get a luscious red color.

An infusion of sage leaves (steep in boiling water, then strain) makes a good skin lotion, a hair conditioner, and a mouthwash that is also good for the gums. The next time you have a sore throat, try this old remedy: pour boiling vinegar on sage leaves in a large saucepan, then lean over and inhale the vapors. Some gardeners claim that fresh leaves laid about the house will keep ants away.

The leaves of sage are larger than those of many herbs, and so they are often used in herb wreaths and tussy-mussies to form a background. Dried sage, especially pineapple sage, is used in potpourri.

Sage is an attractive plant that deserves more attention in gardens. The handsome foliage of common garden sage is a good contrast in flower gardens, adding a soft green base to the brightness of the blossoms. If you have the room, try a whole bed of sage in different varieties: variegated sage (yellow tones), purple (dark red tones), and tricolor (pink and white). Long after your summer flowers have faded, you'll be able to enjoy the rich colors of these beautiful plants.

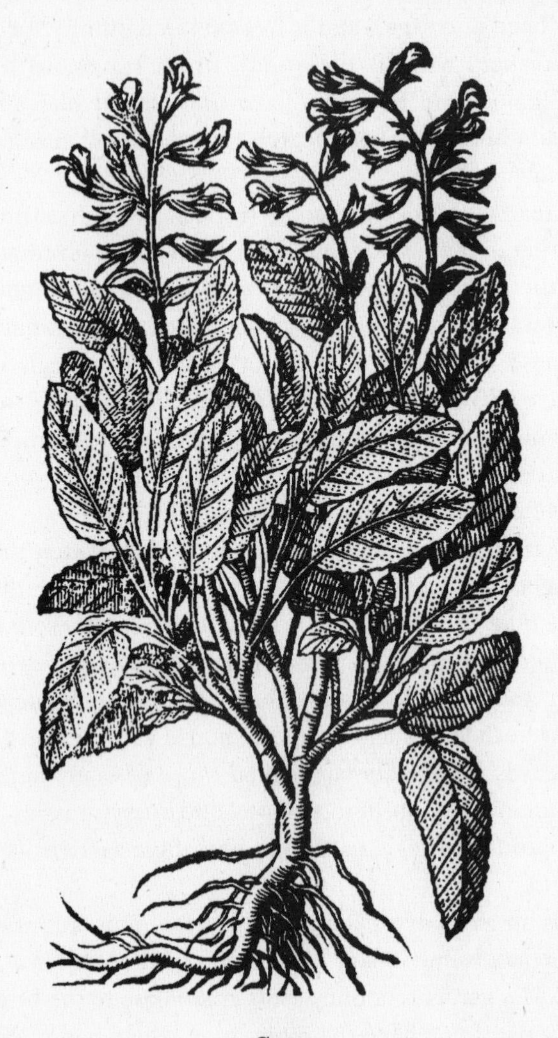

Sage

Traditions: The Latin name of this genus comes from *sal-vare,* which means "to save," a reference to the plant's strong tradition as a healing herb. Hippocrates used sage tea as a general tonic, and it has been used for centuries to ease indigestion from heavy meals (sage's popularity in turkey stuffing is no accident).

After a plague hit ancient Egypt, women were urged to drink lots of sage tea in the belief it would increase their fertility, and the villages would be able to replenish their populations. In ancient Rome, people who felt their memory was diminishing in old age ate lots of sage to revive it. The best known tradition, however, is that people who eat enough sage will be immortal. The old saying is, "How can a man die who has sage in his garden?"

Salad Burnet *Poterium sanguisorba*

PERENNIAL

SIZE: 1 foot

GARDEN: Sun or partial shade; average soil

USED FOR: Cooking, ornamental

AVAILABLE COMMERCIALLY: No

Description: Stems sprout in a rosette form from the base, giving the whole plant a rounded but airy shape that's usually about 1 foot in diameter. Small bright green leaflets have jagged edges, as if someone trimmed all around them with pinking shears. Single round flower heads, green with a reddish tinge, form at the top of long brown stalks. In the early stages the flower too has a brown cast, which is the source of the plant's name: "burnet" is a version of "brunette," French for brown. The scientific name of this plant used to be *Sanguisorba minor,* and you will still find it listed that way occasionally.

Gardening: It's easy to start burnet from seed. If you have several plants, you might want to let one of them flower and go to seed; the following spring you will have a crop of baby plants. Burnet prefers alkaline soil and seems to flourish in very poor soil that is sandy and dry.

Harvest the leaves anytime; for best flavor, keep the flower heads picked off. The leaves do not dry well but retain most of their taste when frozen.

Uses: How would you like to walk outside and pick fresh cucumbers in December? With salad burnet, you can, for its leaves, which stay on the plant most of the year, taste just like cucumber. Use the whole leaves in a green salad or in light soups; chop them and mix with cottage cheese or cream cheese, or salad dressings. Young

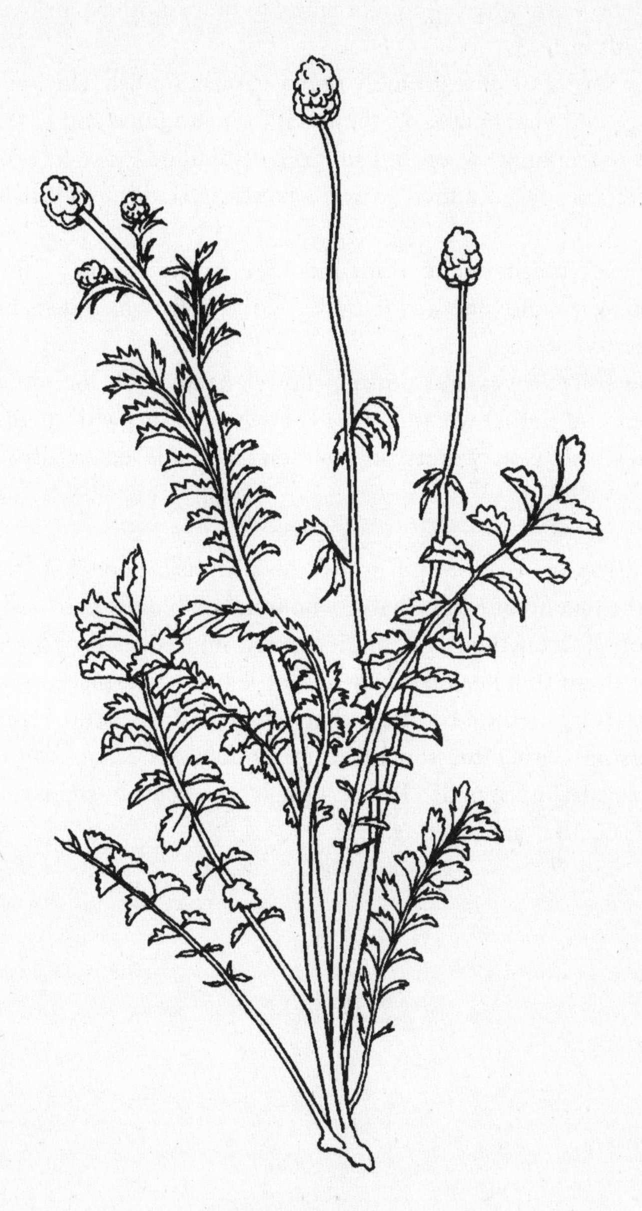

Salad Burnet

leaves are best; when the plant starts to flower, the flavor becomes rather bitter.

The leaves are an extremely pretty garnish for fish, chicken, fruit platters, and vegetables; try them with tomato juice and other cold drinks that are not sweet. In Europe several hundred years ago, burnet was very often added to wine punch, a tradition worth trying anew.

Herbal vinegar made from salad burnet is excellent in salad dressings; it is also one way to preserve the herb, which does not dry satisfactorily.

The frilly leaves and unusual flower heads look nice in tussy-mussies and herbal wreaths. And the whole plant, with its delicate and lacy look, is very pretty in a garden landscape, especially in borders.

Traditions: In eastern Europe, this plant is called Chaba's salve, after the legend of King Chaba, who fought a bloody battle with his brother. Fifteen thousand soldiers were injured, and every single one of them was healed when burnet leaves were placed on their wounds. Old medical books, perhaps copying this legend, often suggest using burnet to stop bleeding; indeed its name *sanguisorba* means "soak up blood." In the past it was used to treat wounds, diarrhea, and hemorrhaging.

Santolina *Santolina chamaecyparissus*

PERENNIAL

SIZE: 1 to 2 feet

GARDEN: Sun; sandy, well-drained soil

USED FOR: Ornamental, crafts

AVAILABLE COMMERCIALLY: No

Description: One common name of this herb is lavender cotton, and indeed it does look somewhat like lavender in the way it grows and to some extent in its leaves: gray-green, rather short, and needle-shaped. The foliage of the main species has a gnarled look that resembles a delicate form of undersea coral; it has a pungent aroma. The flowers are small, intense yellow buttons at the top of long stalks that sit up above the highest leaves.

Gardening: Santolina is easy to grow, for it tolerates almost any kind of soil as long as it has good drainage. It withstands serious pruning, which is one reason it was so popular in knot gardens. It's also easy to propagate by tip layering: take a long branch, bury the middle part underground with something heavy to hold it down, and it will root there; cut the rooted segment away from the mother plant.

Uses: Santolina was one of the favorites of those patient gardeners who created the elaborate knot gardens in Elizabethan England, because it could be pruned and shaped without damaging the plant, and because its gray foliage provided a good contrast for dark green plants. Even though knot gardens are out of fashion at the moment, the plant still has the same virtues and so makes an excellent plant for borders and hedges.

Another quality makes santolina a worthwhile addition to your garden: it is a good moth repellent. Include it as part of a mixture for

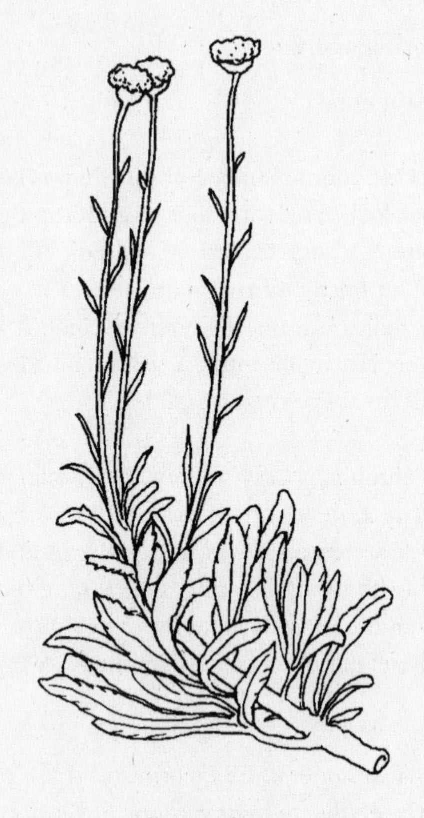

Santolina

closet sachets, or simply put sprigs of it in among your closets and bureau drawers.

The unusual foliage dries very well, and so santolina is especially attractive in herb wreaths and dried arrangements.

Traditions: Santolina is native to the dry countries of southern Europe, and it was included in the "medicine chest" of ancient cultures, primarily to cure intestinal worms. When the plant was introduced to northern Europe in the sixteenth century, it was immediately taken over by the royal gardeners for its ornamental value, and medicinal use faded. One story told to explain its name is that Spanish priests in early California planted it at the missions; so impressed were they by its ability to survive the dry soil and salty air, they named it to honor the saints.

Savory *Satureia*

PERENNIAL/ANNUAL

SIZE: 6 to 18 inches

GARDEN: Sun; average soil

USED FOR: Flavoring

AVAILABLE COMMERCIALLY: Yes

Description: There are two kinds of savory. Summer savory, *Satureia hortensis*, is an annual. *S. montana*, winter savory, is a perennial. Both are small plants with small leaves and flowers; they look something like thyme plants, except with larger leaves. Overall, winter savory is darker green, smaller, and more spreading.

Gardening: Summer savory, being an annual, must be started from seed each year. It transplants easily, and so you can start seed indoors early if you wish; it also self-sows, so if you had some last year and left it to flower, you may have new plants this year without doing anything at all. It needs more water than the winter type. Winter savory is started from seed or a rooted cutting.

Summer savory develops a tendency to flop over as its top branches get heavy with leaves. Some gardeners plant them close together so they hold each other up; others add a low fence or string support to keep the leaves up out of the dirt. Because they stay quite small, both savories are good plants for growing in patio containers.

Uses: Savory is a cooking herb; both types have a spicy, peppery taste. Although summer savory is milder than winter, the taste is similar enough that for all practical purposes they can be used interchangeably. The classic use for savory is in bean dishes and bean and lentil soup. Some say the herb helps with the intestinal gas so often associated with bean dishes; in any case, the two have been

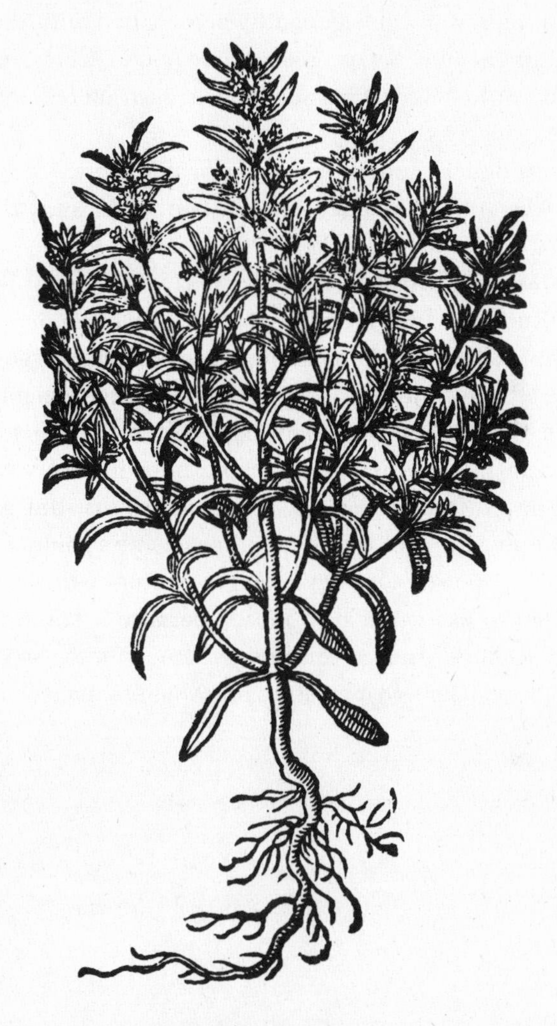

Winter Savory

used together for so long that they taste right together. In Germany savory is called *bohnenkraut*, meaning "the string bean herb."

It is also good with strong-tasting vegetables like brussels sprouts, turnips, and cabbage, and when cooked with them keeps down the strong odor. Savory goes well in potato dishes, in beef and lamb stew, and chicken fricassee, and it is an ingredient in many recipes for country sausage.

Many gardeners report from personal experience that fresh savory leaves, rubbed on bee stings, instantly take away the pain.

Traditions: Roman soldiers brought savory to Great Britain and northern Europe, where it quickly became established as important in both the kitchen and the sickroom. One herbalist suggested pouring "juice of savory" into the ears to stop them from ringing. A poultice made from savory was used externally for arthritis and other inflamed joints. The American colonists brought savory with them, and tea brewed from it was said to lift the spirits. But perhaps its most enduring virtue (or vice, depending on one's point of view) was its aphrodisiac power. One seventeenth-century writer warned: "It is forbidden to use it much in meats, because it stirreth him that useth it to lechery." In fact, this herb is named for the satyr, the legendary half-man, half-goat creature renowned for its lechery.

Sorrel *Rumex scutatus*

PERENNIAL

SIZE: 1 foot

GARDEN: Sun; average soil with good drainage

USED FOR: Cooking

AVAILABLE COMMERCIALLY: Occasionally, in the produce section

Description: There are two kinds of sorrel, similar in taste but different in appearance. *Rumex scutatus,* called French sorrel, is a small plant, not much over a foot high, with light green leaves shaped something like an arrowhead. *Rumex acetosa,* usually called garden sorrel, is a much bigger plant, up to 4 feet high, with bigger leaves, oval shaped but with a squared-off base. Tall, thin flower spikes are green with a reddish cast.

Gardening: In many places sorrel is considered a weed—which should tell us that it's very easy to grow. In fact, it spreads so easily it soon takes over unless you keep after it. Plant seeds one year, and after that you'll always have more. It seeds itself quite easily (sometimes in the same season); and it also sends up new growth from underground runners. Keep the flower heads cut back, for best quality leaves. Every three or four years, dig up old plants and put in new ones.

Uses: We grow sorrel for the leaves, which have an acidic, somewhat lemony taste that is best known in the French cream-based sorrel soup. Its tangy taste is strong, best enjoyed in combination with other herbs. Some cooks add it in with spinach leaves for a cooked vegetable dish with extra piquancy. And chopped fine, sorrel leaves give a tangy flavor to sauces for fish, meat, and vegetables. Usually it is a part of cooked dishes, but sorrel leaves can also be added—sparingly—to green salads.

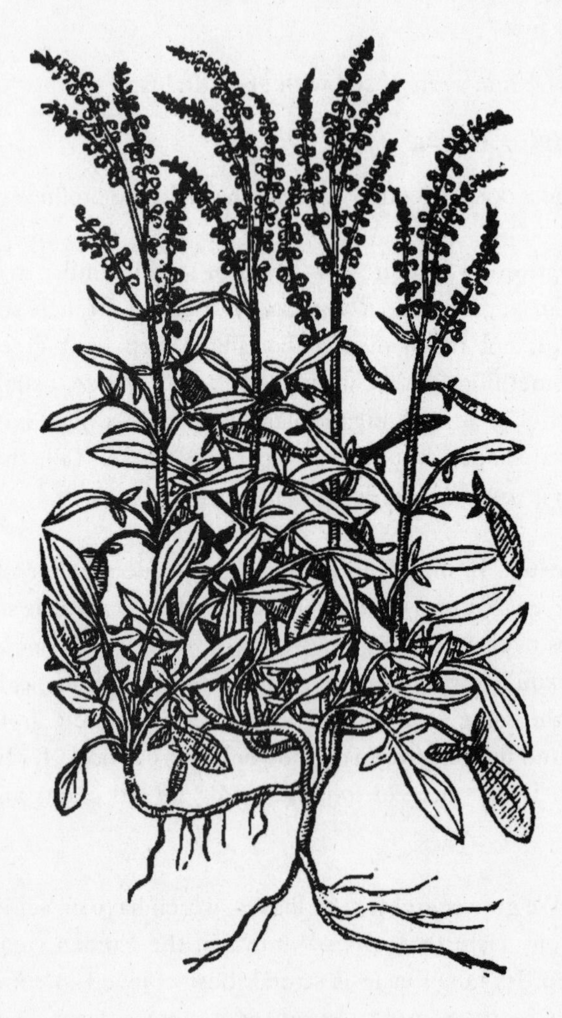

Sorrel

The acidity in sorrel leaves will react with iron pots and will turn knives black; use aluminum or stainless steel pots and stainless steel knives. An English gardener, writing around the time of World War II, said that her housemaid used it to polish the copper pots. Heat the pot in boiling water, she instructed, and rub the outside all over with the sorrel leaves.

Traditions: Four thousand years ago, the Egyptians used sorrel just as we do today: in combination with other greens, to improve their flavor. Its sour flavor probably convinced early herbalists that sorrel was good medicine, for it was used to treat a long list of ills. And it was said that its taste saved "sallets [salads] from vapidity and renders not only plants and herbs, but men themselves and their conversations, pleasant and agreeable."

Southernwood *Artemisia abrotanum*

PERENNIAL

SIZE: 2 to 3 feet

GARDEN: Sun; light, well-drained soil

USED FOR: Crafts, ornamental

AVAILABLE COMMERCIALLY: No

Description: Southernwood is one plant in the genus *Artemisia*, which also includes tarragon and the ornamental plants called artemisias (plant names can be confusing). This particular artemisia shows its family resemblance in the leaves: fragrant, feathery, and silver-green. It grows as a loose and airy-looking shrub. Actually, there are three varieties of southernwood, with names reflecting the fragrance of their leaves: lemon (the most common), tangerine, and camphor. Among the *Artemisia* genus, southernwood has one of the laciest leaves.

Gardening: Southernwood is a hardy plant that grows on most any kind of soil. About all it asks from you is a regular haircut in the spring, to keep it tidy looking as the new growth starts. The foliage dries easily; tie bundles and hang upside down.

Uses: Mostly we grow southernwood because it's so pretty; its lacy gray-green foliage makes a handsome accent plant in the garden, among the stronger hues of flowers and dark greens of other shrubs. Add it to cut-flower bouquets and small nosegays.

The aroma of southernwood is strong but not unpleasant—except to moths. It has been used as a repellent for hundreds of years, and today it is a major element in potpourri mixtures that are intended for closet sachets. Another way to use it is simply to lay branches of it on shelves where clothes and linens are stored. In France people call it *garde robe* and lay it on the floor of clothes clos-

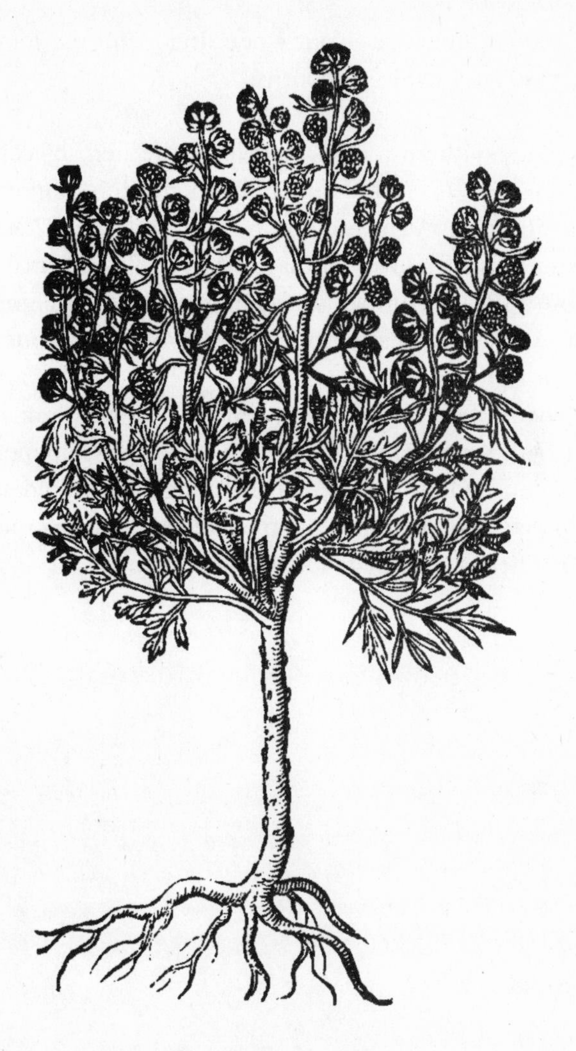

Southernwood

ets. Where ants are common, many people cut southernwood stems and lay them on windowsills and doorsills, to keep ants from entering the house.

Southernwood retains its scent when dried, and the lemon and tangerine types are used in potpourris.

Traditions: Southernwood is known as the herb of constancy. Along with rue, it was used by judges in England to counteract any germs that prisoners might bring into court with them. One of its common names is lad's love; for many years adolescent males, anxious to grow up faster, rubbed southernwood on their chins in the belief it would hasten beard growth. It also had the reputation of restoring hair lost to baldness.

Perhaps both these beliefs originated with (or were reflected in) this recipe from the seventeenth-century herbalist Culpeper: "The ashes [obtained by burning the leaves] mingled with old salad oil helps those that have their hair fallen or are bald, causing the hair to grow again either on the head or as a beard."

Sweet Cicely *Myrrhis odorata*

PERENNIAL

SIZE: 3 to 4 feet

GARDEN: Shade; rich, moist soil

USED FOR: Cooking, ornamental, crafts

AVAILABLE COMMERCIALLY: No

Description: A rather tall, striking plant with extremely frilly leaves that look like fronds of fern and flowers like Queen Anne's lace, sweet cicely could easily be mistaken for chervil. If they were side by side, you could observe two differences: sweet cicely is much taller, and its foliage is finer and lacier. If you tasted each one, you'd find another difference: sweet cicely is, well, sweet. In fact, its other common names are very descriptive: anise fern, sweet chervil, and candy plant. The plant does have a very sweet licorice (anise) taste. The leaves are very soft to the touch. The flower heads produce long, thin seeds almost an inch long, which also have the anise taste.

Gardening: Trying to grow sweet cicely from seed can be a frustrating experience; you're better off to start with a small plant. Even then, be patient; this is a slow-growing herb. Although it will tolerate sun if necessary, sweet cicely is happier in shade. The soil should be rich (with lots of compost worked in) and kept moist. Before you plant, work the soil deeply, for sweet cicely grows a very long taproot.

Uses: Many people grow sweet cicely for the soft, lacy leaves and don't care at all about the taste. The delicate foliage is pretty both in the garden and in cut-flower bouquets, and it forms a lovely background layer in tussy-mussies.

However, the sweet flavor of the leaves deserves our attention.

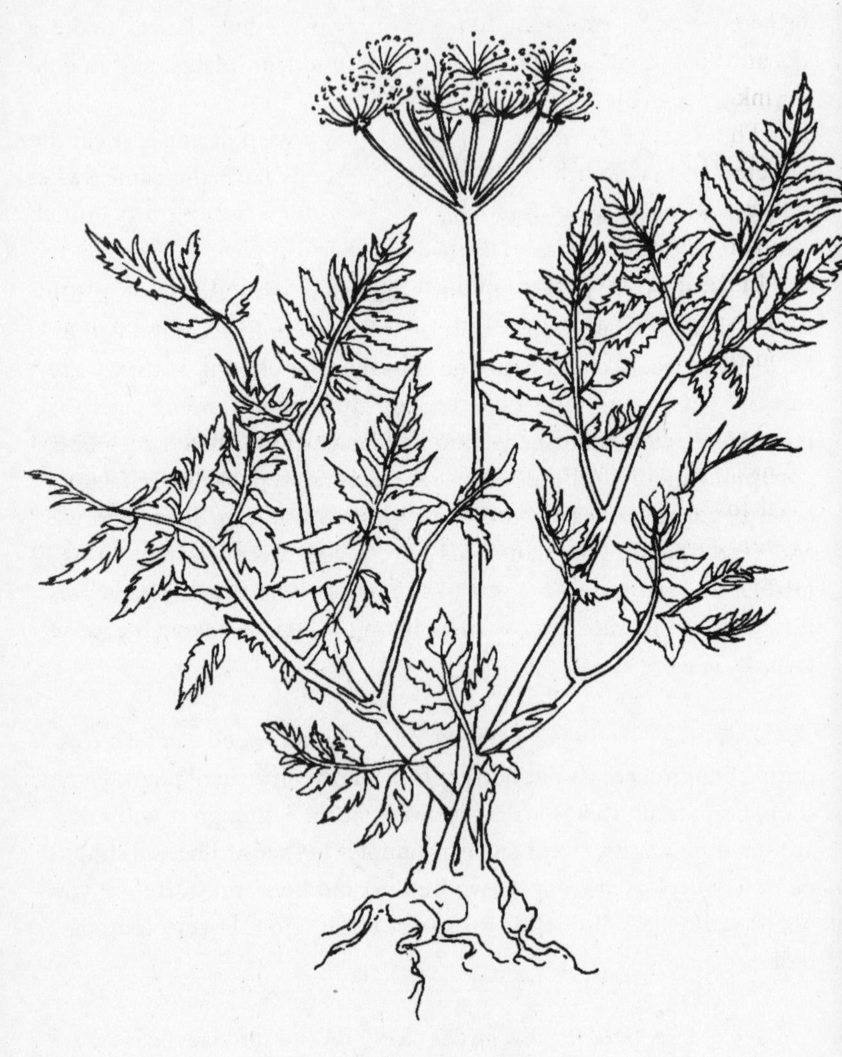

Sweet Cicely

When chopped fine and cooked with tart fruits like rhubarb, sweet cicely adds a natural sweetener so you can use less sugar. Fresh leaves go well in fruit salads, and the hint of sweetness is nice with cooked carrots, cabbage, and cream soups. Whole leaves make a beautiful garnish for fish dishes, soups, and fruit plates, and in cold drinks.

The flesh of the thick root also carries a wisp of anise; it can be peeled and cooked like potatoes. The seeds have the same sweet taste; add whole green seeds to fruit salad for a sweet, nutty crunch and crush ripe (brown) seeds for flavoring fruit pies.

In the past, seeds were pounded into a paste and used as a furniture polish. The aromatic seeds and dried leaves can be used in potpourri.

Traditions: Sweet cicely was used in ancient times as a general tonic. Tea made from the leaves was considered particularly beneficial for young women aged fifteen to eighteen. Old people were given cooked root, in the belief it would strengthen them. And everyone drank the tea as a prevention against the plague.

Sweet Woodruff *Galium odoratum*

PERENNIAL

SIZE: 6 inches

GARDEN: Shade; rich, moist soil

USED FOR: Ornamental, crafts, flavoring

AVAILABLE COMMERCIALLY: No

Description: Sweet woodruff is a small, exquisitely pretty plant that hides shyly under the shade of trees. Its light green leaves are rather short (an inch or less) and quite narrow, and grow in a circle of six or sometimes eight at intervals along the stem. In spring, small clusters of white flowers shaped like tiny stars appear up above the leaves. The plant spreads by sending out runners from which new stems sprout, so that a mature bed of sweet woodruff covers the ground the way a fluffy comforter covers your bed. Sometimes you find this herb listed in catalogs as *Asperula odorata.*

Gardening: Sweet woodruff seeds take forever and a day to germinate, so start with small plants or ask a friend to give you some sections when he divides the plants after a few years' growth. In the wild, sweet woodruff grows in the woods, in the shade of trees where the soil is fluffy with decayed leaves and where there's ample moisture but the soil drains quickly. In your garden, try to give it those same conditions. That kind of soil is acidic, so if you have very alkaline soil you'll have to add some compost or peat moss. Do not even try to grow woodruff in hot, dry areas; the plants will burn up.

After a few years, your bed of woodruff will be full and lush, and you'll need to divide the plants so they don't strangle each other. Dig up an entire plant, then tease the roots apart so that you have several little plants each with some root attached. Start a new bed, or give some away to a friend.

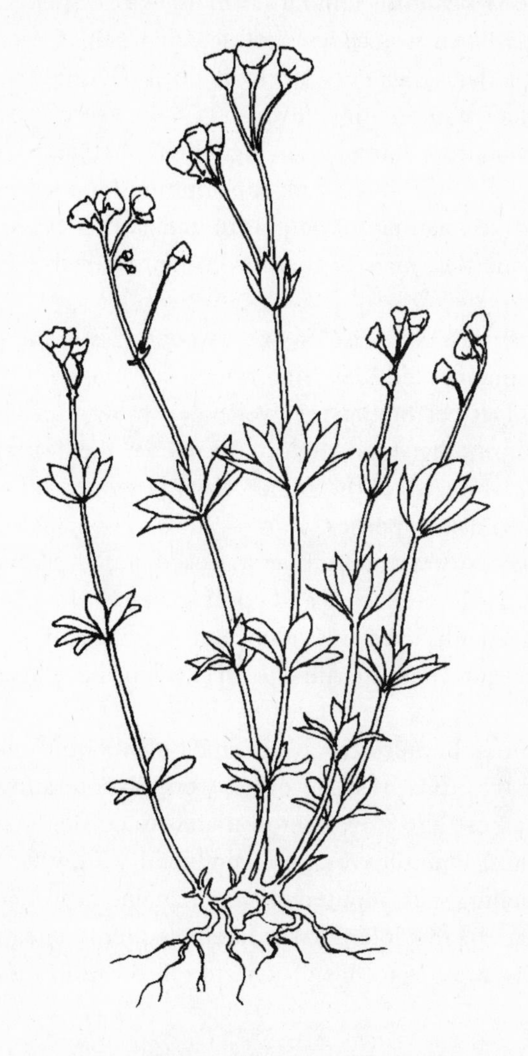

Sweet Woodruff

Uses: Sweet woodruff is a special plant for those who love herbs but are short on sunny locations. It loves shade and dampish soil, and thus is a beautiful ground cover for those spots under trees where other herbs won't grow; and it's a natural for woodland gardens. The foliage goes very nicely in small bouquets and in tussymussies, along with the tiny flowers.

Sweet woodruff contains an ingredient that has a very sweet vanillalike fragrance, and it isn't apparent until the leaves are dried. That makes it a natural for potpourri; in fact, the leaves have some fixative properties, making them even more valuable in potpourri mixtures.

The most traditional use of sweet woodruff is in the preparation of a wine punch called May wine, which in Europe is served as part of the May Day celebration that welcomes spring after a long winter. Woodruff sprigs are dried slightly (to release the sweetness), then steeped in white wine; the punch bowl is topped off with champagne and wild strawberries.

In the past, sweet woodruff tea was used both as a beverage and a home remedy for headaches and upset stomach. However, new laboratory research has shown evidence of toxicity, and now the FDA considers sweet woodruff safe only in alcoholic beverages.

Traditions: Because the sweet smell of woodruff is found only in dried leaves, this was one of the very favorite strewing herbs. Sprigs of it were also woven into garlands to decorate (and deodorize) churches. Dried leaves were combined with other herbs for a kind of smelling salts, reputed to ease migraine headaches. Both for the sweet aroma that it lent to the linens and for its alleged ability to keep moths away, branches of it were often laid in the linen cupboard.

Tansy *Tanacetum vulgare*

PERENNIAL

SIZE: 4 to 5 feet

GARDEN: Sun or shade; average soil

USED FOR: Ornamental, crafts

AVAILABLE COMMERCIALLY: No

Description: Tansy grows in upright clumps. The stems have lots of branches; the leaves are frilly and fernlike and have a strong and bitter smell. The flowers are button-shaped, up to ½ inch across, and a very intense yellow; they are in loose clusters at the outer ends of the stalks. A variety called curly tansy has daintier foliage and is smaller overall.

Some of the common names that have been given to tansy over the years convey a sense of its qualities: bitter buttons (leaves and flowers have a bitter taste); stink fern (for the foul-smelling ferny foliage); and ant fern (because the ants climb all over it).

Gardening: Tansy is a rampant grower that sends out underground runners from which new stems sprout; it also self-sows with a great vigor. In other words, once you have one tansy plant, watch out—it will take over the world. It grows in almost any exposure from full sun to part shade, and in just about any soil except mud.

Uses: In much of the country tansy is considered a weed, and many people would shake their heads in dismay at the thought that anyone would deliberately plant it in a garden. Yet it does have a kind of blowsy charm as a garden plant, with its lush growth and bright flowers. The flowers dry extremely well and keep their color, and so are favorites for those who make wreaths and other floral crafts. It is mostly for those flowers that people grow tansy.

Snip off flower clusters and hang them upside down to dry; use

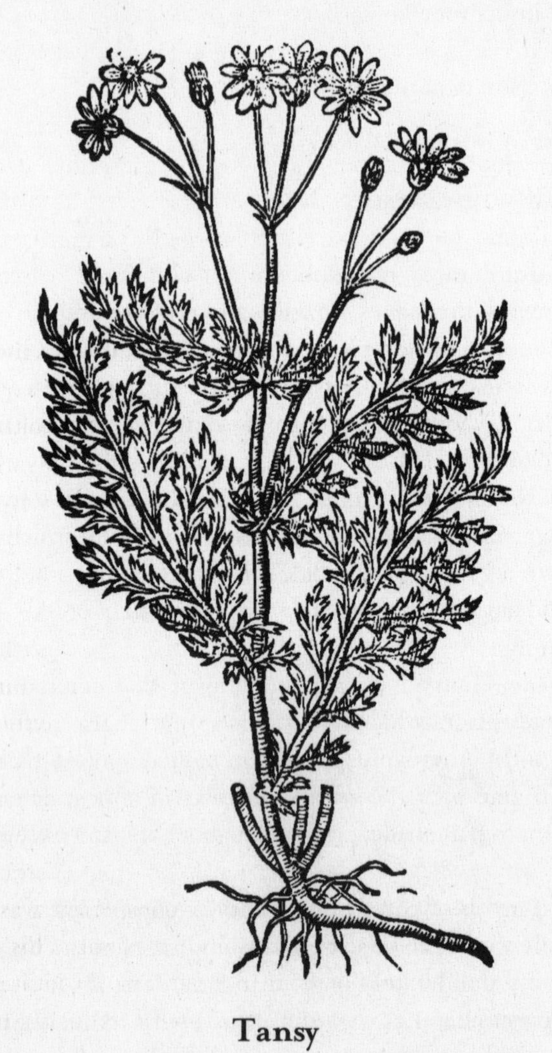

Tansy

the whole cluster in a wreath, or individual flower buttons to give color to potpourri.

The strong aroma of the foliage has been used for centuries as a moth and insect repellent—because it works. Dried tansy leaves are a main ingredient in most recipes for moth-repellent sachet mixtures; and some people just cut off the branches and lay them on the closet shelves. Many rural families hang sprigs of tansy in a window to keep out flies and spread branches across the threshold to keep out ants; they say that although ants crawl all over the plant while it is growing, they don't like the cut pieces and won't cross over them. This is one of those bits of folklore that's hard to prove, but if the ant and fly population is lessened, who cares what caused it?

Tansy was once taken internally as a medicine and used (albeit sparingly) in cooking. Now we know it is poisonous; an overdose can be fatal. Although you may still find recipes and cookbooks that suggest adding "a modest amount," common sense tells us it's not a good idea. Even if some say it's safe in moderation, why toy with something that's known to be toxic, especially since you can achieve the same effect with other, safer herbs.

Traditions: In ancient Greek culture, tansy was thought to make people immortal, a belief that probably originated in the legend of Ganymede. Zeus, the supreme god in Greek mythology, saw the handsome young man in the hills one day and decided to change him into a god. So he gave Ganymede a drink of tansy juice, which made him immortal, and swept him up in a whirlwind to Mt. Olympus, where he served ever after as Zeus's cup bearer.

From then up through the Middle Ages, tansy was used in funeral ceremonies to prepare the body for burial. This no doubt conferred immortality on the spirit of the departed, but it also had a practical purpose: to help prevent spread of fatal disease. It was one of the stronger strewing herbs and was administered as medicine for intestinal worms, cramps, and gout. American colonists continued the European practice of rubbing fresh meat with juice extracted from tansy, for it was said that flies would not light where tansy was.

Up through the fifteenth century, a special bread called tansy cake was served at Easter services; some say this recalls the Jewish custom of eating bitter herbs at Passover, and of course it may simply be a symbolic recognition of tansy's powers of immortality. In later centuries, the tradition evolved from tansy cake to tansy pudding, also served at Eastertime.

WARNING: Tansy is not safe for internal consumption.

Tarragon *Artemisia dracunculus*

PERENNIAL

SIZE: 2 to 3 feet

GARDEN: Sun or part shade; rich soil with very good drainage

USED FOR: Flavoring

AVAILABLE COMMERCIALLY: Yes

Description: Tarragon belongs to the same genus as southernwood, wormwood, and the decorative artemisias such as Silver King—but it is quite different from them in one important way: it's the only one that tastes good. Tarragon grows as a low, shrubby plant; it has very narrow leaves an inch or so long, and clusters of small flowers that most gardeners never see, because they keep them clipped off.

There are two types of tarragon: French and Russian. French tarragon, *A. d. sativa,* is the one with the best flavor; it does not produce seeds, and so you can only buy young plants. Russian tarragon can be grown from seed and is somewhat hardier, but it has very little of the flavor we recognize as tarragon. Unfortunately, you can't recognize the difference by looking at the seedling, and the scientific names are so close they can be misleading—or misspelled. Your best bet is to get a root division from a friend (so you can taste it), or buy a started plant of French tarragon from a reputable nursery.

Gardening: Tarragon does best in full sun in a somewhat protected spot, such as against a wall. It will survive weather a few degrees below freezing, but needs protection in colder winters. Some cold weather is necessary, however, if the plant is to go dormant, which it needs for healthy growth the next spring. Soil with good drainage is critical; otherwise roots will rot.

Tarragon spreads by underground runners. Every three or four years dig up mature plants in the early spring and divide them, roots and all, into separate small plants. Don't let flowers develop; the taste of the

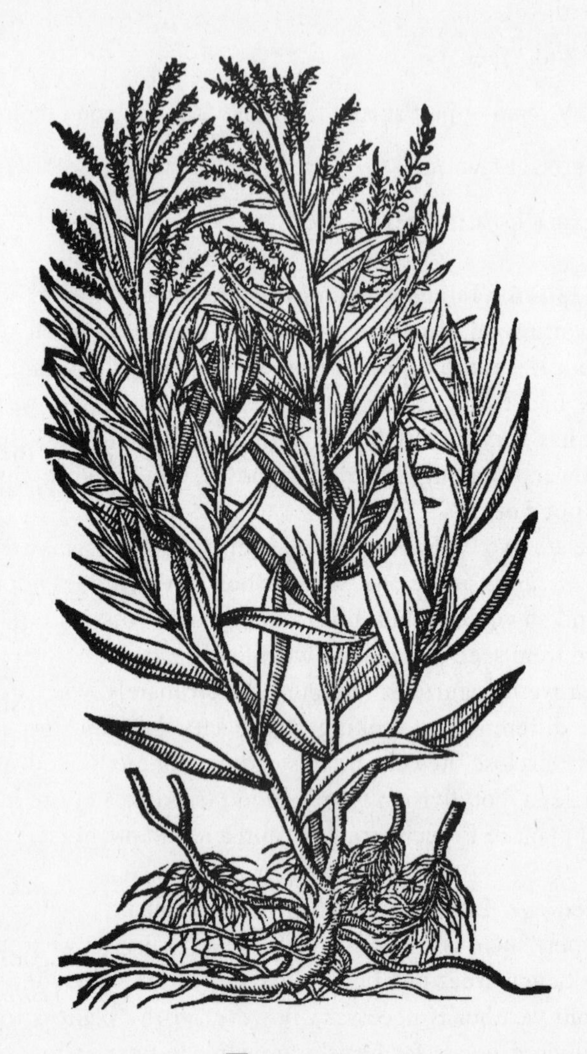

Tarragon

leaves deteriorates. Pinch off any flower buds that the plant tries to produce. In fall, cut stems back to about one-third the total length.

Harvest leaves all year long to use fresh; home-dried tarragon is disappointing, so freeze it or preserve its wonderful taste in vinegar.

Uses: Today we use tarragon only as a seasoning for food—but what a seasoning it is! The warm, spicy, vaguely sweet taste gives a special flair to many, many foods. It is the primary herb for many classic French sauces: béarnaise, tartar, ravigote, and remoulade; and it is often included in the mixture called fines herbes. It goes well with deviled eggs, omelets, cucumber salad, potato salad, fish, and especially chicken; and it adds a richness to mild vegetables, either sprinkled over the top with a little butter or in a sauce.

The taste is not overpoweringly strong, but it is distinctive, and so tarragon is often used by itself. It should be added near the end of cooking, so that its flavor remains light; some cooks add it after the cooking is finished, and allow the dish to rest for a few minutes while the tarragon does its magic.

One of the most familiar—and best—uses of tarragon is in flavored vinegar. Tarragon does not dry especially well, so this is an excellent way to preserve its special flavor if you have a large crop. Pack a jar with fresh leaves, pour white vinegar to cover, let sit in the sun for a couple of weeks, then strain. Makes the best salad dressing in the world.

Traditions: Tarragon was well known in ancient Greece and Egypt, where it was used to treat, among other things, dragon bites; we don't know for sure what these "dragons" actually were (scorpions, maybe) but the species name *dracunculus* means "little dragon." Even today in France, where it is very popular, tarragon is called *estragon.*

In the Middle Ages, people believed that tarragon would give stamina and keep them from getting tired, and those who had a long journey ahead put tarragon leaves in their shoes.

French tarragon, fresh, will cause your tongue to go slightly numb temporarily, and doctors used to give a patient a leaf to nibble before they had to take unpleasant-tasting medicine.

Thyme *Thymus vulgaris*

PERENNIAL

SIZE: 2 to 12 inches

GARDEN: Sun; light, dry, well-drained soil

USED FOR: Flavoring, ornamental, crafts

AVAILABLE COMMERCIALLY: Yes

Description: If you're looking at a plant that grows in a small, low mound and has teeny-tiny leaves, ninety-nine times out of a hundred it's a thyme. There are two general kinds of thyme—upright and creeping—and several dozen varieties, but they all have those tiny leaves in common. They produce tiny flowers in a large (well, large compared to the size of the plant) vertical cluster; the flowers are sometimes white, occasionally yellow, but mostly some shade of pink.

Thymus vulgaris, known as common or garden thyme, is the one most often grown and most often used in cooking (*vulgaris* here means not vulgar but common, as in *everyday*). It is the basic upright species, and from it many varieties have been developed; the uprights are usually 8 to 10 inches high. The "basic" creeping plant is *Thymus praecox arcticus*, known as wild thyme or mother of thyme; this subspecies used to be called *Thymus serphyllum*, and you may still find that name used. There are also quite a few varieties of creeping thyme, many with variegated or scented leaves; most of the creepers stay low, 2 to 4 inches tall.

Gardening: After a while, people who have the space for it tend to become thyme collectors; there are many interesting types, they're not overwhelmingly large, and they work nicely planted together. Here are some possibilities:

- Lemon thyme, with very lemony taste and smell; there is both an upright lemon and a creeping lemon, and there is also one called lemon curd thyme.

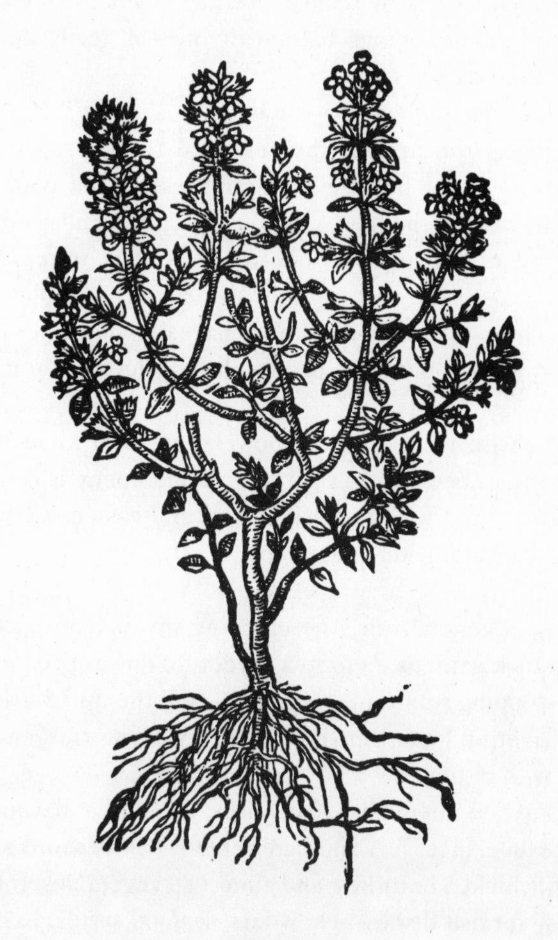

Thyme

- Those with variegated leaves: silver thyme (white and green), golden thyme (yellow and green), woolly thyme (gray-green and fuzzy).
- Those with unusual scents: nutmeg thyme, caraway thyme, oregano thyme, orange balsam thyme—all really do have the smell their names suggest.

Each spring, the upright thymes need to be pruned. Cut the stems back to about half their length to keep the plant full and bushy; otherwise all the new growth is out at the ends and the middle of the plant is bare. Even so, you may want to replace plants after a few years as they get scraggly. You can buy new plants, or start new plants from the ones you already have. Thyme lends itself well to tip layering, or you can divide the plant at the roots or make stem cuttings.

Thymes, with their aromatic flowers, are well known for their ability to attract bees to your garden; thyme honey is considered a gourmet treat. And with their small size and easy care, thymes are good candidates for patio containers.

Uses: As a general rule, the creeping thymes are used decoratively—in rock gardens, to form a border for flower beds, or planted between stepping stones in a walkway—and the upright thymes are used for flavoring food. But there is no law about this, and you can do either with either.

In the kitchen, thyme has many uses. Its familiar flavor enhances spaghetti sauce, meat loaf and hamburgers, hearty soups and stews, stuffing for chicken or turkey, and almost all vegetables. It has a special affinity for fish dishes—chowders, seafood salads, baked fish—but it has a powerful taste, so always add it lightly. Fresh thyme, especially lemon thyme, makes a very good flavored vinegar.

Thyme is a common ingredient in potpourri mixtures, especially where a spicy, rather than flowery, aroma is the goal. The ones with the scented leaves work particularly well. The flower heads, dried, add a special note to potpourri, and help keep moths and other insects away from linen closets.

Dried thyme is refreshing when added to the bathwater or a face wash, but if you have sensitive skin, test it first. Thyme leaves and flowers contain an oil called thymol, which is used commercially in many pharmaceutical and cosmetic products. However, pure thymol has been known to cause negative reactions both internally and externally, so you should be cautious about trying home remedies.

Traditions: Thyme is known as the herb of courage. In ancient Greece, it was believed to confer strength and bravery on all who used it; tired soldiers took a bath in thyme water, and later were massaged with thyme oil, to give them renewed strength for the battlefield. Departing knights and crusaders were presented with scarves that their ladies had embroidered with pictures of thyme.

In the Middle Ages thyme was used as a strewing herb, for which it no doubt worked extremely well, for we now know it has antiseptic and disinfectant properties. It has a long history as a medicinal herb: it has been said to cure fevers, digestive problems, asthma and other respiratory illnesses, to relieve headaches and hangovers, to dispel melancholy, and to prevent nightmares.

Wormwood *Artemisia absinthium*

PERENNIAL

SIZE: 2 to 3 feet

GARDEN: Sun or partial shade; average soil, well drained

USED FOR: Ornamental, crafts

AVAILABLE COMMERCIALLY: No

Description: All the artemisias except tarragon look much alike: full, bushy shrubs with gray-green foliage that flashes silver in the moonlight or in a light breeze. The leaves are all frilly and feathery, although wormwood is somewhat coarser than some other artemisias. The flowers are small, yellow-green, and not especially noteworthy.

Gardening: If you want to grow wormwood you would probably start with a young plant or a root division. Choose a spot just for this plant, for wormwood contains a water-soluble substance that keeps other plants from growing nearby. On the positive side, it does keep down the weeds. Wormwood will grow in either sun or part shade, is not fussy about soil, and requires little care.

Uses: With this plant, we learn an important lesson: just because an herb was once grown for a certain purpose does not mean it is wise to continue that use. Wormwood is known for its bitter taste, and it was the principal flavoring agent in a liqueur called absinthe. That beverage is no longer manufactured, because it is extremely harmful; it causes convulsions, paralysis, even death. But many older references refer to the now-illegal absinthe, and books published as recently as World War II suggest wormwood tea as a remedy for headaches and for intestinal worms (from whence comes its name).

Wormwood is in modern herb gardens for two reasons: its foliage

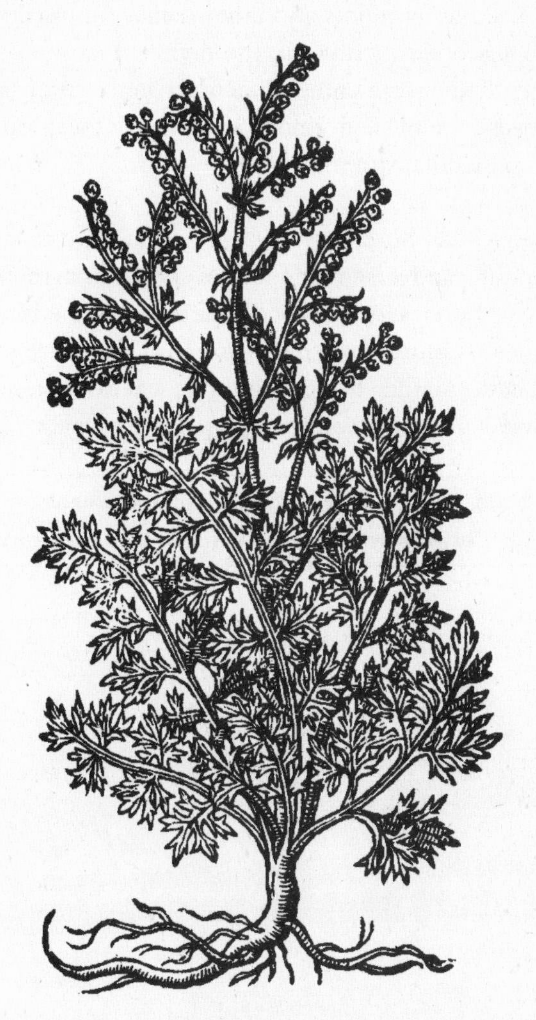

Wormwood

is very lovely, especially to provide a contrast to the darker greens that predominate in most gardens; and it is a superb moth repellent. Dried leaves added to mixtures for sachets, or simply hung in the closet, will keep away moths and other damaging insects. Indeed, the Greek Dioscorides, writing in the first century A.D., suggested this use, and a famous seventeenth-century herb writer said, "This herb wormwood being laid among cloaths [clothes] will make a moth scorn to meddle with the cloaths."

Traditions: The bitterness of wormwood is often noted in ancient literature, and it is mentioned several times in the Bible: "In the end she is bitter as wormwood, sharp as a two-edged sword." That bitterness is probably also the source of the old legend about the serpent in the Garden of Eden: after he was cast out, the serpent slithered away and wormwood sprang up along his path.

CAUTION: Wormwood should not be used internally; don't drink it, don't eat it.

Yarrow *Achillea millefolium*

PERENNIAL

SIZE: 2 to 3 feet

GARDEN: Full sun; average to poor soil

USED FOR: Crafts, ornamental, cosmetics

AVAILABLE COMMERCIALLY: No

Description: Chances are good you've seen yarrow at some point in your life; it grows wild over much of the United States, and in fact many people consider it a weed. It grows in clumps with tall stems, proportionately small leaves that are very feathery, and broad, flat clusters of flowers at the ends of the stems. The flowers of the "weed" variety are white, but cultivated varieties have very pretty shades of pink and a strong mustard yellow.

Gardening: You can start yarrow from seed, or get a friend to give you a start, which no doubt she will be happy to do because the plant produces lots of babies. And if you find it growing by the road (in a place where it's okay to do so), dig it up and bring it home. It needs full sun but will be happy in just about any soil and will tolerate drought quite well. Yarrow spreads by underground runners, sending up little plants all around; if you want a full bed, leave them in place, but every four or five years you should divide the clump.

Many gardeners are convinced that having yarrow nearby gives other herbs a richer flavor and makes vegetables grow better. While this has not been scientifically verified, it certainly couldn't hurt.

Uses: Yarrow is grown mostly for its flowers—to be enjoyed either as a garden perennial, as a cut flower, or dried for wreaths and floral arrangements. If you've seen only the white or yellow varieties, you're in for a surprise: the pink and red flowers are very pretty, and much softer looking.

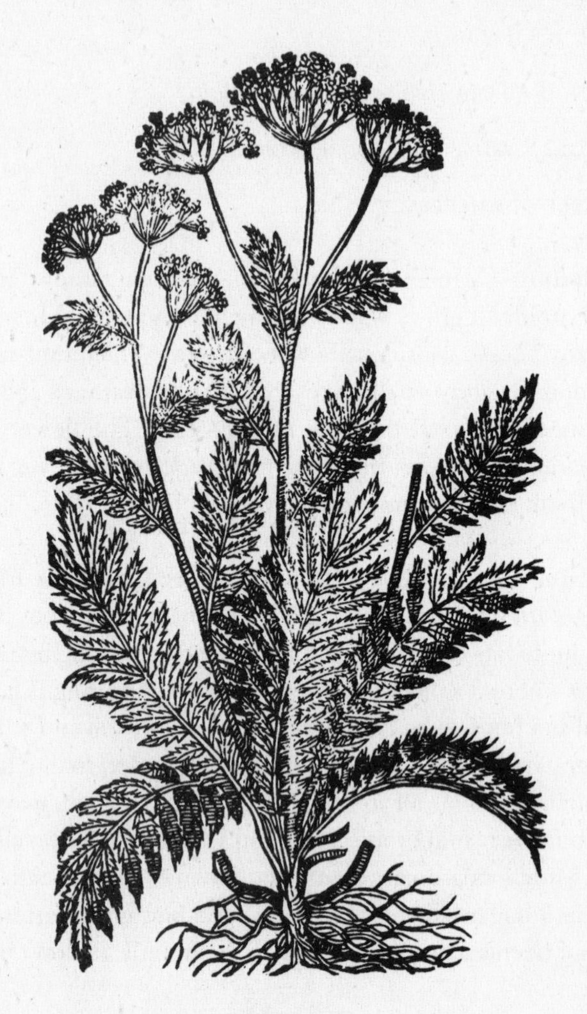

Yarrow

To dry the flowers, cut long stems when the flower is at its peak and hang them upside down individually. The white and yellow flowers keep their color well, but unfortunately the reds and pinks do not.

There are other garden yarrows, including one that's worth growing just for the fun of its name, sneezewort: the white flowers are fragrant, but sniffing them makes you sneeze. Other varieties are low, creeping plants that are appropriate to use as ground covers or in rock gardens.

Yarrow has antiseptic and astringent qualities, and a herbal water made from it is a good face wash, especially for oily skin. However, some people have a mild allergic reaction (a skin rash) to the leaves, so test before using. It also makes a relaxing bath that is good for the skin (assuming you're not one of the allergic ones).

Traditions: According to Greek legend, yarrow gets its scientific name from the great warrior Achilles. At the battle of Troy, in which many Greek soldiers were wounded, a Greek god appeared and showed Achilles how to stop the bleeding by applying leaves of a plant growing nearby, which thereafter bears his name.

That ability to help blood clot has been noted since the very first writings about herbal healing, and up through the American Civil War yarrow was grown and shipped to the front for treating wounds. American Indians used yarrow extensively, and so did the colonists.

Outside its medicinal uses, yarrow is accorded mystical qualities in some cultures. The Druids (ancient England) used stems of it to help forecast weather changes, and in China, the "sticks" that are an important part of the I Ching ceremony for understanding the meaning of life and seeing the future were actually very straight stems of yarrow, cut to exactly the same length.

On a level somewhat more prosaic but no less significant for its believers there is this bit of folklore, presumably chanted by young girls: "I will pick the smooth yarrow, that my figure may be more elegant, my voice be like a sunbeam, my lips be like the juice of strawberries."

PART TWO

Herbs Through Time

CHAPTER ONE

The Romantic History of Herbs

- Company's coming for dinner and you've made your special chicken dish. "What's that flavor?" someone asks. "Tarragon," you answer. "Oh, no wonder it tastes so good."
- A group of people at a neighborhood party are talking about their lawns. When you mention that you have a small herb garden, all the others get a kind of dreamy look in their eyes.
- You come across some lavender soap in the drugstore and hold the package up to your nose; the smell takes you back to your grandmother's house, and you smile at the memory of her.

Why are herbs so appealing?

Partly because they have the ability to enrich everything they touch—both the tangible item and our experience of it. In the garden, herb plants are not particularly flashy; in the supermarket, they come in little glass jars that are no more dramatic than baking powder. Yet their contribution is rather magical. And in a world so full of glitz and flash, that is part of our pleasure in herbs: the continual sense of wonder that something so modest could have such a big impact.

In part, our attraction to herbs stems from a yearning for old-fashioned pleasures that take us back to a time when the pace of life was slower and the world was easier to understand. Your enjoyment of herbs may come in the form of a relaxing cup of chamomile tea, or a hair rinse made from rosemary, or lavender-scented bathwater, or any one of dozens of ordinary uses. But no matter what form it takes, every time you do something with herbs, you are for a short time transported to a gentler way of life.

Sometimes, to be sure, that nostalgic feeling is not realistic. None of us really wants to live without electricity or telephones, and washing a month's worth of clothes by hand with homemade lye soap is not the least bit romantic. But trimming that little basil plant on the balcony, or adding an herb to a recipe that doesn't call for it, gives us a feeling of creativity and satisfaction too often missing from a high-tech, high-convenience world.

Once you learn that people have been using herbs for thousands of years, you have another reason for appreciating them. It is a way to reach back through time to earlier generations, to feel the continuity of human experience.

When you give a cup of soothing mint tea to a child who has a tummyache, you can symbolically stretch your hand back through three thousand years to the mother in Greece who is worried about her feverish child. She too is giving her baby mint tea; it is all she knows to do. From your vantage of antibiotics and modern technology, you sit down beside her, put your arm across her shoulders, and comfort her.

Herbs Through History

We know for sure that families have been using herbs for some 5,000 years, and there is some archaeological evidence that herbs were part of life many thousands of years before that.

Throughout all that time, herbs have been used in many ways:

to enhance the flavor of food

to treat illness

to protect linens and winter wools from insect damage

to make colorful dyes for home weavers

to honor outstanding achievement, in ceremonial wreaths and garlands

to create beauty lotions and ointments

to perfume the air

to create love potions and witchcraft charms

Mystics, Witches, and Saints

Herbs have always been associated with religion. In Greek and Roman mythology, herbs play a main part in some of the legends about the gods, and individual plants were dedicated to certain gods. Many of today's common names reflect these myths: Jove's flower, the herb of Jupiter, and so on.

Then there is the group of plants named for Old Testament characters: Solomon's seal, Aaron's rod, Adam's needle, for example. Later still, herbs were given names that honor the saints and apostles: St. John's wort, St. Anthony's turnip, St. Andrew's cross; and most of all, the Virgin Mary: Our Lady's mantle, Our Lady's bedstraw, Our Lady's glove, Our Lady's thistle. Angelica, named for the highest archangels, is the most sacred of all, so powerful it could keep away the dreaded plague.

In the Middle Ages, religion held a central place in people's lives. Rituals, many of them incorporating herbs, were daily events in those pious times. Sometimes herbs were burned in churches like incense. This also had the effect, coincidentally, of cleaning the air of germs, since the herbs had disinfectant qualities. The medieval priests, lacking our knowledge of chemistry, did not know why this practice worked; they knew only that it seemed to help.

This is one of the fascinating things about herbs—thanks to modern science, we now know that often these ancient practitioners were right.

History's Medicine Chest

From the standpoint of history, the most important trait about herbs is their long tradition of use as medicine. Until very modern times, when we figured out how to create drugs in a laboratory, the only way people could treat disease was with some formulation made from the things in the world around them—animals and plants. Some animal concoctions were used, but mostly—fortunately—healers turned to the plants growing in their area.

As new plants were studied, new formulas attempted, these healers began to write down what they learned. These precious medical records were passed down to the next generation and were added to as new knowledge was accumulated. This cumulative written record of herbal information is a very important part of how we know what we know about those ancient times.

Most of the herbs we know today are native to the hot, dry regions of the Mediterranean. That region is also the home of two of the most important cultures in the history of the world: the Greeks and the Romans. Each civilization contributed to our history of herbs in its own way: the Greeks, a culture of scholarship, philosophy, and art, studied the plants and wrote about them. The Romans, a culture of commerce and warfare, took the Greek knowledge of plants with them as they marched across Europe and brought back new plants they encountered along the way.

Hippocrates, the Greek physician who is known as the father of medicine and who gave us the Hippocratic Oath, described uses of some four hundred herbs. Dioscorides, a Greek doctor who traveled with the Roman armies, wrote extensive descriptions of about five hundred plants; his book formed the basis for the practice of medicine for the next fifteen hundred years.

During the medieval period, the treatment of the sick was in the hands of religious leaders. The first actual herb gardens in Europe were planted in the sixth century by Benedictine monks; in Italy, Switzerland, France, and England, monks began collecting herbs and planting cloister gardens, to have at hand the herbs needed to treat the sick. They laboriously wrote down, by hand and in Latin, the uses of the plants they grew.

Some of the prescriptions were, to say the least, bizarre. This was the time of the great plagues that terrified all of Europe; there was no real cure, so people were advised to try to keep from getting it by carrying in their hands certain herbs believed to have magic powers. Some very elaborate formulas were concocted for treating the sick, with more than a hundred ingredients, including some that were definitely weird; only the rich could afford them.

Did these concoctions really work as medicine? Yes and no. Some herbs, we now know, do indeed have properties that work against disease. And in a broader sense, any medical doctor will tell you that your body will heal itself more rapidly if you have faith in the treatment you're getting. But the herbal formulas did not save people from the plague, did not instantly mend broken bones. If a certain remedy seemed to help with a certain illness, the monks recorded it as successful and used it with other patients; if the patient died, it was considered God's will.

In the monasteries, monks continued to experiment with combinations of herbs. Today some of the most famous liqueurs echo these formulas. Benedictine, for instance, originally produced by the Benedictine monks as a tonic, is said to contain angelica, thyme, hyssop, mint, and many others; the exact formula is a secret. The small glasses in which cordials are generally served today are said to represent the small glass in which the medicine was dispensed to patients.

Then, in a relatively short period, three things happened:

1. Medical books using everyday language, instead of Latin, were produced, so that the information was available to everyone instead of an educated few.

2. The printing press was invented, and soon it became possible to have many copies of books instead of a few hand-lettered editions.
3. The great monasteries began to break up, and the care of the sick passed to the parish priest, who continued the tradition of growing herbs at his door for the benefit of the parishioners.

All this led to the phenomenon during the Renaissance years of the special kind of book known as a *herbal.*

A herbal is a book that describes herbs, usually with illustrations of some kind; presents information about the healing properties they have; explains what diseases they are effective against; and tells how they should be administered. (By the way, herbals are still being produced by practitioners of herbal medicine.)

Among the writers of herbals are several whose names you will encounter often if you read more about herbs, for they are oft quoted, even today—if only for the novelty value:

- William Turner, a clergyman who was forced to flee England for his religious beliefs and took advantage of his time in Europe to study with botanists there.
- John Gerard, a leading apothecary in the late 1500s; apothecaries grew herbs, prepared formulas to a physician's prescription, and treated the patient.
- John Parkinson, who was apothecary to King James I of England at about the same time.
- Nicholas Culpeper, who produced a book for the commoners: medical herbalism mixed with astrology.

All the herbal writers perpetuated the monks' treatises and added some of their own new "discoveries," some of which are nothing short of outrageous.

Soon, the great age of exploration brought the colonization of the

New World. The colonists carried with them the herbs they depended on so heavily, carefully guarding the seeds during the long sea voyage. At the same time they found new plants in the colonies and sent them back to Europe.

As new immigrants arrived in America from different regions of Europe, each group brought the herbs of its homeland. Then, in the 1800s, Shaker communities developed commercial herb farms to supply city dwellers who had no garden space. The old patent medicines, sold door to door by traveling salesmen, were basically syrups made of herbs and spices.

Gradually, with new discoveries in the laboratory and the commercial manufacture of synthetic drugs, the use of herbal medicines declined. Only now are we finding that some of the old cures are pharmacologically sound.

HOUSEHOLD NECESSITIES AND LUXURIES

But through all those years, herbs were used for more than just medicine. Just as we do now, people in earlier times used the plants growing right around them in ordinary, everyday ways. For instance, there is the custom of *strewing herbs*.

Room Deodorizer

In the Middle Ages, churches, monasteries, and great halls of the castles did not have floors as we know them today. They were made of dirt or paved with flagstones, and in either case were difficult to sweep. Instead, it became customary to strew certain herbs over the floor; as people walked on them, the herbs would release their fragrance and the sweet aroma would help counter any musty odors. It just so happened that many of the special strewing herbs also had natural astringent qualities (although of course this was not known at the time), and in addition to the sweet smell, they helped kill germs.

In homes, hay and grasses were generally used, but on important occasions, as when a member of the aristocracy came to visit, special sweet-smelling herbs were used; then the old herbs would be swept up and replaced with new ones. Even into the early 1800s, royal families in Europe had a Court Strewer, who went in front of the king and queen on ceremonial occasions and strewed herbs in their path.

Food Flavoring and Preservative

Today, we add herbs to foods to give them an extra zing of flavor. People did the same in centuries past, but for a different reason. In those days before refrigeration, meat tended to go rancid before it was all eaten, and about the only way to make it palatable was with a heavy dose of herbs and spices.

Meats and any available vegetables were cooked into huge meat pies, meant to last several months. Toward the end of that time, the food had begun to deteriorate, and the herbs helped disguise the foul taste.

Herbs were also used as substitutes for vegetables. There was no such thing as pulling a bunch of fresh spinach from the refrigerator or a package of beans from the freezer, so households had vegetables only in their season. The rest of the year, any greens had to come from the edible plants that still had leaves on them: the herbs. The old term *potherb* refers to those leafy herbs that were added to the pot—that is, cooked like a vegetable.

And there is one other way that herbs played an important part in the kitchen, although indirectly: they were very valuable for their ability to attract bees. Before the days when you could go into a supermarket and buy cane sugar in five-pound sacks, households depended on honey for sweeteners, and so beekeeping was an important skill. Plants that attracted bees were thus especially prized, and the aromatic flowers of certain herbs are bee favorites. From the Greeks to the American colonists, families made sure to grow the herbs that the bees loved.

Perfumes and Deodorants

For many centuries, herbs have been made into lotions, body ointments, and perfumes. As far back as ancient Rome, women and men perfumed their bathwater with lavender flowers, giving the plant its name: lavender comes from *lavare*, meaning to wash.

In a rather less romantic mood, the fragrance of herbs served as a kind of deodorant. Taking a shower every day is a fairly new idea, as civilization goes. For centuries, it was common that people washed their bodies once a month and their clothes once a year. Fragrant herbs were used to cover up odors in the meantime.

Herbs were used as stuffing for mattresses, to create "sleep pillows" for insomniacs, and to keep moths and other insects away from linens and winter woolens. Certain herbs were found to be natural repellents, and sprigs of them were laid in the closets along with the clothes. This was the beginning of today's potpourris and sachets.

The Gentle Escape

Around the time that Elizabeth I was queen of England, gardening as a hobby became popular in Europe. At first it was a hobby for rich people; all the families of the aristocracy had chief gardeners, and competed with each other for the most elaborate garden designs. This was the period of the *knot gardens*, when herb gardens were planted in complex patterns meant to be looked down on from a castle window, and the plants were painstakingly shaped to maintain the pattern.

But it wasn't long before all kinds of people began to take pleasure in growing flowers for beauty. They found, as has every gardener before and since, that growing herbs produces more than seasoning for food or fragrance for the home; it also produces a way to escape from the stress of the day.

In 1657 William Coles wrote: "If a man be wearied by over-much study, there is no better place in the world to recreate himself than in a garden. Neither do the herbs only feed the eyes, but comfort the wearied brain with fragrant smells, which yield a certain kind of nourishment."

Today we no longer depend on herbs to cure us when we're sick; we have pills and hospitals for that. We don't stuff our mattresses with herbs; we have fiberfill and foam rubber for that. We don't crown our athletes with garlands of herbs; we give them gold medals and endorsement contracts. But we do continue to grow and enjoy herbs, for we need that gentle respite as much as the overwearied Mr. Coles—perhaps more.

In the middle of World War II, one of America's great gardeners, Helen Noyes Webster, wrote a small book on herbs. In its preface she spoke of the "renewal of interest in those ancient plants called herbs." Noting that many gardens had been neglected during "the warring years," the author closed with this plea: "In times of truer peace than that of today's they [the gardens] may be built again by our children who seek, as did their forebears, the joy and happiness this pastime has ever created in man."

Nothing changes. Now, fifty years later, we have another renewal of interest in herbs, another generation seeking the serenity to be found there. The world has not found true peace, sad to say, but in our herb gardens (even those confined to balcony or windowsill) we can find a teaspoonful of tranquil beauty.

PART THREE

Growing Your Own Herbs

Time spent working in your garden
will not be deducted from your life.

Introduction

It is not necessary to grow your own herbs in order to enjoy cooking with them or making your own herbal products or gifts—but it is sort of inevitable. If you have any sort of yard at all, the day will come when you'll dig a hole and put in one herb plant, just to see how it does. And then you're hooked.

Even if you don't have a yard, if you love herbs chances are you will eventually want to grow some on your balcony or your windowsill.

When you do, this gardening section has the information you need. It rests on several assumptions:

- you don't know very much (or anything) about gardening
- you want to start small
- you approve of reasonable shortcuts
- you know where the closest large garden center is

Growing herbs is easy, because the plants are not fussy:

- they don't need constant watering or fertilizing
- they grow in less than perfect soil
- bugs don't bother them because they don't like the taste
- pruning takes care of itself (almost)

And that is the joy of herb gardening: that you get so much pleasure from so little effort. Enjoy!

CHAPTER TWO

Basic Gardening Principles

Note: This chapter is written for beginning gardeners. It covers the fundamentals, explains some basic terms, and strives always to present the easiest way of doing things. Experienced gardeners and botanical purists, if they feel a gurgle of protest at these simplified instructions, are encouraged to remember their own early feelings of confusion. The goal here is maximum success, via reasonable shortcuts and common sense.

Are you ready for some good news? Growing herbs is *easy.* Probably easier than growing anything else, except weeds and maybe grass. It is only a slight exaggeration to say that all you do is put them in the ground, then stand back and smile.

It's only when you've passed beyond the beginning stage that it gets complex. Buying one lavender plant is easy; evaluating the differences among fifty different varieties is not so easy.

Best to take it slow, and slide into herb gardening gradually. Let's start at the beginning.

Scientific Names

One of the first things you will notice as you browse through a garden center or a mail-order catalog is that each plant is shown as having two names: one in English and one in Latin. The English name is what is called the *common name*, and the Latin is the *scientific name*.

A problem with common names is that they are inexact. The same plant is called by two very different common names in different parts of the country, and the reverse also happens: the same common name is applied to two different plants. This can create confusion, as you may imagine.

However, there seems to be less confusion with herbs than with other kinds of plants. In point of fact, common names are used quite frequently with herbs, and in this book you will not find anyone insisting that you *must* learn the scientific names of all the plants. You should be aware of them, however, because you will encounter them in the catalogs and well-run garden shops; and if you ever want to track down a very specific variety, you'll need to know the Latin name. So here's a short course.

The Latin name has two parts (sometimes more, but always at least two):

Genus the first part of the name, always capitalized

Species the second part of the name, not capitalized

It's a bit like people's names:

Johnson, Jeremiah

Johnson, Alicia

The genus (pronounced JEAN-us) is a grouping of plants that are botanically similar to one another in some way; sometimes those similarities are obvious and sometimes not. The species is one distinct group within a genus.

To refer to a specific kind of plant, you use both names:

Artemisia dracunculus = tarragon

Within the *artemisia* genus there are other kinds of plants, so if you were to refer to "artemisia" alone, no one would be sure which plant you meant. But you would not say just "dracunculus," because by itself it has no meaning: it must be joined to the species name.

A third word in a Latin name denotes a subspecies; for instance:

Artemisia dracunculus sativa = French tarragon

Sometimes a plant has a third name that is in English, written in quotation marks; this is a new variety, developed in a greenhouse and given a name that honors a person or reflects some quality of the plant. Let's switch over to lavender for examples.

Lavendula = the lavender genus

Lavendula angustifolia = English lavender (a species)

Lavendula angustifolia "Hidcote" = Hidcote lavender (a popular variety)

When several Latin names are written close together, they are usually abbreviated after the first time, like this:

Lavendula angustifolia nana = compact English lavender

L. a. Munstead = Munstead lavender

One species name you will encounter often is *officinalis,* or *officinale.* It means "official," as you probably guessed, and it refers to the fact that that particular plant was once listed in official medical books as the species to be used for medicine.

Three Kinds of Plants

One basic concept you need to have under your belt is that plants have different lifespans: annual, biennial, and perennial.

- *Annual.* The plant lives its entire life cycle in one year. It grows from a seed into a full plant, flowers, then dies, all in one growing season. Next year, you have to plant new seeds. However, many plants drop their seeds to the ground, where they germinate the next spring without any assistance from you; gardeners refer to this as "self-sowing."
- *Biennial.* A plant that lives two years. The first year, it starts from a seed and develops leaves and a strong root system that carries it through the winter; the second year, it flowers, produces seeds, and then dies.
- *Perennial.* In theory, a plant that lives forever. In practice, most herb plants (especially the ones that develop woody branches, like a small shrub) tend to get bare down in the center, or scruffy looking overall, and so herb gardeners plan on putting in new plants every three or four years.

You'll need this information when you're shopping through the catalogs, planning what to plant and where. Most people find it easier to group perennials together in one spot and annuals in another. Each spring there is a certain amount of work to be done to get the soil ready for planting annuals, and it's more difficult to do that when you have to work between perennials, being careful not to damage their roots.

Another set of terms relates to how tough the plant is, primarily in terms of ability to withstand cold temperatures.

- *Hardy.* A plant that will survive harsh growing conditions, like extreme cold.
- *Tender.* Will not survive cold winters.
- *Half-hardy.* An in-between condition.

When used in combination with lifespans, these terms give us important information about the plant in question. For example:

Tender perennial	This plant needs extra care to make it through a winter, so you would either plant it in a very protected spot or plan to bring it inside in the winter (and plant accordingly).
Hardy annual	Botanically, this is an annual, but in a warm climate (or an unusually mild winter) it will live through to next spring.
Tender annual	This plant, on the other hand, is extremely sensitive to cold, more so than most annuals, and will die at the first hint of frost.

The U.S. Department of Agriculture has divided the country into eleven "hardiness zones," grouped by average coldest temperatures; eastern Canada is zone 2, southern Florida is zone 10. It is useful to know what zone you live in, because much written information about plants refers to it; seed catalogs, for example, will say that a certain plant is "hardy to zone 7."

To find out what zone you're in, ask your neighbors who do a lot of gardening or a local garden club, or check the USDA map on the following page. But remember that the map is just a general guide; very specific conditions in your neighborhood may create a microclimate that is significantly different. That's why in this area, as in so many others, a neighbor who is an experienced gardener is a gold mine of good information.

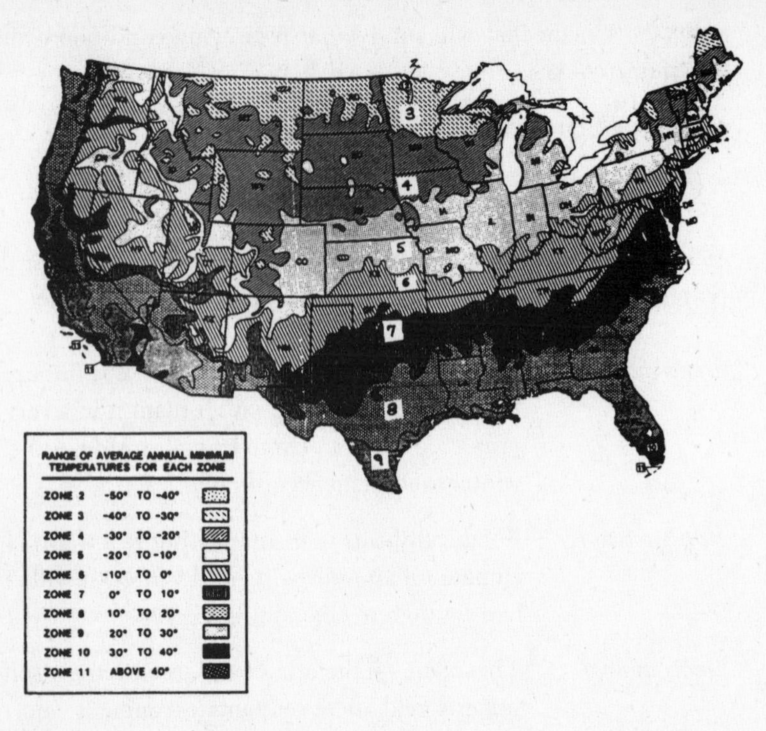

USDA map shows eleven temperature zones; many seed catalogs use the zones to indicate a plant's hardiness.

A Plant's Basic Needs

All species in the plant kingdom, from dandelions to giant sequoias, need four fundamentals:

1. Sunlight, which is essential to the process of photosynthesis, by which plants manufacture their food.
2. Water, so the roots can take in water-soluble nutrients, and so the plant doesn't flop over.
3. Soil, which serves as a medium for storing water and nutrients, and gives the plant something to stand up in.
4. Nutrients, which are various minerals that keep plants healthy.

But not all plants need the same amounts of those four things, and many will adapt to situations that provide less than optimum proportions of these basic needs. The finesse of gardening lies in knowing the relative needs of any one plant, and knowing when you can successfully cheat a little.

What about herbs? How much of those things do they need?

Sunlight

Most herbs—a large majority—need full sun. That means that for at least five hours each day, full sunlight (with no shade) needs to fall on the plants. A few herbs must have shade and will shrivel in full sunlight. Quite a few of the sun-lovers will adapt successfully to partial shade (less than five hours of sun), and some actually prefer it.

So, look at your space—either garden plot or balcony—and take note of how much sun it gets. Then choose plants accordingly. In chapter 3 you will find several lists of herbs grouped according to sun needs.

One aspect of available sunlight is *exposure*, which means the compass direction; if your balcony faces south, we say it has a southern exposure. At different points along the sun's arc, the angle and intensity of sunlight vary; you get more oomph from four hours of southern sun than four in a northern exposure. The four exposures rank this way:

South	the most sunlight
West	next most
East	next
North	least sunlight

Every exposure gets less intense light in the winter than in the summer. Overall, the exposure is not as important as whether the sunlight is blocked by a tree or a nearby building. But it is something to be aware of.

Water

Most herbs grow wild in hot, dry climates (many of them are native to the Mediterranean), so they can withstand periods of drought much more successfully than most garden plants—it's in their genes. But that doesn't mean you never need to water them. When plants are actively growing, they need more water than when they are resting (termed *dormant*). The active growth period for most plants is summer, a time when the weather is usually drier.

Here's a general rule of thumb: in the summertime, water your herb plants about half as often as you water vegetables or flowers. In spring and fall, water only when it hasn't rained for two weeks; in winter, after a month without rain or snow.

Soil

Two qualities of soil are important: its physical characteristics, and its pH value. Of those two, the first is the more important.

One thing you will read and hear consistently about herbs is that they need "well-drained soil." Good drainage means that water passes freely down to and through the plant's roots. Soil that doesn't drain well usually has a high proportion of clay; the soil particles bond tightly together, and water doesn't easily move through. Gardeners call this type of soil "heavy," and the good stuff is called "light."

Why is drainage important? Because herb plants are especially vulnerable to damage if their roots are in standing water. To tell if you have clay soil, dig a small hole and pour water in. If it drains right through, no problem; if water is still sitting in the hole after a minute or so, you have poor drainage. And you need to do something about it.

One solution is to "lighten" the soil by adding various things to it. Some of the common additions are:

sand

compost

shredded peat moss

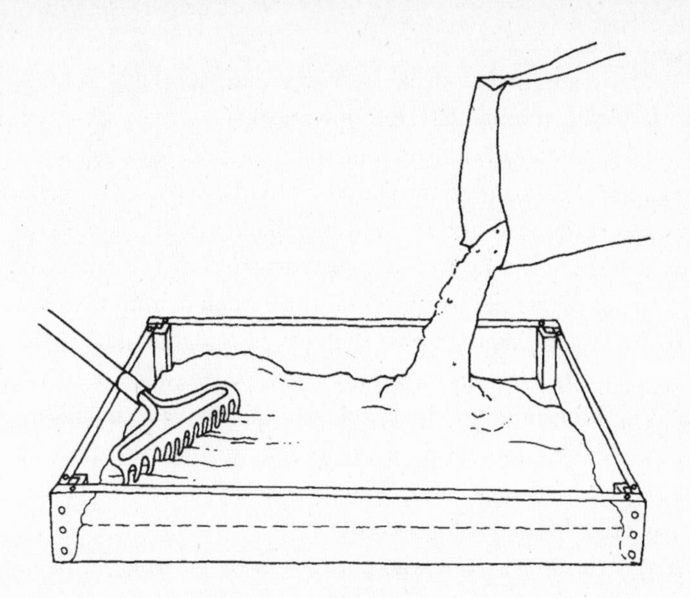

Raised beds are a very effective way of improving drainage and soil conditions. Build a bottomless box of outdoor lumber, reinforce the corners, and add in new soil up to the top of the box.

All these things can be purchased at your local garden center. With a pitchfork or small tiller, you work them into the soil early in the spring, or late fall for next year's garden. It's hard work, but dedicated gardeners consider this kind of soil improvement a major investment that pays off in the future. Also, if you're just starting a small herb garden, you'll be working with a manageable area.

Another way to improve drainage is to build (or have someone build for you) *raised beds*. A raised bed is a bottomless box, built of treated wood or metal, set down partway into the soil and then filled with topsoil that you bring in from another source, like a garden supply store. The soil in the raised bed is thus higher than the surrounding yard, which in itself automatically improves drainage. Also, the topsoil that you add will be lighter, better-draining soil; you wouldn't fill it in with clay soil, or you'd defeat the purpose.

Both these solutions represent a significant investment in time or money. A third approach is to forgo the yard altogether and grow your first herb garden in containers. (See chapter 5 for details.) Then you'll know whether you like growing herbs enough to make the necessary adjustments for the following year.

Now, the second factor of your soil: pH. Soil scientists have created a numerical scale to measure how acidic soil is. The scale runs from zero at the acid end to 14 at the alkaline end; 7 is neutral. For herbs, soil should be neutral—between 6 and 7.5. You can check this out yourself with a pH test kit from the garden center, which is simple to do, or you can ask a neighbor, which is a great deal easier.

Overly acidic soil can be modified, or "sweetened," as it's called, by adding limestone; too little acid can be corrected by adding sulfur or a sulfate compound, or organic matter like compost or peat moss. All these things can be purchased at your garden center; follow package directions for quantity.

Or you can bypass the whole question by growing herbs in containers. Generic potting soil that you buy to fill the containers will be the appropriate pH.

Nutrients

The nutrients that plants need to stay healthy and grow strong are already present in well-tended garden soil, but after a while they need replenishing. That's where fertilizer comes in.

Broadly speaking, herbs don't need much fertilizing; in fact, it's easy to overdo it, which gets you lots of green leaves without much aroma or flavor. In the first year or so, it won't hurt to add organic material such as manure or compost, or a commercial fertilizer made with organic ingredients, such as fish emulsion. But once a perennial herb plant is established, you don't really need to fertilize it.

On the other hand, if you're growing herbs in containers, that soil will become depleted, and you'll need to add a balanced fertilizer a couple of times during each growing season. At your garden center, look for fertilizer that says "organic" on the label, and one in which the three large numbers representing the principal nutrients are in approximately equal proportions: such as 10/10/10. Follow the directions about how to apply it. If it's the kind you mix with water, do *not* make a stronger dose; you'll burn the roots.

Getting Started with the Plants

Where do baby plants come from? They grow from a seed, or from some part of a mature plant that is cut off and started as a new plant. The collective term is *propagation,* and it's why commercial greenhouses are sometimes called nurseries—it's where new plants get born. All the techniques that commercial nurseries do can be done at home, but some are not worth the effort.

Seeds

Look through large seed catalogs, and you will see that almost all herbs can be started from seed. Growing plants from seeds is rewarding but can be slow. When you're first starting out, especially if you're unsure of your commitment level, it is much simpler to buy small plants rather than trying to start from seed. This recommendation applies to annuals as well as perennials. Later on, when you have some experience under your belt, it makes excellent sense to buy seeds; for large gardens, you'll save money. Any of several dozen general gardening books can show how to work successfully with seeds and seedlings; some of the seed catalogs also have good directions, along with all the accessories you need.

Cuttings

This propagation technique, on the other hand, does make sense for your first garden. A cutting (sometimes called a *start* or a *slip*) is a piece of plant that is removed specifically for the purpose of starting a new plant. You can do it with a plant you already have or with one from a friend.

Gardeners are a very friendly bunch and usually delighted to share their knowledge with others. If you have a friend who has an established herb garden, you are definitely in luck. Just show the

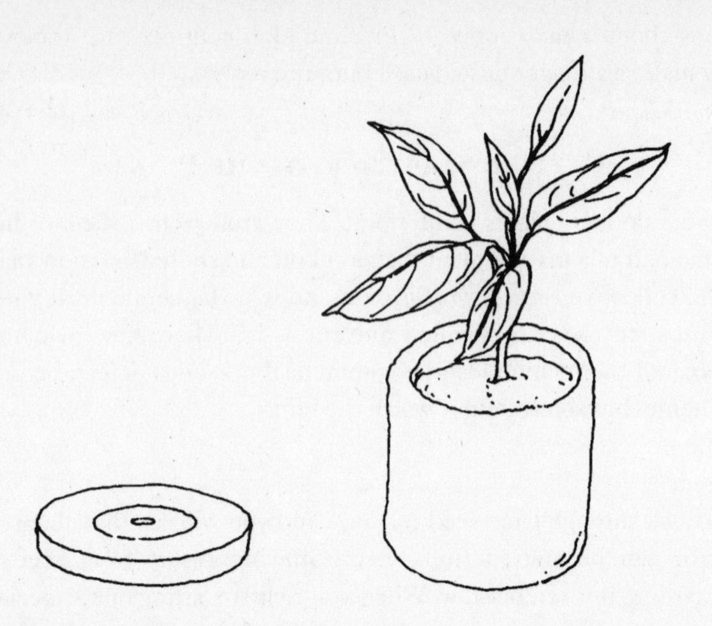

Peat pellets, flat and dry when you buy them, expand in water to form a sterile mini-pot in which to root cuttings. When roots have formed, plant the whole thing in the garden.

slightest bit of interest, and you'll find yourself with an unending supply of information, advice—and cuttings. In fact, it's a good bet that half the herbs growing in home gardens came from someone else's garden, friend to friend.

So now you're back at home, with cutting in hand. What next? If it's a mint, just stick it in the ground (or your big container) and stand back out of the way. For everything else, you'll be more assured of success if you root the cutting before you put it in the ground.

Rooting a cutting means that you help the cutting grow roots. Trim off the bottom leaves up to about the halfway point; the roots will form at the point where the leaves were attached to the stem. If the stem is very hard and woody, dip the cut end in rooting hormone (which you buy at the garden shop); this is not essential but will speed up things. If the stem is soft, you can skip this step.

Now plant the stem in a small pot filled with one of these ingredients or a mixture: potting soil, vermiculite, perlite, or sand. (Don't use dirt you dig up from the backyard; it's not sterile.) The solid material provides something moist for the stem to stand in while the roots are forming.

Set the pot in a warm, sunny window and keep the rooting material lightly damp. The rooting process can take anywhere from one week to one month, depending on how tough the stem is. After a week or so, pull very gently at the base. If it comes right up, it hasn't rooted yet. If you feel resistance, it's ready.

And here's a terrific shortcut: at your favorite garden shop or catalog, buy a package of peat pellets. These are flat circles of compressed peat moss encased in netting, about the size of a silver dollar, that when wet expand to about 2 inches in height. To use, soak one thoroughly to make it expand, then poke the stem of your cutting down into the middle hole. Keep the peat moist until the cutting is rooted, then plant the whole thing, netting and all, into the ground.

Root Division

This propagation method is even easier. You (or your generous friend) dig up a plant that has grown full and bushy, then with your hands or a sharp knife pull the whole thing apart—roots and all—so that you have two plants.

This is done all the time with plants that have outgrown their space. Try to get yourself invited when your gardener friend is dividing plants; she'll put one (now smaller) back into the garden and give you one to take home. Keep the roots moist until you get home, and plant it directly into the ground. That's all there is to it.

Layering

This technique is rather like rooting a cutting before you cut it off the plant. It can be done only with plants that have flexible stems, and it's especially easy with those that have a low, spreading growth pattern.

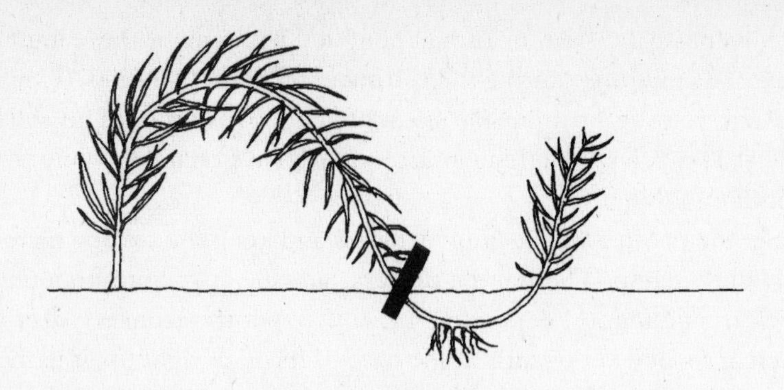

Tip layering is a way of propagating new plants without taking a cutting first. Bend the steam down and bury part of it underground (or use a rock to hold it down). After roots form, slice through the stem where indicated; now you have two plants.

Take a long stem and bend it down to the ground. Make a small ditch and bury part of the stem that has a node (the bulge on the stem where leaves are attached), but leave the outer tip unburied. Add a small rock or a bent piece of wire to hold the stem buried. Roots will form underground. Then you come along later and cut the rooted part away from the parent plant. Now you have a new plant.

Season-by-Season Maintenance

Spring

- If you're using seeds and want to get a head start, plant them indoors in shallow containers in the spring; thin the little seedlings and move them outside when all danger of frost is past.
- If this is your first year with a garden, start preparing the plot as soon as the ground is no longer frozen: weed, turn the soil over and over, break up clumps, work in some compost or manure, add other soil amendments if needed to improve drainage or pH.

- Check the perennials from last year. Most will need trimming, even if you cut them back last fall as you were supposed to. New growth starts from the tip, not the soil level. If your plant has lost some leaves down at the bottom (which is normal), it will never fill in with leaves there, and you'll always have a bare center. The only way to have a nice shape and full look is with careful pruning.

Summer

- Don't put basil plants into the ground until the weather, and the soil, are really warm.
- Watch for flower buds to form on perennials; just before flowering is the best time to harvest herbs for preserving.

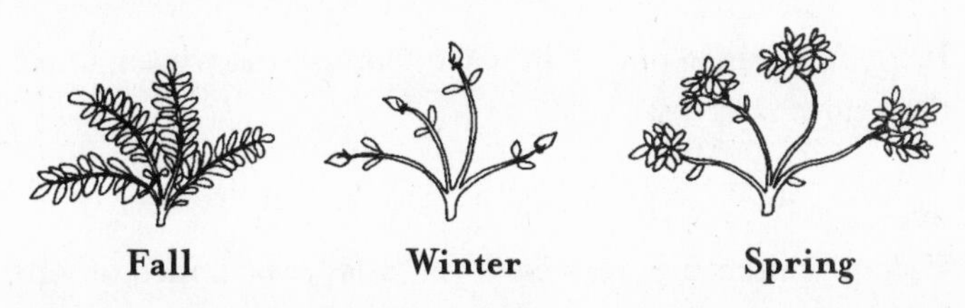

Failure to prune in the fall produces an unsightly plant in the spring. Although the plant looks fine in the late summer (left), in winter it will lose most of the lower leaves (middle), and then new growth next spring (right) will be limited to the very ends of the branches, leaving the middle bare.

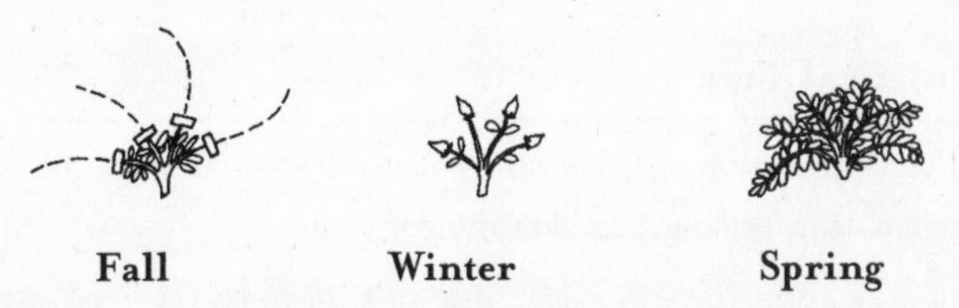

Good pruning in the fall produces nice, bushy plants in the spring. Cut back each branch to about one-third its length (*left*), then the length of bare stem in the winter will be shorter (*middle*), and the new springtime growth (*right*) will be much fuller.

- Watch for flower buds on annuals and pinch them off, to keep leaves from becoming bitter. Exception: if you're growing the plant for its seeds, let the flower form and then turn to seed.
- Water the plants during summertime dry spells.

Fall

- As soon as the weather forecaster even whispers "frost," pull basil plants out of the ground; they turn black at the first cold night.
- All perennials should be pruned back to get ready for winter. Don't cut off all the foliage, though; leave about one-third.
- Tender perennials like rosemary and lemon verbena should be put into pots (if they're not already) and brought to a protected porch or indoor spot.
- If you want small pots of herbs indoors for the winter, make cuttings now.

Winter

- If your winters are very cold, put a layer of mulch around the herb plants: pine needles, hay, leaves, or other organic material is best.
- Make yourself a cup of herb tea and snuggle down with the catalogs for next spring's order.

Practical Tips

- Remember: growing herbs is easy. They can withstand drought, they seldom need fertilizer, bugs don't bother them.
- Buy plants, not seeds, for your first herb garden.
- Watch the sun pattern and plant accordingly: put sun-lovers in areas of full sun, shade-lovers in the shade.

* If your soil doesn't have good drainage and you don't have the time or money to correct it, plant your herbs in containers.

* Cultivate the friendship of an expert gardener, preferably one who lives nearby and has the same gardening conditions to deal with.

CHAPTER THREE

Planning Your Herb Garden

When it comes to herb gardening, it seems that most people sort of tiptoe in. Maybe they decide to tuck in an herb plant or two among the flowers, just to see how they'll do. Or they buy a pot of chives on impulse in the supermarket, and then realize they have to *do* something with them. Or they're visiting a friend, admiring her herb garden, and before they know it they're heading home with a mint cutting in hand.

But few people can stop with just one plant. Growing herbs is so easy, and so satisfying, that pretty soon, most of those accidental herb gardeners get hooked. They add a few more plants, and then next year still more. And it isn't long before they are dreaming of a full-fledged herb garden.

Whether you're coming to herb gardening gradually, or have simply said to yourself one day out of the blue, "I want to have an herb garden," it's a good idea to do some planning before you start digging.

The Process of Planning

Planning starts with two basic questions:

1. Where should the herb garden be located?
2. Which herbs should be included?

Obviously these two questions are closely interlocked, so which do you tackle first? My suggestion is that you look first at the space you have available, and then choose herbs that will grow in those conditions. After those two fundamentals are settled, then you can think about the finer points, such as the layout of the garden and the specific varieties you wish to plant.

Where, and How Big, Is the Herb Garden?

Walk around your yard and think about where you could plant herbs. The main consideration should be sunlight. Of all the conditions that plants need in order to grow well—soil texture and acidity level, nutrients, minerals, water—the amount of sunlight is the one thing you cannot change.

If you have several possible spots to choose from, pick one that gets sunshine most of the day. Most herbs grow best in full sun. So if you have a sunny spot, you have lots of choices of plants to put there. But if all you have is a shady spot, then so be it—that's what you have to work with.

Then you have the question of size. Often this question is answered for you by circumstances: the place you have available is just so big. But let's assume you're lucky enough to have a large area: how big should the garden be? We want your first herb garden to be a success—a source of pleasure, not aggravation. So we'll start small.

There are countless designs you can use to give your garden an attractive layout, but every possible design (including no design) is basically either a square, a rectangle, or a circle. To keep things manageable, consider these guidelines:

Square	6 feet by 6 feet, with a walkway up the middle
Rectangle	3 feet by 10 feet
Circle	6-foot diameter, with one or two walkways

These dimensions (which produce approximately 30 square feet of usable space) will give you enough room for a good beginning set of plants, yet each is small enough that you can easily maintain it.

And they can all be expanded. Add more rings to your circle; make your rectangle longer; or double the square. Just remember that 3 feet is about as far as you can reach, so for any distance greater than that, you'll need to plan a path or stepping stones.

Which Herbs to Plant?

Knowing the location of your herb-garden-to-be will tell you whether you are limited to shady plants or have the much broader range of sun-loving herbs to work with. That's the first step.

The next step is deciding which herbs to plant. If you have a sunny location, this might seem an overwhelming task, since there are so many to choose from. How to go about it?

First, make up a rough list of the herbs you might like to grow. One way is to browse through the first part of this book, noting the plants that appeal to you. Another approach is to think in terms of your general interests. How do you think you'll be using the herbs?

- Are you mostly interested in herbs to cook with?
- Would you like to grow plants to use in crafts, such as dried arrangements or potpourri?
- Do you want to develop a garden around a particular theme, such as a "moonlight garden" or a fragrance garden?

Then read about the various herbs and start to narrow your list down. To help you with this part of the process, this chapter contains many different kinds of lists: herbs categorized by size, color, what kinds of light conditions they need, and so on, along with some suggestions for theme gardens. Later on you'll narrow things down even more and select the specific varieties that are compatible with your plan.

Garden Design: Three Basic Shapes

You have picked a spot for your herb garden, evaluated its sunlight, and decided which herbs you want to include. Now you are almost ready to start planting. The last step is to decide on a layout, the overall design of the garden.

If you want to design it, that is. There's absolutely nothing wrong with just putting the plants in willy-nilly (except that if you mix annuals and perennials in a jumble they'll be harder to take care of). But if you do take the time to plot out the relationship of one plant to another, being aware of leaf and flower color, texture contrasts, and the like, you can create something that is pretty to look at as well as useful.

It is reasonable to think of herb gardens as being one of three basic shapes: circle, square, or rectangle, with variations. The art comes in the variations.

Circle Gardens

With a circle design, you can get a lot of plants in a small space. Just remember that you'll need to be able to reach all the plants, to cut off pieces to use and to weed around them. If your circle is more than three feet in diameter, you'll need to put in a walkway or some stepping stones, otherwise you won't be able to reach the plants in the middle.

The two basic designs built around a circle are (1) concentric rings or (2) pie-shaped segments. With the concentric design, it is easy to expand next year to a larger garden: just add more outer rings. In the pie-shaped style you can make the pie pieces any size you want, but you should have a minimum of four.

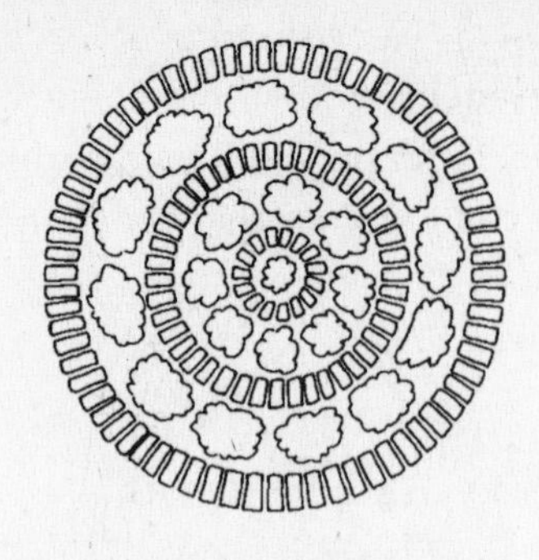
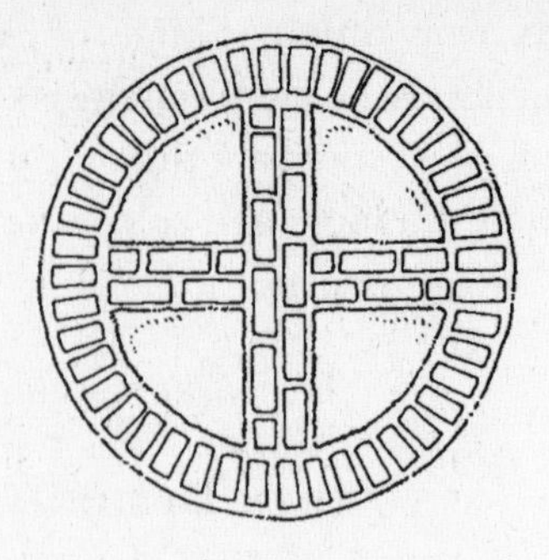

Circle designs for herb gardens can be divided into wedges like a pie (*left*) or into concentric rings (*right*). Bricks or stepping stones contain the edges and give you something to walk on.

The circle is the basis of one of the most familiar herb garden plans, and one of the most charming: the wagon wheel design. We might call this a settler's garden, for it calls to mind the homesteads of the pioneer days. The rim of the wheel defines a round space, and the spokes separate the overall shape into segments, each one planted with a separate herb.

The original settlers used wagon wheels because they were handy and cheap (they probably used damaged wheels that could no longer be repaired). Today, not many of us have old wagon wheels lying around, but we can still use the basic idea. Use bricks or flexible edging material to make the outer ring (and the round center, if you want one); use bricks or wood for the "spokes."

Plants for the settler's garden should have similar needs for sunshine and water. Beyond that, planning the wagon wheel garden is mostly a matter of esthetics. If you recreate a true wagon wheel shape, with a round space in the middle, put something tall in that center spot. Then in the pie-shaped sections you can put your choice of plants. You can reserve some sections for annuals, or plant the whole garden with perennials.

Think about colors. You might alternate dark green foliage plants with gray-green; or plan according to flower color, with blue-flowering sage next to oregano, with its pink blossoms, for instance.

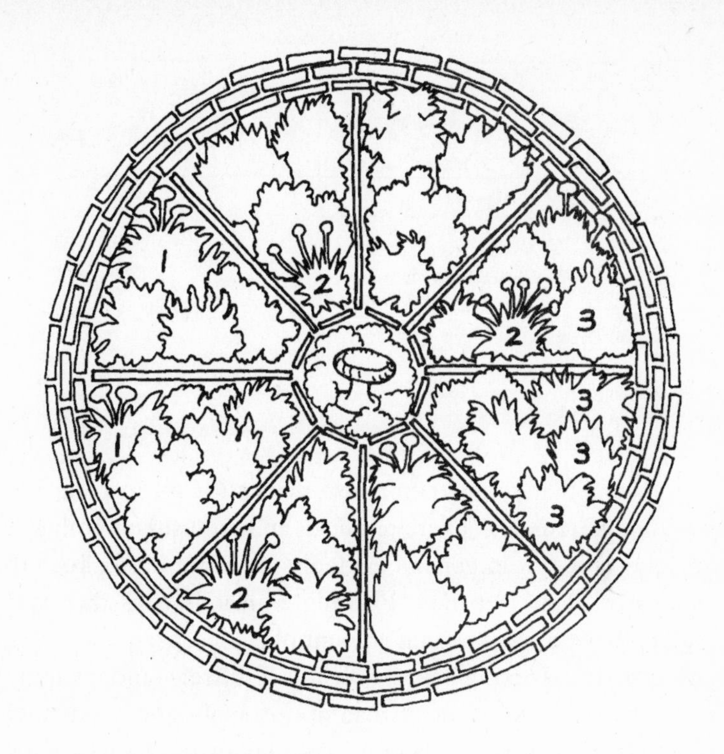

Wagon wheel design mimics the old settler's garden that used a real wheel to separate garden sections. Bricks and boards substitute for rim and spokes. Design your garden on paper first, using code numbers for the herbs.

Think about size. If you put one vigorous plant next to a low-growing plant, you'll have to keep the bigger plant well trimmed so it doesn't overtake the smaller one. And if you want mint in one of the sections, be prepared to keep digging it out of the others.

Rectangular Gardens

The rectangle is one of the easiest shapes to work with, because you can make a garden narrow enough to reach across and thus avoid having to build a path. If you want to expand next year, just make your rectangle longer. But if your space won't permit that, add a path (or paving stones) along one long edge of your first rectangle and add the second, so that the new garden is twice as wide.

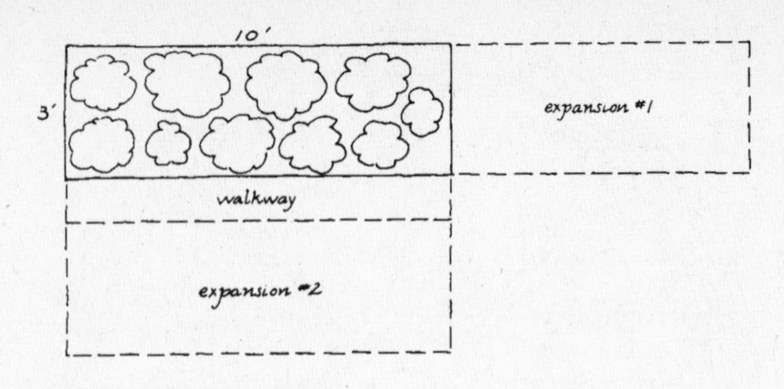

Rectangular designs are easy to expand.

The rectangular configuration also makes it easy to plant both annuals and perennials. There're pluses and minuses on both sides of this question, but in general gardening is easier if you keep the two types of plants separate. Planting annuals means that every spring you have to do a certain amount of soil preparation—tilling, weeding, maybe working in some organic fertilizer—and it's simply easier to do this in a big chunk than in tiny spots where you might accidentally cut into the roots of nearby perennials. So, with a long skinny garden, you can devote one or both ends to annuals, and the midsection to perennials. Or vice versa.

Square Designs

The square is the basis of many different designs, including that favorite of the Elizabethans, the knot garden. If we can expand our definition to include squarish rectangles, slightly longer in one dimension, we can say that the square is the most versatile shape of all, for it lends itself to so many variations.

Pictured above are just a few of the possibilities.

One popular style that is both attractive and easy to maintain is the checkerboard: a series of small squares, some with plants and some paved with bricks or stepping stones. The paved squares provide a way to walk among the herbs and also serve to keep weeds down; the plants spill over into the "blank" squares as they grow,

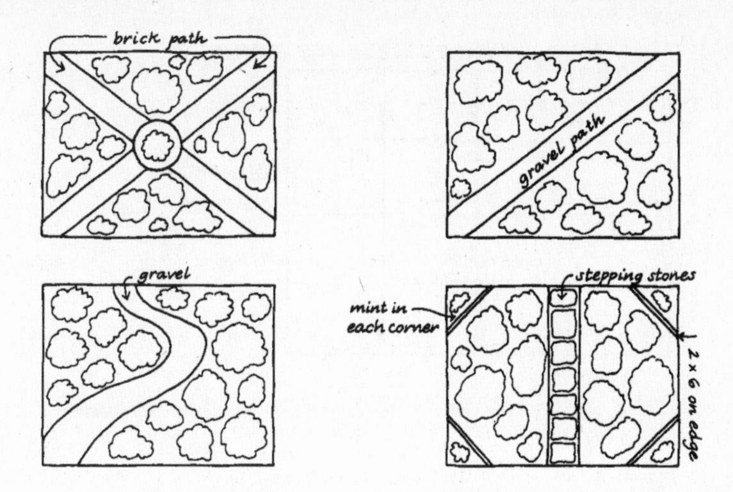

Square designs permit many variations; be sure to plan in some kind of walkway so you can reach all the plants.

softening the edges. It's easy to expand this garden: just add another row of squares.

And finally, a word about knot gardens. In these elaborate designs, herbs were planted in interweaving and often intricate patterns. This style originated in Europe in the seventeenth century and was popular with aristocratic families, who had the two prerequisites for gardens of this type: large castles, and full-time gardeners. The first is important because these gardens are meant to be looked down on from above—that's when their design becomes apparent—and the second because they require a great deal of maintenance, with constant pruning and shaping to maintain the patterns.

Twentieth-century herb gardeners with a feel for history and an appreciation of herbal traditions sometimes enjoy planning a knot garden, but the truth is, this kind of garden is for people with lots of time on their hands.

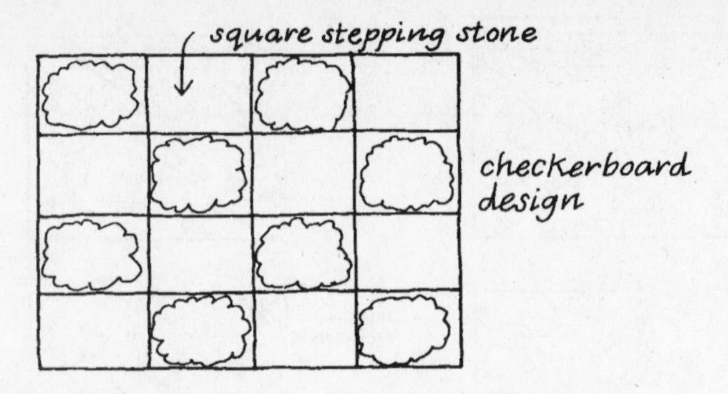

Checkerboard design can be expanded indefinitely, yet provides plenty of room to work among the plants.

The Esthetics of Design

Within the general layout you have settled on, you now have other decisions to make: exactly which varieties are you going to include, and exactly where will each one go? Those decisions have a lot to do with the overall look of your garden.

At the moment your herb garden exists only on paper, so you can play with different combinations. Be aware of:

- *Size.* When the plant is two or three years old, how tall will it be? How wide does it get? Don't put a tall or a fast-spreading plant in a spot right next to a low or slow-growing one, or pretty soon it will block out its neighbor.
- *General shape.* Is it tall and spiky? Low and spreading? A two-foot mound?
- *Leaf color.* The prettiest gardens are planned for visual contrast. If you put a plant with dark green leaves next to one with silvery foliage, both will look better.
- *Leaf texture.* Contrast is also achieved through texture. Something feathery and lacy looks more attractive if it's next to a

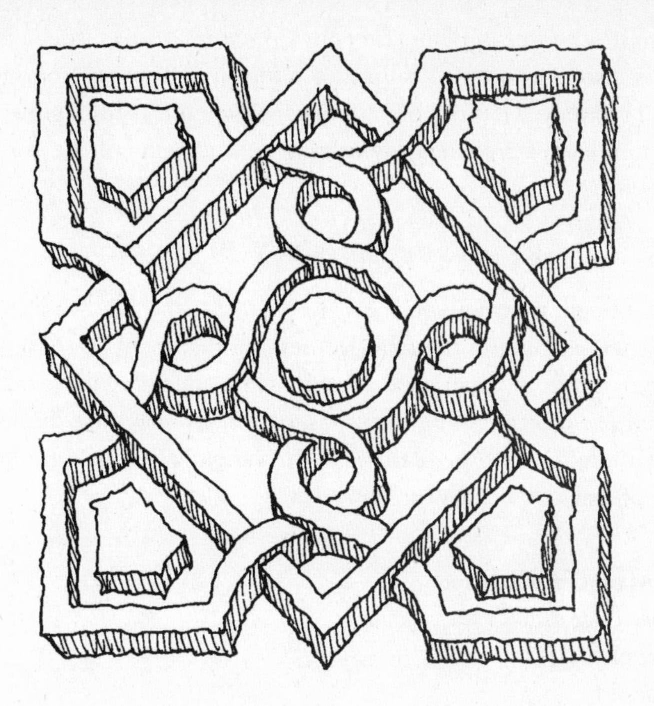

Knot gardens, where plants of different foliage are entwined, require continual maintenance.

plant with dense, solid-looking leaves; each one enhances the other.

- *Flower color.* The color of the flowers gives you another range of possibilities to work with as you plan for visual appeal.

If you're lucky enough to live near a nursery that grows herbs, by all means visit. Browsing among the many varieties in the company of a knowledgeable grower is the best way to fully appreciate the fine points: the different colors of variegated sage, say, or the difference between apple mint and pineapple mint.

The next best thing, in terms of learning about varieties, is reading the catalogs of mail-order nurseries (see Appendix). Pay attention to information about size, leaf color, and color of flower (if any).

Another source of plants for your garden is cuttings from a friend; this is also a wonderful source of education. You can see in your friend's garden what the plant looks like when it is fully grown, and no doubt learn a great deal about growing and using the herb as well.

Resource Lists for Planning

As you begin plotting your new herb garden, the following lists are presented as food for thought. Remember that many of these plants come in different varieties; that's why some appear on more than one related list. For planning purposes, especially planning the look of the garden, some of the features of the varieties may be significant—color of leaf, color of flower, and so on.

Growing Conditions

Shade: These actually prefer shade

- angelica
- chervil
- sweet cicely
- sweet woodruff

Shade: These will tolerate shade or partial shade

- bergamot
- catnip
- chamomile
- comfrey
- coriander
- costmary
- dill
- fennel
- feverfew
- germander
- hyssop
- lady's bedstraw
- lemon balm
- lovage
- mint
- parsley
- rosemary
- salad burnet
- tansy
- tarragon
- thyme
- wormwood

These will grow in damp areas

- angelica
- bergamot
- lovage
- marsh mallow
- mint
- parsley
- sweet woodruff

Size

Tall (more than 3 feet)

- angelica
- comfrey
- dill
- fennel
- lemon verbena
- lovage
- marsh mallow
- rosemary
- rue
- salad burnet
- southernwood
- sweet cicely
- tansy

Medium (2 to 3 feet)

- bergamot
- borage
- chamomile, German
- chervil
- coriander
- costmary
- feverfew
- germander
- horehound
- hyssop
- lady's bedstraw
- lavender
- lemon balm
- parsley
- santolina
- savory
- scented geraniums
- tarragon
- wormwood
- yarrow

Short (up to 2 feet)

- anise
- basil
- calendula
- caraway
- chamomile, Roman
- chives
- coriander
- nasturtium
- oregano
- parsley
- sage
- savory
- sorrel
- sweet woodruff

lavender, dwarf
marjoram
tarragon
thyme

Life Cycle

These are annuals

anise
basil
borage
calendula
chamomile, German
chervil
coriander
dill
nasturtium
summer savory

The following two, which in botanical terms are perennials, are effectively annuals:

- fennel (to eat the base of the plant, you must harvest the whole plant, so it becomes an annual by default)
- marjoram (in northern areas, this should be treated as an annual)

These are biennials

angelica
caraway
chervil (often used as if it were an annual)
parsley

Flower Color

If the same plant appears in more than one list, this means that there are different varieties, with different colors.

White

angelica
anise
caraway
chamomile
chervil
horehound
hyssop
marjoram
salad burnet
sweet woodruff
thyme

Yellow/Orange

- calendula
- costmary
- dill
- lady's bedstraw
- nasturtium
- tansy
- yarrow

Pink/Red

- bergamot
- hyssop
- yarrow (red varieties)
- oregano
- thyme

Blue/Purple

- borage
- hyssop
- lavender
- rosemary
- sage
- savory
- thyme

Theme Gardens

The Good Cook's Garden

- basil
- chive
- coriander
- dill
- mint
- oregano
- parsley
- rosemary
- sage
- tarragon
- thyme

A Tea Garden

- angelica
- anise
- bergamot
- borage
- calendula
- caraway
- catnip
- chamomile
- fennel
- horehound
- lemon balm
- lemon verbena
- mint, apple
- mint, orange
- peppermint
- spearmint
- rosemary
- sage
- sweet cicely

A Fragrance Garden

angelica
basil
bergamot
chamomile
costmary
hyssop
lavender
lemon balm
lemon verbena
marjoram
mint
rosemary
sage
scented geraniums
southernwood
sweet cicely
sweet woodruff
thymes

A Salad Garden

borage, chervil, sorrel, sweet cicely, chives *(use young leaves as salad greens)*

lovage *(leaves are a substittue for celery)*

salad burnet *(leaves taste like cucmber)*

fennel *(throw in a bit of the ferny foliage)*

nasturtiums *(leaves and flowers both taste peppery and the flowers add that incomparable color)*

The Herb Sampler

This garden will give you a little bit of everything. It is built around the herbs that are not so easy to find commercially (or so satisfactory); notice, too, that some are in the garden for two purposes.

For cooking
basil
chives
parsley
thyme

For fragrance	lavender
	lemon verbena
	scented geranium
For color	bergamot
	calendula
	pineapple mint
	tricolor sage
For tea	fennel
	lemon balm
	peppermint

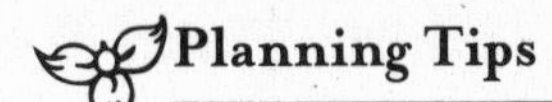

Planning Tips

* Decide where your herb garden is going to be, then choose plants that are compatible with the amount of sun in that spot.

* Make your first herb garden small; you can always expand next year.

* Put tall plants in the back, medium plants in the middle, low-growing plants in front.

* Put annuals in one place and perennials in another place; they're much easier to maintain that way.

* Plant some things purely for their beauty.

* Visit as many herb gardens as you can; observe what the plants look like when they are fully grown.

CHAPTER FOUR

Herbs in the Landscape

From a gardener's viewpoint, there are few things in the world more rewarding than growing herbs. But a full-fledged herb garden—a separate garden area with nothing but herbs—is not the only way to experience the pleasure of growing herbs.

You can incorporate herb plants into your flower gardens, your vegetable garden, or your general landscaping. In fact, whether you live in a house, condominium, or garden-court apartment, wherever there is a bit of ground, you can grow herbs.

HERBS AS LANDSCAPE PLANTS

The practical uses of herbs are so valuable that sometimes we forget how beautiful they are. With their delicate flowers and interesting and unusual leaves, many types of herbs make a wonderful addition to any landscape. They serve admirably as ornamental plants, either to be enjoyed for their own beauty or to create a background or contrast for other plants—and every one comes with a bonus: its utilitarian role.

To incorporate herbs into your general gardening, take a few minutes to look through the lists in chapter 3. You will want to familiarize yourself with the plants' size and shape, the color and texture of their foliage, and the colors and blooming period of their flowers.

Some of the best herbs to use as ornamentals are those with silvery or variegated leaves (colors other than plain green); for example:

Herbs for Colorful Foliage

- Silver King or Silver Queen artemisia
- purple basil (an annual, but worth the extra work for the rich wine-red color)
- tricolor sage (white, magenta, and green)
- variegated sage (yellow and bright green)
- green or gray santolina
- silver or golden thyme

To perk up your flower beds, you might consider adding some of these:

Herbs for Flowers

bergamot	rich red flowers with an unusual shape
chives	pink puffball flowers are edible as well as cute
feverfew	masses of tiny white daisylike flowers
yarrow	tall plants for the back of the flower bed; flowers are pink, yellow, creamy white

Hedges and borders

The great majority of herbs are perennials, and so among them you can find several that will produce an unusual low hedge. Here are just a few suggestions:

- germander (nice dark, shiny leaves)
- hyssop (added bonus: its lovely flowers)
- rosemary (unless your winters are very cold)
- rue (leaves have a blue cast)
- santolina (either gray, or green, or both in combination)

And then there is lavender, with its gray-green spiky foliage and haunting sweet scent. Line the walkway to your front door with lavender, and keep it thick and luxurious. Visitors will brush against it, releasing into the air a swish of fragrance that serves as a special welcome to your home.

Ground covers

A ground cover is a low-growing plant that spreads out in all directions and covers an area like a green carpet, one that may be accented with flowers in season. They are useful wherever you can't grow a lawn—or don't want to. Herbs that work as ground covers are the ones that spread out to form a mat; for example:

Ground Cover Herbs
Roman chamomile
Corsican mint
pennyroyal
sweet woodruff
creeping thyme

One that is not so well known as it deserves to be is sweet woodruff. It has much to recommend it: charming little leaves, tiny white flowers, and a light vanilla fragrance, plus the fact that it grows happily in the shade and so works beautifully under trees where other ground covers will not grow.

Another use of these carpeting plants is to fill in the spaces between stepping stones or bricks. They will all survive being walked on occasionally—in fact, Roman chamomile grows better—and it's much prettier than having weeds grow up between the bricks on your walkway.

HERBS IN THE ROCK GARDEN

Many of the lower-growing herbs that form a mat on level ground will spill down attractively when grown on a slope, and this makes them perfect for adding to rock gardens. Any plant that has "creeping" or "prostrate" in its common name grows this way; the terms *repens* or *recumbens* in a Latin name also indicate this kind of growth pattern.

In addition, many of the common herbs are available in dwarf varieties—just the same as the regular herb, but in miniature. These are also lovely in rock gardens. Look for varieties named *compacta* or *nana*, or labeled "dwarf." And of course the regular variety of plants that never get very tall work well in rock gardens too; chives, with its unusual flowers, is an example.

Here are some ideas for rock-garden herbs:

- chamomile, Roman
- chives
- lavender, dwarf
- mint, Corsican
- mint, pennyroyal
- parsley, curly
- rosemary, creeping
- sage, variegated
- thymes (especially, for their color, those with variegated foliage)
- winter savory

HERBS IN THE VEGETABLE GARDEN

Another painless way to add a few herbs to your life is to plant them in with your vegetables. They get to piggyback on your tilling, soil preparation, and watering (although they need all three less stringently than vegetables). And here too you get a bonus: certain herbs are believed to be effective in repelling from the garden insects that would otherwise damage your vegetables.

This way of growing vegetables is known as "companion planting." Some of the beneficial effects have to be considered folklore, but why not try it? You have nothing to lose except your bugs.

Another aspect of companion planting is positive: some plants appear to help others grow more lustily if planted in close proximity.

Herbs for Companion Planting

anise	encourages growth of coriander, and vice versa
basil	seems to make tomatoes grow better
bergamot	also helpful for vigorous tomatoes
borage	contributes to overall health and disease resistance in neighbors
calendula	keeps bugs away from tomatoes
catnip	repels squash bugs
chamomile	good neighbor for cucumbers and onions
dill	makes cabbage and lettuce grow better
garlic	repels aphids; controls cutworms and hornworms that can ruin tomatoes
hyssop	protection against white fly; try with cabbage
mints	repel aphids, cabbage worms, and beetles
nasturtiums	keep white flies and aphids away
oregano	helps beans grow
parsley	keeps asparagus beetles away
rue	said to repel beetles
sage	good for carrots, cabbage, tomatoes
santolina	aphids hate the smell

southernwood, camphor	repels cabbage moths
tansy	used to ward off ants, flies, cabbage worms, squash bugs, and potato beetles
thyme	discourages cabbage worms and white flies, encourages tomatoes, potatoes, and eggplant

Landscaping Tips

* Add perennial herb plants to your flower beds; the foliage contrast is stunning.

* Hate mowing grass? Put in a chamomile lawn. Or flagstones with creeping herbs between them.

* Mix herbs with vegetables, to help control harmful insects and to promote growth—the zen of vegetable gardening.

CHAPTER FIVE

If You Don't Have a Garden

You live in an apartment, you say, or a condominium, or a houseboat . . . with no bit of yard to call your own. Can you still grow herbs? Sure you can. It will have to be on a smaller scale, and you may have to be a bit resourceful, but if you live in an apartment you're used to that, right?

Let's look at two general ways to have a no-garden garden. The first assumes you have some kind of outdoor space, no matter how tiny: a patio, a balcony, a front porch, a fire escape, whatever. For the sake of simplicity, let's call this patio gardening. The second we'll call indoor gardening: growing herbs in pots inside your apartment.

Patio Gardening

The idea here is that you attempt to recreate, as much as possible, the growing conditions of a yard-based herb garden—except that your "yard" is a container. You will walk through the same steps: evaluating your space, deciding which herbs to grow, preparing the soil, and caring for the plants. One thing is different, and you might as well get used to it now: you will have to do more watering.

How Sunny Is Your Space?

Most herbs need sunshine—at least six hours a day. That is the number-one fact that determines planning for all herb gardeners, whether they're working with two hundred square feet of earth or two small patio pots.

So your first step is to take note of how much sunlight there is on your patio (or whatever it is). And that's determined by two things: the exposure, plus or minus any shade-making obstruction.

Figure out which exposure you have—east, west, north, south—and then make allowance for anything that would block out light: nearby trees, adjoining buildings, roof overhangs, and so on. Remember this sequence: south has the most sun, then west, then east, then north. A south-facing balcony blocked by a tall building counts as east, maybe north.

What Herbs Can You Plant?

In very general terms, we can say that you can grow in a container anything you can grow in the ground, as long as you are able to make certain adjustments, and as long as you are willing to accept the fact that you won't always get the same results.

Being confined in a pot is not a natural condition for a plant; the net result is that it will grow more slowly and less vigorously. Instead of a six-foot dill, you may get only a two-foot plant. But it's still dill, with the pretty feathery foliage and unique taste.

On the other side of the coin, life in a container is just what some herbs need. Even people who have large outdoor herb gardens grow lemon verbena and sweet bay in large pots, so they can move them into protected spots in the winter. And what better way is there to contain the invasive growth of lemon balm or the other mints?

The amount of sunlight available is the key factor that determines which herbs you can grow successfully. If you have a shady area, you should stick to shade-loving plants; check the lists in chapter 3. If you have a spot that gets a mixture of sun and shade, you have a wider range of possibilities. And if you have full sun, you have even more choices.

Planting Your Garden

If you spend some time browsing through your local garden center, it's easy to feel overwhelmed by the merchandise. So many different kinds and sizes of pots . . . gizmos for watering . . . fertilizers and other mysterious stuff in bottles—not to mention the enormous variety of plants themselves.

First, let's learn about pots.

What Kind of Container?

Clay The familiar brick-colored terra-cotta that has been around forever is still the favorite of many gardeners. The material is porous, which means that it lets air into the soil and the roots, which is good. It also lets moisture out, which is both good (it helps prevent waterlogged soil) and bad (it dries out faster). Clay is heavier; it is also brittle, thus more easily broken.

Plastic Plastic pots are lightweight, nonporous, and come in several different colors. Soil moisture is retained, which means (1) you need to water less often, and (2) you are more apt to overwater if you're not careful.

Ceramic Hand-painted and brightly colored ceramic pots are pretty but expensive. They are usually intended to serve as an outer pot, covering a more pedestrian pot down inside.

Fiber Fiberboard pots are grayish brown and have a pebbly texture. They look like cardboard—which is what they are: dense paper fibers pressed into the shape of a flowerpot. They work just fine, but they are not permanent. On your patio, they will certainly last one year, maybe two.

Which should you use? You'll get lots of recommendations from gardeners, nursery owners, and garden center staff. My suggestions:

- plastic, if expense is a concern, or if you're away from home a lot, or both
- clay, if you can be conscientious about watering (or if you're a classicist)
- fiber, if you're trying to save money or if you're not sure you'll want to have a garden next year

There is only one absolute: Whatever pots you choose *must* have a drainage hole in the bottom. This is important for all plants in containers, and it is essential for herbs, which have a particular need for good drainage.

If you have enough room, you might want to consider wooden planter boxes. They are not cheap, but they do look wonderful. The disadvantage of wooden planters is that eventually they will rot from the wet soil, although many will last for several years. Perhaps the best way for you to use them is as an outer container, disguising homelier pots put down inside.

Finally, look around to see if you have any place you can put a hook for a hanging planter. It's a good way to make the most of a small space.

What Kind of Soil?

This question is much simpler to deal with. In the garden shop, buy a big bag of houseplant mix. It's ready to use, right out of the bag. If you're going to have just one or two pots and want to create as little bother as possible, this is the easiest way.

The other approach is to buy what is generically referred to as potting soil and add other things to it: perlite or vermiculite to keep it loose and fluffy, peat to improve water retention, sand to improve drainage. This approach makes sense if you plan to have lots of containers with different kinds of plants. The problem is that if you don't use up all the soil materials, then you have half-empty bags of stuff sitting around, which is a nuisance in an apartment.

Mixed Containers

A very attractive technique, which also maximizes limited space, is to have just a few very large containers, and to plant several different herbs in each one. Put one herb that grows upright and tall in the middle, surrounded by smaller plants, including some that will cascade down over the edge. Mix annuals with perennials, and next year you can put in some different annuals.

And where is it written that you have to restrict your containers to herbs alone? Add in flowers for a bright splash of color: alyssum (white), lobelia (intense blue), and petunias (many colors) tumble prettily over the side.

Here are some suggestions:

Container Combinations

- rosemary (tall), parsley (medium), thyme (trailing)
- tarragon, marjoram, and nasturtiums
- chives, basil, parsley, oregano—an Italian collection
- sweet bay with sweet woodruff in its shade
- pineapple sage, tricolor sage, gold variegated sage, green sage
- sweet cicely (tall), calendula (medium, yellow flowers), lemon thyme (creeping)
- salad burnet, creeping savory, woolly thyme (tiny pink flowers)
- rose-scented geranium, spearmint, and Roman chamomile
- lemon balm, peppermint, and pennyroyal

- sweet bay (tall), parsley (medium), thyme (creeping)—a bouquet garni pot

Large garden centers carry a special kind of planter called a strawberry jar, an urn-shaped container with several "pockets" in the sides. They're usually made of terra cotta and come in several sizes; try to find one at least two feet tall. They were originally designed to grow several strawberry plants in a compact space. (In the garden, strawberries spread all over the place by sending out runners, which root and make new plants.)

We can use that same principle for herbs. In fact, it almost seems the strawberry jar was actually invented for herbs, for you can grow a different herb in each pocket and so have an entire herb garden in something that takes up about two square foot of floor space.

The secret to success with these planters starts with a trip to the hardware store. Buy a piece of PVC pipe (the lightweight white

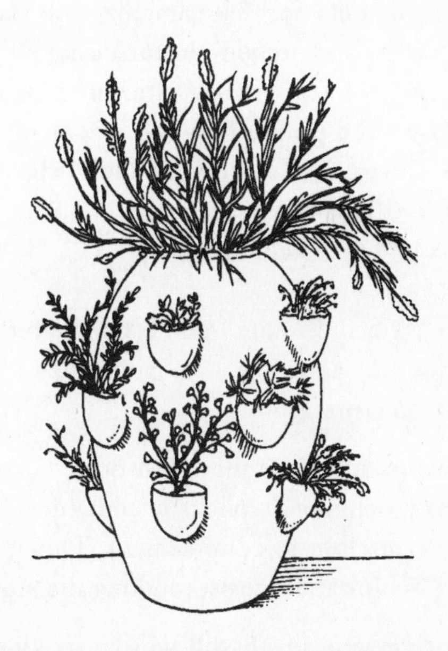

Strawberry pot, with its many separate pockets, is an ideal way to grow several herb plants in one small space.

plastic pipe) about 2 inches in diameter and approximately as long as your pot is tall. Drill small holes all around it, and sink it down into the soil before you add the plants. This will ensure that water gets evenly dispersed to all the plants.

Now you're ready for the fun part: adding the plants. In the top of the planter, put things that grow upright. In the pockets, put herb plants that creep and dangle downward. Flowering plants like nasturtiums are nice for a splash of color.

Aesthetics of Patio Gardening

You don't have lots of space to work with, like traditional garden designers, but you can still approach your project with an eye for how it all looks. In fact, because your miniature garden is so concentrated, it's even more important to plan the visual aspect.

If all other things are equal (that is, if you don't have to think about where the sun is), put containers in carefully planned groupings. Two or three coordinated clusters is more appealing than ten individual pots. Plan a cluster that capitalizes on the plants' visual qualities. For example, a kitchen cluster designed around foliage contrasts: parsley (rich forest green), variegated sage (which is yellow and chartreuse), and purple basil. Or mix shapes and textures: the thin strips of chives, the feathery mound of chamomile, and the free-form oregano with its tiny leaves.

Here are some points to keep in mind:

- Use just one style and color of pot. It takes a bit of discipline to maintain this, but allowing a hodgepodge to develop is the quickest way to visual clutter.
- Keep the plants nicely pruned and dead flowers picked off. Untidiness is much more obvious in containers because people want to move in close to admire them. This is particularly so with herbs; people cannot resist fondling the aromatic foliage.
- Think about viewing level: will you be looking down on the plants (if they're on the floor), from below (if they're in hanging

pots), or at eye level? Try to match the plant's best angle with the viewing angle.

- Vary the height in your garden by putting some pots on pedestals: turn an empty pot of the same or larger size upside down and set the plant on top.

Caring for Your Patio Garden

Like all plants, herbs have just a few basic needs: sunlight, water, and the right kind of soil; herbs, in fact, are much less fussy about these things than other kinds of plants. If you can provide those necessities, there's no reason you can't grow herbs in containers.

Light

As to sunlight, there's not much you can do to change existing conditions. But there are a few possibilities. To stretch limited sunshine:

- If you have a mixture of sun and shade, rotate your plants. You don't have to do it every single day, but once a week at a minimum move some pots into the sun. Make it part of your regular plant maintenance. If you have very large containers this will be easier if they're on wheels, so think about this when you're planning your containers.
- If you can, paint the nearest wall white; it will reflect light back onto the plants. If you don't have permission to paint, maybe you can put up a white screen.
- Do the same with the floor area: lay white tiles around the plants. You don't even need to glue them in place—just lay them down on your patio.

If you want to grow shady-area plants and have to contend with blasting sun, try these ideas:

- Put the pots under a table or bench.
- Grow your plants in very large containers and put a picnic shade umbrella in the center.
- Build a very simple trellis arrangement, train a vine like ivy or honeysuckle to grow on it, and position your smaller pots in the shade it creates.

Water

This is the one part of container gardening that is very different from "earth" gardening. The soil in containers dries out much faster, and you will have to compensate by regular watering. Fortunately, as a general rule herbs are more drought-tolerant than most flowers and vegetables, but that does not mean that you can forget about watering altogether.

It is impossible to give a cut-and-dried rule about watering, since so many factors come into play. Whether any particular pot needs watering will depend on how big that pot is, what material it is made of, what the weather has been like and, to a lesser extent, what kind of plant it contains.

The best thing for you to do is check the soil by poking down into the pot with your finger. If it is dry as far down as you can reach, it needs some water. Another quick rule of thumb: if you are also growing flowers or cherry tomatoes on your patio, water your herbs one-half to one-third as often as you water your petunias.

If you're going to be away during the summer and can't get anyone to water your plants for you, here's a trick: Water the plant very thoroughly, then cover the top of the pot with several pieces of plastic wrap, worked in tight against the stem. When the moisture evaporates, it will condense on the underside of the plastic and drip back down. You don't want to leave this in place forever or you'd rot the stem, but it will get you through a two-week vacation.

Fertilizer

In the greater scheme of things, fertilizer is not a major concern with herbs. In fact, unless you're growing them strictly for looks, you're better off not fertilizing herbs heavily; you'll get vigorous leaf growth, but the oils that give flavor or fragrance will be spread disappointingly thin.

By the end of the summer of the first year, and several times during the growing season each year after that, add a light application of all-purpose fertilizer. Most herb growers recommend that you use an organic kind such as fish emulsion. Follow the label instructions about how strong to make it. *Do not* give your plants a double dose; you'll just burn them.

Pest control

You'll need to check for bugs every once in a while, although one of the great things about growing herbs—as opposed to, say, brussels sprouts—is that insects and other critters pretty much tend to leave them alone.

If you do have a major influx of insects, *do not* rush off to the garden store for a chemical insecticide. Remember, you are planning to eat these leaves someday, so you don't want to spray poison on them. Instead, use a mild insecticide such as rotenone or pyrethrum, which are made from plants; or try one of these organic controls:

- Mix up a solution of dishwashing detergent and spray it all over the plant; then spray several times with clear water to wash off.
- Grind up garlic cloves and mix with water (one clove to one cup of water); strain and spray on plant. Good for aphids.

Pruning

When you grow herbs, pruning—which means trimming the plant so it stays in a tidy shape—pretty much takes care of itself: as you snip off pieces to cook with, you are pruning at the same time.

But it's a good idea to stand back now and then and take an overall look at the shape of your plants. If things are getting lanky, do a little judicious pruning to neaten up the form. Or make a mental note that one side is too long, and plan to cut there during the next harvest.

Pruning is *good* for the plants. When you take off the end of a stem, it will send out side shoots. And if you later take off the ends of those stems, they will branch out again. And that's the way you end up with a plant that is full and bushy, instead of tall and lanky. This is especially important for the plants you are growing for their leaves (which is the case with most herbs). If you don't keep pinching out the growing tip, you'll end up with something that has two or three long spindly stems with no leaves on the bottom.

And it's doubly important with annuals (basil is the most popular one). The plant, with a natural urge to procreate, is doing its darnedest to flower and make seeds; you want to prevent that. Once a basil plant flowers, the leaves lose quality. So keep pinching off the flower head, and you can keep your basil tasty up until frost. You can cook with the part you pinch off.

Seasonal Care

Your big concern here will be helping your perennial plants survive through the winter. In a garden, plants have the insulating factor of all that soil to protect against bitter cold. In a container, a plant has only a few inches of soil between its roots and the outside world.

When the weather becomes extremely cold, move your containers to the most sheltered spot you have. Even if all you can do is tuck them up against the outside wall, that's a help.

What about bringing them inside? That's a bit tricky but can work, as long as you plan ahead. One thing most plants hate is sudden change. If you leave your plants on the balcony through the early winter and then bring them inside because the weather report predicts a hard freeze, the abrupt change from cool atmosphere to the heated apartment will throw the plants into shock. If your area is subject to really cold winters, you should plan for a gradual transition: first move them to a sheltered outside spot for several weeks, then to the coldest indoor spot you have, then to a more moderate spot.

If you're growing rosemary, it *must* come inside; it's so tender it often doesn't survive a winter even in an outdoor garden. This pretty plant makes a nice houseplant, and so it's worth the effort to acclimate it to an indoor environment for the winter.

When warm days of spring trigger new buds, do a thorough pruning job so that the new growth comes in in a nice shape. Then, in the hot days of summer be watchful of watering needs. The rest of the time, just enjoy.

Window Boxes

If you have no outdoor space at all, but a window with a sunny exposure, you can still grow herbs: plant a micro-garden in a window box.

Window boxes—long and skinny—come in several sizes and several kinds of material. The two main kinds are plastic (which is lighter and lasts longer) and wood (which is usually more attractive). As with planter boxes, however, wooden window boxes will eventually rot from your watering. One way to use them is to put individual pots down inside; then you can easily remove one pot at a time for maintenance, or replace a plant if it becomes sickly.

If you plant the herbs directly into the window box, be sure it has drainage holes.

The general guidelines about planning and aesthetics apply here too. Read up on the plants you're interested in, especially their mature size and growth pattern, and think about color and texture when planning your combinations.

Here are two suggestions:

A Summer Herb Window Box

basil
calendula
chervil
chives
dill
summer savory

A Winter Herb Window Box

parsley
rosemary
sage
salad burnet
thyme

If your only window is in the shade, all is not lost. Make up a window box with several kinds of mints and enjoy the luscious aroma all winter.

Indoor Gardening

Yes, you can grow herbs in pots inside your apartment; no, you won't get huge amounts of produce.

Let's be clear about this: no herb grows *better* indoors than it does outdoors. There is no such thing as a houseplant herb. But some of them will do reasonably well on a windowsill if it gets good light. And, if you have an outdoor space available, many herbs can be used as indoor plants on a rotation basis: a few weeks indoors, a few weeks outside, then back in again.

You probably will not get a large crop from your windowsill garden, but if you enjoy the idea of growing herbs in your apartment and like the looks of the plant, it's definitely worth trying. You will have fresh sprigs of mint or thyme to use as a garnish or a conversation piece—both of which have value—and then there is that wonderful aroma when you rub the leaves.

These Can Be Grown Indoors

basil

bay (grow it as a shrub in a patio pot, bring pot indoors in winter)

chives

scented geraniums

lemon verbena (grow it in a tub, bring indoors in winter)

marjoram

spearmint, peppermint

oregano

parsley

rosemary

sage (dwarf variety)

pineapple sage (not hardy outside in winter)

winter savory

tarragon

thymes

Caring for Your Indoor Garden

The techniques of indoor gardening are much the same as described for patio gardening. To repeat the most important points:

- Be sure every pot has a drainage hole.
- Remember that clay pots dry out faster than plastic.
- When you first bring a plant home, water it thoroughly and slide it gently out of its pot. If the roots are growing around in a tangled mass, repot into a pot one size larger.
- The plant will grow toward the sun. To maintain an even shape, give the pot a quarter turn every week.
- If you also have foliage houseplants, you need to be especially watchful for insects.

- Fertilize with a weak solution of organic fertilizer when the plant is actively growing; in winter, water less often and don't fertilize at all.

Patio Tips

* Take note of how much sunlight you have available; don't forget to allow for tall buildings and the shade they create.
* All pots must—repeat, *must*—have a drainage hole in the bottom.
* Large containers planted with several different plants look very nice, especially if one of the plants is a flower.
* Plants in containers need more frequent watering; be especially watchful if the weather is hot and windy.
* Give your pots some kind of protection in winter.
* Herbs grown as indoor plants never get as big as in outdoor gardens; enjoy them for their aroma and consider anything else a bonus.

CHAPTER SIX

Harvesting, Preserving, and Storing Your Herbs

If you get infected with Herb Fever (and it's easy to do), pretty soon you'll be adding lots of herbs to your garden, or creating a special garden just for herbs. Then, because they're so very easy to grow, before you know it you have a *lot* of fresh herbs on your hands.

What to do? Cook with them, yes; give bunches to friends, of course. But if you still have excess, why not preserve some for use later in the year. As the farmer said, when asked about his bumper crop of tomatoes, "We use what we can, and what we can't, we can." Well, you can't really can herbs, but you do have several options for preserving them.

WHEN AND HOW TO HARVEST YOUR HERBS

What Time of Day

If you're getting herbs to use immediately, it doesn't matter when you do it. Just step outside and snip off what you need for the salad or the stewpot. But if you're harvesting—taking a lot off the plant to preserve for later in the year—it does matter.

The best time is midmorning; that's when the oil content is highest. You want to be sure of two things:

1. The plant is dry—no dew, no raindrops.
2. The afternoon sun hasn't yet had time to dissipate the oils into the air.

If you have to choose between those two conditions, the first one is more important. You don't want to start out with wet herbs, especially if you're going to be drying them: they could mold before they dry. So you want to wait until any dew has dried. And if it's raining, wait till tomorrow.

What Time of Year

The season for harvesting in quantity depends on what part of the plant is going to be used.

If what you want is the leaf (and this is the majority of herbs), the general rule of thumb is: harvest herbs just before the plants flower. At that point the plant has in its cells the most of the oils that give it the characteristic aroma.

How do you know when that is? Easy: just watch for the flower buds. It will probably be late spring or early summer. If for some reason your attention should be diverted and you don't notice the buds, the very first open flower is your signal. Time to get to work.

You can also take a middle ground: leave some stems to make flowers, and harvest others. The flowers of most herb plants are small and dainty, and many are quite pretty. And they have other virtues as well. They are an unusual addition to small bouquets. They attract honeybees. They add color to the herb garden, and to everything they touch. For instance, make herb vinegar from the rich blue flowers of garden sage, and in addition to the sage flavor you get a beautiful pink color.

If you're growing a certain herb for its seeds, such as caraway or anise, then you let the flowers blossom and leave the dead flower heads in place until the seeds form. When the seeds have reached their mature size, you'll see that they are starting to dry. At that point, you can cut the entire flower head off and dry the cluster.

How to Harvest

This part is not hard. Cut off a section of the stem with garden clippers or a sharp knife. Or, if the stems are soft enough, you can pinch off the pieces with your fingers. The plant will make new growth at the point where you cut, and before long it will be lush and full again. With most plants, you can get two or three harvestings, sometimes more, each summer.

You can cut off a pretty long section, as much as two-thirds of the entire stem. But in most cases you don't want to cut all the way to the ground. A bare stem, with all its leaves gone, won't grow anymore. This is especially important for plants whose stems are very tough and woody.

The one exception is chives. In this case you *do* want to cut down close to the ground. Take some of the blades around the outer edge of the clump, and cut them off with scissors, leaving only an inch or two.

Unless the leaves are dusty or have mud flecks on them, don't wash the cuttings. Check for bugs; if you grasp a clump of stems and shake the whole thing gently, you'll dislodge any creepy-crawlies that came inside with you. One organic herb grower suggests setting your harvest down in a colander for a few minutes; "After a bit," she says, "the little fellows just walk away."

Now you're ready for preserving. You have several methods to choose from.

Drying Herbs

The oldest way of preserving fresh herbs, and still the most popular, is drying. The idea is to promote evaporation of the moisture that is present in the stems and leaves, leaving only the natural oil that gives the plant its distinctive fragrance and flavor. If all the water is gone, things don't rot. So theoretically something that is thoroughly dried can last indefinitely. Unfortunately, with herbs the flavor won't last much more than a year.

The process of drying is simple; the full process can be time-consuming, but it's a pleasant way to spend your time. And there is more than one way to accomplish the task.

Plants have a lot of water in them; it takes anywhere from eight to ten pounds of fresh herbs to produce one pound of dried.

Air Drying

In this time-honored technique, moisture is drawn out by warm, circulating air.

The Right Location

Search through your house for a spot that is:

- dark (or at least away from direct sunlight)
- warm, not cool
- dry, not damp or humid
- drafty (you want circulating air)

What works very well for many people is an attic, especially if it has a window they can open to get some air movement. You could also use a basement, if it's not damp. You don't want to use a space that is naturally humid, like most kitchens, because that defeats the whole idea. And although things will eventually air-dry in cool rooms, a warm area is better because the drying will occur faster, which is to the good.

If it's warm enough you can use an outdoor garden shed, if you have one, but don't use your garage: you don't want carbon monoxide around herbs you're going to cook with. Of course if you're one of those people who use the garage to store stuff in—everything but the car—then that's a good place too, as long as it meets the other requirements.

Occasionally you see in home design magazines pictures of "country" kitchens featuring woodstoves, with baskets and dried herbs artfully hanging nearby. It makes a nice picture, but what a fire hazard! Dried plant materials are *very* flammable. So even though it seems tempting because it's so warm, don't dry your herbs right beside the stove.

And don't hang them in the window. Even though the sunshine is warm coming through the glass, direct sunlight will dissipate the oils. You'll end up with something that's very dry and quite flavorless.

Few people have a separate room in their home that they can dedicate just to drying herbs; it's a matter of searching around for a corner you can use in season.

You can either hang bundles of herbs by their stems, or lay them flat on some kind of drying rack. Remember, in either case you have to make sure that air can circulate all around.

Flat Drying

How much preparation? You can start with either the whole stem (with leaves still intact) or strip the leaves off before drying. Be guided by common sense and your tolerance for detail work. For herbs with large leaves (like sage), it's just as easy to take the leaves

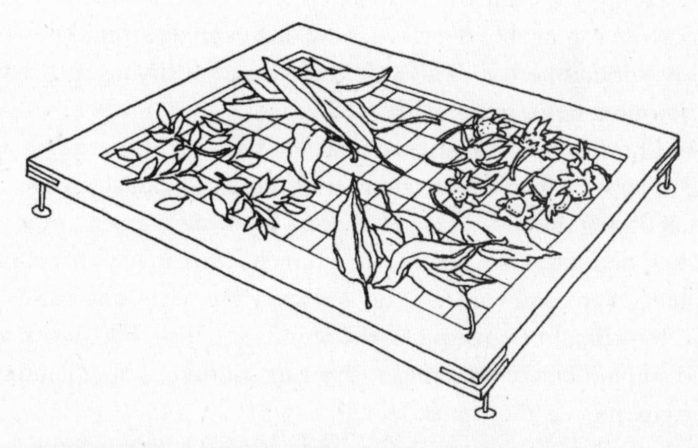

Drying tray for herbs can be made from an old window screen; add nails to the corners for "feet" to increase air circulation.

off first. If the leaves are minute (like thyme), you'll probably want to dry the entire sprig.

What to use? You need some kind of material that lets air through. You probably have something in the house or garage that you can use; look creatively. Possibilities are:

- a flat basket or wicker tray
- a sweater dryer (the kind with short metal legs and mesh surface that you set down into the bathtub)
- nylon net or cheesecloth stretched over a storage crate
- an old window screen, which you can improve by driving a large nail partway into each corner, creating "feet" to elevate the screen so more air circulates underneath

How long does it take? It varies, but usually not more than a few days. The herb is ready when it's crisp-dry and scrunches when you squeeze it.

Hanging Herbs to Dry

Gathering cut stems into a bunch and hanging them in some warm room is probably the classic way that everyone thinks of when we say "drying herbs." The advantage over flat drying is that you can dry more herbs in a smaller area.

Start by stripping off any leaves at the bottoms of the stems; you need at least an inch of bare stem. (Put those individual leaves onto a small drying tray.)

Then tie four or five stems into a bunch. You can use twine, pipe cleaners, or any soft cord. But far and away the best—and easiest to come by—is rubber bands. As the stems dry, they will shrink and could slip out of a bundle tied with string. But the rubber band will just tighten up as the stems dry.

Now the bundles have to hang somewhere. There're a lot of ways to accomplish this.

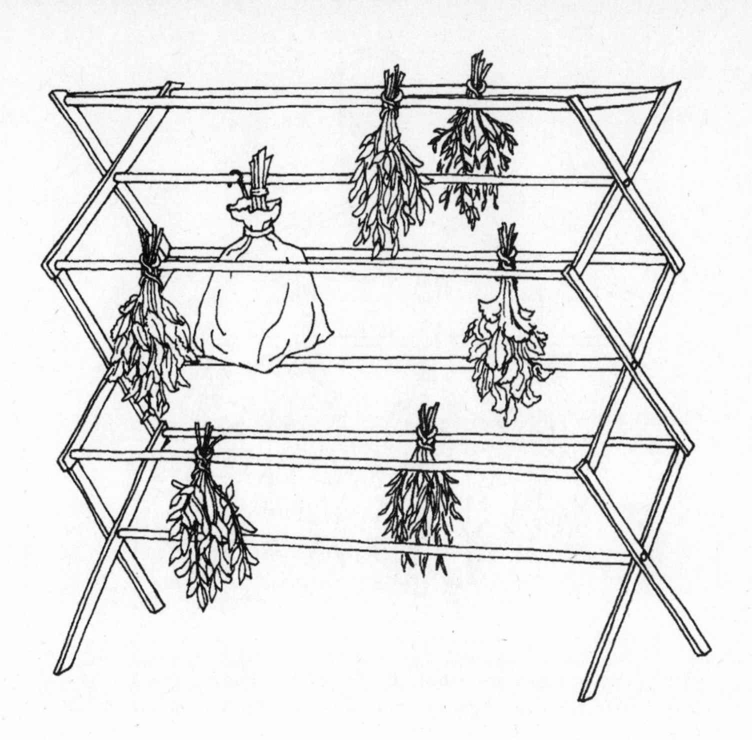

Drying rack originally meant for clothes works very well for herbs; it provides lots of drying space in a very small area. Tie on a bag to catch small seeds.

- Stretch a rope or wire between two ceiling joists, or across a corner of a room, and tie the bundles on.
- Multiply your drying space by tying the bundles onto coat hangers, then hang those from your rope.
- Nail up a temporary drapery rod, clothes rod, or dowel.
- Find one of those folding clothes-drying racks with the wooden crosspieces. You can fit a lot of herbs into a very small floor area.

In a pinch, you could even lay a broom across the backs of two chairs and tie your herb bunches to the handle.

If you're using rubber bands, here's a nifty way to tie the bundles and hang them all at the same time: Wrap the rubber band around

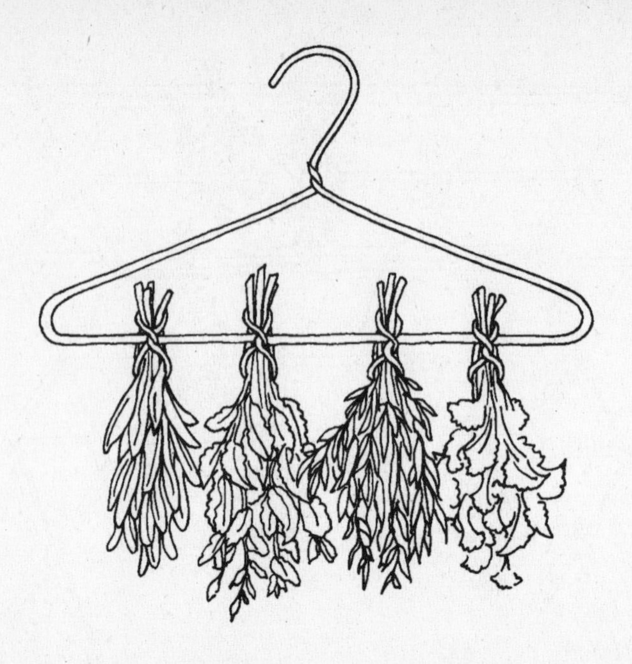

Quick drying technique uses something that every household has—tie herbs to a clothes hanger, put the hanger in a hot, dry spot with good air movement.

until it's moderately snug but still has some slack. Hold the bunch on one side of the horizontal span (the curtain rod, the bottom of the clothes hanger, or one of the rungs of the clothes dryer). Pull the slack part of the rubber band underneath the rod, up the other side, over the top, and loop it back over the stems.

The herbs are dry enough when they're crisp and crunchy, usually a week or less. Try not to leave them longer than necessary; they'll start to get dusty.

Drying Seed Herbs

If the part you want to dry is the seeds, hang-drying is a good way, but you have one extra step. Slip a paper bag around the herb bundle and tie it at the top. When the seeds dry they will fall from the upside-down flower heads, and the bag will capture them.

When the seeds have fallen (shake the bag and listen for the rattle), remove them from the bag and rub between your palms to get

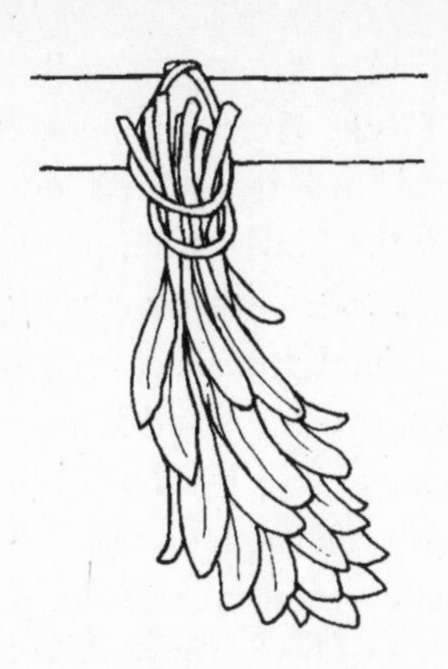

Rubber bands are the simplest and best way to tie together bundles of herbs for drying; at the same time, they also provide a quick way to fasten the bundle to the drying rod.

rid of the chaff. Then spread the naked seeds on a paper bag and dry for another week, until they are thoroughly dry, before storing them.

Other Ways to Dry Herbs

Air drying is convenient, if you have the right space and enough of it. But it's not the only way.

Oven Drying: You can also dry herbs in your oven. The trick is to keep the temperature *very* low—100°F to 150°F. If yours is a gas oven, the pilot light produces a perfect temperature. Strip the leaves, if you have the patience; the drying will go faster. Use cookie sheets lined with paper towels or brown paper bags from the grocery; or just put the bags directly onto the oven racks. Spread the herbs just one layer deep. Drying should take just a few hours; check progress periodically.

Food Dryer: A food dehydrator, either commercial or homemade, is excellent for drying herbs—if you happen to have one. If not, don't go out and buy one, since there are so many other good ways to dry your herbs.

Microwave: This modern kitchen miracle can be used to dry herbs. It's a bit tricky, for they burn like *that.* But if you have just a little bit to dry, it's worth a try. Here's how to do it: Cover a microwave-safe plate or flat bowl with a paper towel or paper napkin; lay in the herbs, one layer only; cover with another paper towel or napkin. Microwave on high for 30 seconds; open the door and let the steam escape. Check the herbs and if necessary add more time, 30 seconds at a time. Stay close by. These things will burn faster than you can believe, and can catch on fire.

Microwaved herbs keep their green color much better than any other kind of drying. Some herb growers feel that the microwave action is detrimental to the taste (one says it "blows out the oils"); others think the taste is quite satisfactory. Try an experiment, and decide for yourself.

Storing Dried Herbs

When your herbs are completely dry, strip the leaves from the stems. At this point you can either crumble the leaves or not. If you leave them as whole as possible, the flavor will be better preserved, but crushed and powdered leaves take up less storage space.

As an extra precaution, put throughly dried herbs in a 200 F. oven for 10 minutes; any insect eggs that happen to be caught in with the leaves will be killed. Then proceed to storing.

Put herbs into a storage container that is airtight and, if possible, opaque. Glass is better than plastic, for plastic sometimes imparts an odor to the herbs, and colored glass is better than clear, for the flavor of herbs deteriorates in sunlight. But make sure you can close it tight, to keep the moisture in the atmosphere from being reabsorbed.

Don't forget to label the jars. All dried herbs look alike, especially if they are crumbled. Include both the name of the herb and the date. As a general rule, well-dried herbs are good for a year.

Store your jars in a place that is dark and cool. You will be tempted to keep them on a windowsill, for display, or on a shelf above the stove, for convenience—both bad ideas. Heat and light are detrimental to quality of dried herbs.

Other Preserving Methods

Freezing

Most of the leafy herbs take well to freezing. Some turn dark, and they will be limp when defrosted, but the flavor is very close to fresh. Use in the same quantities you would use fresh herbs.

The easiest method is to spread the fresh herbs, thoroughly dry, on a cookie sheet or pie tin, and put in the freezer for a few hours. Then, once they are frozen, transfer to freezer bags or containers. Mason jars work well; they help prevent freezer burn. Don't forget to label.

One technique that works well is to make up small packets of herbs, just enough for one recipe, and store several packets together in a container. For these individual packets you can use sandwich bags or make bundles out of aluminum foil.

You can also make up packets of herb blends, ready for use. Think about what you like to cook, and what you have growing, and create your own blends, using these suggestions as idea starters.

Spaghetti blend	marjoram, oregano, thyme, parsley
Meat loaf blend	parsley, sage, savory, oregano
Fish blend	chives, fennel, lemon balm
Soup blend	basil, thyme, marjoram, rosemary
Chicken blend	chives, tarragon, lemon thyme, savory

Another nifty technique is herb ice cubes. Put the fresh herbs in a blender container with a little water, and buzz the blender on and off till the leaves are chopped. Pour the green slush into ice cube trays, then freeze. Pop the frozen cubes out of the trays and transfer to freezer boxes or bags. Don't forget to label. Now you have little rectangles of herbs in a handy size, all ready to throw into the soup pot.

Frozen Butters and Oil Mixtures

Another way to freeze a healthy crop of herbs is to make a dense mixture with butter or oil and freeze in small portions. It's like making herb butter (in the case of butter) or pesto (in the case of oil), only more so: the butter or oil acts as a "carrier" for the herbs.

Chop the fresh herb (or herbs; blends work well here too) into tiny pieces, and mix with softened butter or oil. The general proportions are 2 cups chopped herb to ½ cup oil or butter.

Freeze in small batches and label; here again an ice cube tray produces a good size. When you are making a dish that needs both herbs and the flavor of butter or oil, take out a portion and add directly to the recipe. Oil doesn't freeze solid, so you can spoon out the amount you need. Remember, the herb flavor is very concentrated; start with a small amount.

Herb Vinegars

In another section of this book (see chapter 14) you will find information about making herb-flavored vinegars. Here we are using the natural preservative qualities of vinegar as a way to save the flavor of fresh herbs.

The process is the same; the only difference (as with herb butters) is that here you will use a much higher proportion of herbs. Remember, you're not making a salad vinegar lightly flavored with an herb; you are using vinegar as a preserving agent.

Start with a clean jar of whatever size will hold the amount of herbs you have. Fill it to the top with the sprigs or leaves of fresh herbs, pressing down lightly as you go. Then pour in enough vinegar to completely cover the herbs. Use red wine or white wine vinegar, or good-quality white distilled vinegar. If the lid to your jar is metal, use an inner liner of plastic wrap or waxed paper.

Place in a dark cupboard and leave undisturbed for several weeks, then strain off the herbs. For a really clear finished product, pour the strained vinegar through a coffee filter to get rid of any small flecks. Put the herb-infused vinegar into a clean jar and label it.

Now what you have is a very concentrated form of herb vinegar. It will taste like vinegar, of course, but also very thoroughly of the herb you used. To use it in salad dressings, you will want to dilute it with plain vinegar. Use it full strength in recipes where you want the taste of the herb and where the vinegar undertone would be appropriate, such as pot roast or stews.

Preserving Tips

- Harvest herbs for preserving in the morning after the dew has dried and before the sun is really hot.
- Dry them in a spot where air circulates and there is no direct sun.
- Store in airtight glass jars; don't forget to label.
- Leafy herbs freeze well.
- After a year on your shelf, dried herbs have lost most of their flavor.

PART FOUR

Cooking with Herbs

Introduction

Today's interest in herbs as elegant seasonings may seem modern, even trendy, but it is not new. Archaeologists tell us there is evidence that prehistoric cultures used herbs many thousands of years ago to flavor their food.

The traditions are rich, and the creative possibilities for new taste combinations are unlimited. Here we can only scratch the surface.

In nine brief chapters, you will find recipes and suggestions for using herbs in your family meals. The goal is to show you examples, not to present a complete cooking course. There are so-called basic recipes, in which any herb (or combination of herbs) that you happen to like can be used.

The hope is that the general ideas presented here will make you more aware of herbs so that, as you thumb through your cookbooks and collected recipes looking for something for tonight's dinner, you will be more interested in the contributions of the herbs. Some assumptions in this section are:

- You can use whatever you have—fresh herbs or dried. As a general rule of thumb, it takes three times as much fresh to give the same flavoring as one amount of dried herb.
- Creative experimentation is encouraged. Substitute to your heart's content.
- If you already know you don't like the taste of a particular herb, for heaven's sake leave it out.

CHAPTER SEVEN

Cooking with Herbs

Just like everything else in life, our taste in seasonings changes. For a while one particular herb or spice will be popular, then it seems to pass from favor. In 1971, just twenty years ago, a cookbook writer described sage as the most widely used culinary herb in America. In 1992, herb growers who supply fresh herbs to restaurants and supermarkets reported that their most requested herb, by a long shot, was basil.

The moral of that story is, there are no rules about herbs. The decision of what to use with what dish, and how much, is in your hands—or rather, your taste buds.

General Guidelines

- If the taste is new to you, start by adding a small amount; you can always add more, but you can't take it out.

- Note that some herbs lose their flavor quickly when they are subjected to heat, and should be added near the end of the cooking process. See lists below, and be aware of this when following recipes.

- When you add an herb to something you're cooking, you should bruise (yes, that's the term for it) the herb first to release the oils that give it the flavor. If it's a dried herb, crumble it into the pot. If fresh, tear or mash with the back of a spoon first.
- Don't hold the jar right over the saucepan while you pour out the herb. Steam from the pan will get into the jar and be absorbed by the herbs.
- Even though it seems convenient, don't keep your herbs right over the stove; heat is bad for them. So is sunlight. Best storage place is in a cool cupboard.
- Dried herbs lose most of their flavor after a year. This is one advantage to growing and drying your own; you know how old it is.

What Goes with What

The following two sections summarize culinary uses of the main cooking herbs, from two standpoints: first, groups of foods and the herbs that complement them, then the herbs and the foods they work well with.

Note that here we concentrate on the herbs that are most commonly used. You will find more detailed information in the encyclopedia section of this book. There, each herb that can be used in cooking is identified as such in the "Used for" heading. Then, the text for that herb gives cooking suggestions.

Choosing Herbs for Your Dishes

Meats

Sage	rosemary
marjoram	oregano
dill	bay
savory	garlic
thyme	parsley

Chicken

Tarragon
basil
thyme
dill
marjoram
chives
rosemary
sage

Cheese and egg dishes

Chervil
chives
dill
tarragon
basil
oregano
parsley
fennel
savory
thyme

Fish and seafood

Fennel
basil
bay
dill
tarragon
oregano
thyme (especially lemon thyme)
chives

Vegetables

Basil (especially tomatoes)
savory (especially beans)
chives
parsley
rosemary (especially winter squash)
oregano
marjoram
thyme
dill

Salads

Salad burnet
chives
parsley

Fruits and drinks

- Angelica
- lemon balm
- lemon verbena
- mint
- sweet cicely
- sweet woodruff

Breads

- Dill
- caraway
- garlic
- oregano
- rosemary
- sage

Cookies and cakes

- Anise
- caraway
- scented geraniums
- mint
- sweet cicely

Herb tea

- Mints
- lemon balm
- chamomile
- lemon verbena
- lemon thyme
- catnip
- fennel
- anise

Choosing Dishes for Your Herbs

Basil The number-one tomato herb. With fresh tomato salads, tomato sauces, and sphaghetti sauce; in pesto; in minestrone soup; with zucchini; with lamb; in omelets and scrambled eggs.
Medium flavor

Bay In soups, stews, spaghetti sauce, and other long-simmering dishes; part of bouquet garni combinations; in marinades for chicken and meat.
Strong flavor

Chervil	In omelets and other egg dishes; with chicken or veal; in sauces and light soups. Very popular in French cuisine; one of the fines herbes. Add at end of cooking. *Mild flavor*
Chives	In cream soups (traditional garnish for vichyssoise) and sauces; in omelets; with baked potatoes, cottage cheese, cream cheese. Add at end of cooking. *Mild flavor*
Dill	With fish (especially salmon), chicken, or veal; in salads (especially cucumber salads); with cooked potatoes and potato salad; in sauces. *Medium flavor*
Fennel	Foliage: with fish, soups, and sauces; add at end of cooking. Seeds: apple pie, breads, salad dressings. *Medium flavor*
Marjoram	With chicken, pork, and lamb; with hamburgers and meat loaf; with carrots, peas, potato, tomato dishes, and especially with summer squash. *Medium flavor*
Mint	As tea or flavoring for cold drinks; fruit salad; cook with peas, carrots, potatoes, and zucchini; sauce for lamb; with yogurt-based sauces or soups. *Medium flavor*
Oregano	Spaghetti sauce, pizza, and other Italian dishes; meat loaf, hearty soups, and casseroles. *Strong flavor*
Parsley	In soups, stews, and casseroles; with omelets and scrambled eggs; with boiled potatoes and potato salad; fresh in green salads; number-one garnish. *Mild flavor*

Herb Seasoning Chart

SPICE	APPETIZERS	SOUPS	PASTAS	SEAFOOD & POULTRY	MEATS	POTATOES & GRAINS	VEGETABLES & BEANS	SALADS & DRESSINGS	DESSERTS
Basil	Italian tomato toasts	minestrone	pesto sauce	shellfish stew	Italian beef roll-ups	polenta	stewed tomatoes	liced tomatoes & onions	
Bay leaves	marinated mushrooms	bean	tomato-meat sauce	marinades for barbecuing	skewered grilled lamb or beef	Middle Eastern pilaf	steamed peas & lettuce		
Caraway seeds	Liptauer cheese spread	cabbage		chicken paprikash	pork or veal stew	roasted potatoes	sauerkraut	potato salad	spice cookies
Coriander seeds		lentil		curried chicken	pork kebabs	Indian rice pilaf	coriander butter for winter squash	yogurt dressing for fruit	coffee cake
Dill weed & seeds	sour cream & yogurt dips	cream of vegetable	egg noodles	herbed butters	Scandinavian veal meat balls	boiled new potatoes	green beans	marinated cucumbers	
Fennel seeds	pickled shrimp	pasta & bean	Italian tomato sauces	bouillabaisse	beef stew		braised celery	seafood salad	
Garlic	cheese dips	vegetable	all tomato-based sauces	roast chicken	roast lamb	mashed potatoes	sauteed spinach	creamy Italian dressing	

SPICE	APPETIZERS	SOUPS	PASTAS	SEAFOOD & POULTRY	MEATS	POTATOES & GRAINS	VEGETABLES & BEANS	SALADS & DRESSINGS	DESSERTS
Majoram	clam dip	split pea	seafood sauce	poultry stuffings	veal stew	roasted new potatoes	vegetables & bean stews	vegetable salads	
Mint	pineapple juice	chilled fruit			roast lamb	Greek rice	steamed carrots	creamy fruit dressing	chilled summer fruits
Oregano	vegetable juices	bean	Neapolitan pizza sauce	broiled fish	Greek lamb stews	lemon roasted potatoes	crumb-topped green beans	mixed vegetable salads	
Rosemary	marinated artichokes	lentil	vegetable lasagna	chicken saute with olives	lamb kebabs	sauteed potatoes	grilled tomatoes	warm lamb & bean salad	wine-poached fruits
Sage	cheese sticks	bean	browned butter sauce for ravioli	chestnut stuffings	sauteed liver	stuffed peppers	baked lima beans & tomatoes		
Tarragon	marinated mushrooms	shrimp gumbo	tarragon butter for noodles	chicken breasts with wine	stuffed veal chops	rice & vegetable casserole	green beans & onions	chicken & vegetable salad	poached pears
Thyme	cheese-stuffed mushrooms	vegetable beef	pork-filled cannelloni	shrimp creole	boeuf bourguignon	wild rice	yellow & red pepper saute	tabouli	

Courtesy of American Spice Trade Association

Rosemary	With all kinds of meat, especially lamb, pork and chicken; stuffing for turkey; biscuits and bread; with carrots and winter squash. *Strong flavor*
Sage	In stuffings for turkey, chicken, or Cornish hen; in cheese spreads; in bread; in soup and chowder. *Strong flavor*
Savory	The number-one herb for beans. With green beans, peas, or dried beans; with lentil soup; in meat loaf, vegetable soup, and deviled eggs; with potatoes and tomatoes. *Strong flavor*
Tarragon	With chicken and fish; with omelets and other egg dishes; in béarnaise sauce and tartar sauce; best-known herbal vinegar. Add near end of cooking. *Strong flavor*
Thyme	In beef stew, pot roast, and hearty soups; clam chowder; with chicken and fish; many vegetables. *Strong flavor*

Herb Blends

In many cookbooks and articles about cooking, you find references to herb combinations such as fines herbes, bouquet garni, and *ravigote*. These blends are common in French recipes, but don't let that scare you. They are simply combinations of herbs that experience tells us taste good together, and although certain herbs are traditional in these combinations, nobody will put you in jail if you make substitutions.

Fines herbes: A certain combination of herbs is chopped fine (that's what *fines* means) and added toward the end of cooking; when the dish is served, little pieces of the herbs will be present. In many

French dishes, the herbs used are chervil, chives, and one of these: tarragon, thyme, marjoram, or basil.

Bouquet garni: A combination of herbs (and perhaps some spices too) is bundled together and added to the dish while it is cooking. The bundle is removed before the dish is served, so that the taste of the herbs is there but not the herbs themselves. Traditionally fresh herbs are used, since they hold together better, but in practice either fresh or dried herbs can be tied into a cheesecloth bag or put into a tea ball, which is easily removed when ready. A bouquet garni usually contains a bay leaf, thyme, and either parsley or chervil, but other herbs can be used too.

Herbes de Provence is a traditional French blend of basil, thyme, savory, fennel, and lavender flowers.

Ravigote is a blend of herbs used to create a French sauce that is also called *ravigote:* parsley, tarragon, chervil, and sometimes chives.

One of the most satisfying things to do with herbs you have grown and dried yourself is to create your own special blends. Often if you have just one or two plants of a certain herb, at the end of the season you don't end up with enough dried leaves to fill a jar. Combining several into a blend is a good solution to this problem.

It also makes life a little simpler: if you design a blend that you like for chicken, for instance, then whenever you cook a chicken dish you don't have to think—just use some of your special blend. Of course you can also make blends with commercial herbs; in fact, the spice companies have already done it for you. Poultry seasoning, pickling spices, Italian seasoning are all blends.

Here are a few suggestions for blends.

HERB BLEND NO. 1

2 parts marjoram
2 parts savory
1 part basil
1 part thyme
1 part tarragon

An all-purpose savory blend for many meat and vegetable dishes.

HERB BLEND NO. 2

2 parts basil
2 parts thyme
2 parts parsley
1 part grated lemon peel, dried

Delicious on chicken, fish, and many vegetables.

BOUQUET GARNI FOR FISH

2 tablespoons celery leaves
2 tablespoons dried parsley
2 bay leaves, broken into pieces
1 teaspoon dried basil
½ teaspoon dried sage
½ teaspoon dried savory
½ teaspoon fennel seed

Mix all ingredients; divide into three equal portions and tie into cheesecloth bags.

BOUQUET GARNI FOR BEEF STOCK

2 tablespoons dried parsley
2 tablespoons dried celery leaves (or lovage, which has a celery taste)
2 bay leaves, crumbled
1 teaspoon dried marjoram
1 teaspoon dried thyme
½ teaspoon dried savory
¼ teaspoon dried sage, powdered

This makes enough for three garni bags.

SPAGHETTI SAUCE BLEND

4 parts basil
2 parts marjoram
2 parts parsley
1 part oregano

SALAD DRESSING BLEND

1 tablespoon dried marjoram
2 teaspoons dried thyme
2 teaspoons dried savory
2 teaspoons dried basil
1 teaspoon dried sage

Use blender to mix all ingredients thoroughly; store in covered jar. To make salad dressing, combine 2 teaspoons of blend with ¾ cup salad oil and ⅓ cup vinegar. Also good on cooked vegetables and fish.

—McCormick/Schilling

HERB BLEND FOR CHICKEN

1 tablespoon dried thyme
1 tablespoon dried marjoram
2 teaspoons dried rosemary
1 teaspoon dried sage

—McCormick/Schilling

HERB BLEND FOR BEEF

1 tablespoon dried marjoram
1 tablespoon dried thyme
1 tablespoon dried basil
1 teaspoon celery seed

Use in meat loaf, hamburgers, or pot roast.

—McCormick/Schilling

If You're Watching Your Salt

Any of the herb blends in this chapter can be kept in a salt shaker, for use at the table. This makes it very easy for those in the family who are watching their sodium intake to use a healthful substitute without any special aggravation for the cook. And because it is so flavorful, they won't feel deprived.

SALT SUBSTITUTE

This very delicious blend was created by a long-time herb gardener, using her home-dried herbs. You could also use store-bought herbs, substituting regular thyme for the lemon thyme. She runs the whole batch through a food mill, to get everything thoroughly mixed.

2 cups parsley
1 cup oregano
½ cup dill seed
½ cup winter savory
½ cup marjoram
⅛ cup rosemary
2 tablespoons sage
2 tablespoons lemon thyme
½ teaspoon cayenne pepper

Start with dried herbs. Blend well and store in tightly covered container.

—JOYCE LAITINEN, CANBY, OREGON

CHAPTER EIGHT

Appetizers

BASIC HERB DIP FOR VEGETABLES

Dill · Garlic

Substitute your favorite herbs, either fresh or dried, in place of the dill to vary this basic recipe.

1 cup plain yogurt (or half yogurt and half sour cream)
¼ cup mayonnaise
1 teaspoon Dijon mustard
1 clove garlic, minced very fine
¼ cup fresh dill, minced
Salt or seasoning salt to taste

Mix all ingredients; chill in refrigerator 2 hours or more. Serve with carrot sticks, celery sticks, cherry tomatoes, sliced cucumber, or other "dippin' " vegetables.

1 MEASURE OF DRIED HERB = 3 MEASURES OF FRESH

SEAFOOD SPREAD

Mixed Herbs • Parsley

One 8-oz. package cream cheese
1 cup sour cream or plain yogurt
1 cup crabmeat
1 envelope dried onion soup mix
½ teaspoon mixed herb blend (your choice of dried herbs)
2 teaspoons dried parsley
Salt to taste
Shrimp (optional)

Beat together cream cheese and sour cream. Clean crabmeat, watching for bits of shell. Stir in soup mix, crab, herbs, parsley, and salt to taste. Small bay shrimp, cut into bits, may be added. Spread on crackers. —CAPRILANDS HERB FARM

1 MEASURE OF DRIED HERB = 3 MEASURES OF FRESH

BURNET SANDWICH SPREAD

Salad burnet • Chives

This makes use of the wonder salad herb, burnet, which is a hardy perennial and an evergreen. It stays green under the snow and may be picked all winter. It has a real cucumber flavor when left overnight in a mixture. This is a good spread for party sandwiches—very colorful.

One 8-oz. package cream cheese
4 tablespoons fresh salad burnet leaves (chopped or cut fine)
2 tablespoons chives or leeks
2 teaspoons salt
Pepper to taste
¼ cup dry white wine or milk, as needed

Let cream cheese soften, then combine with burnet and chives. Add salt and pepper to taste. Bind with white wine or milk, if needed to hold together. —CAPRILANDS HERB FARM

1 MEASURE OF DRIED HERB = 3 MEASURES OF FRESH

ELLEN OGDEN'S BOURSIN

Garlic • Basil • Dill • Chives

Boursin is generally served as an appetizer spread on crackers, or stuffed into cherry tomatoes, but sometimes we make roast beef sandwiches with a layer of boursin as a base.

MAKES 1 CUP.

8 ounces cream cheese
2 cloves garlic, peeled
1 tablespoon fresh basil
1 tablespoon fresh dill
1 tablespoon fresh chives
6 pitted black olives

Blend cream cheese, garlic, and herbs until smooth, using food processor or electric mixer. Chop in olives. Transfer to a small bowl and keep refrigerated until ready to serve. —THE COOK'S GARDEN

1 MEASURE OF DRIED HERB = 3 MEASURES OF FRESH

HERBED YOGURT CHEESE

Start this homemade version of cream cheese the night before your party.

1 quart plain yogurt
Mixed herbs (about ½ cup fresh or 3 tablespoons dried)
Salt

First, line a colander or large sieve with cheesecloth or a thin cotton dishcloth. Set the colander down inside a bowl; there should be at least an inch of clearance at the bottom. Pour the yogurt into the colander, and set the whole thing into the refrigerator overnight to drain. The liquid whey will drain out, leaving a very thick yogurt about the consistency of soft cream cheese.

The next morning, put the cheese into a bowl and add the herbs of your choice; try dill, tarragon, chives, marjoram, or any combination. Dried herbs should be crumbled, fresh herbs should be chopped very fine. Stir well, add salt to taste, and return the cheese to the refrigerator to firm up.

For a party, you may prefer to put the herbed cheese into smaller containers so that you can prepare several different cheese platters. Garnish with fresh herbs. Serve with crackers or vegetables.

1 MEASURE OF DRIED HERB = 3 MEASURES OF FRESH

TORTILLA CHIPS

Make these healthful dipping chips with any herb or combination; choose herbs that complement the flavors of the dip.

Butter or margarine
Prepared herbs
Flour tortillas
Salt (optional)

Melt butter, adding the herbs you have chosen; dried herbs should be crumbled, fresh herbs should be minced. With knife or kitchen scissors, cut tortillas into pie-shaped wedges. With pastry brush, paint each tortilla segment with herb butter; sprinkle lightly with salt if desired. Lay on ungreased cookie sheet, in one layer, and bake at 375°F until crisp, 6 to 8 minutes.

VARIATIONS

Instead of tortillas, use pita bread. Cut into quarters, then carefully separate top and bottom. Paint with herb butter and toast.

CHAPTER NINE

Soups and Breads

- Next time you make biscuits from a mix, add a pinch of dried herbs.
- Perk up corn muffin mix with a bit of sage or savory.
- Add herbs to the crust of quiches; make sure the flavors enhance, not fight, the seasonings in the egg mixture.
- When you make crust for chicken pot pie, add a bit of savory, tarragon, or marjoram.
- Jazz up canned soup with herbs or top with herb-flavored sour cream; try basil with tomato soup, savory with split pea soup, tarragon with cream of chicken.

CUCUMBER SOUP

Basil • Chives • Mint

SERVES 4 TO 6.

4 medium cucumbers
1 cup chicken broth
2 teaspoons lemon juice
¼ cup chopped fresh basil
2 teaspoons snipped fresh chives
6 fresh mint leaves
2 cups plain yogurt

Peel cucumbers, if desired, or wash off wax. Cut in half length-wise, use the tip end of a spoon to scrape out the seeds. Discard seeds and cut cucumber into chunks. Place broth, lemon juice, cucumbers, and herbs in a blender and blend at high speed until finely chopped. Transfer to a bowl and whisk in yogurt. Chill before serving. Garnish with fresh mint leaves or chive flowers.

1 MEASURE OF DRIED HERB = 3 MEASURES OF FRESH

GREEN PEA SOUP WITH MINT

Mint • Rosemary

SERVES 6 TO 8.

1 cup chopped onion
1 ½ teaspoons dried mint
⅓ teaspoon dried rosemary, crumbled
2 tablespoons butter
Three 10-oz. packages frozen peas, thawed
1 ½ cups milk
2 cups half and half
¼ teaspoon salt

Saute onion and seasonings in butter until onions are tender. Add thawed peas and continue sauteing for five minutes. Puree onion and pea mixture in food processor or blender. Return to pan. Add milk, half and half, and salt. Heat on medium to serving temperature, stirring constantly. Serve immediately, before bright green color fades. Garnish with fresh mint leaf. —ALBERTINA'S II

1 MEASURE OF DRIED HERB = 3 MEASURES OF FRESH

HERBED TOMATO SOUP

Basil • Bay • Oregano

Adelma Simmons of Caprilands calls this "soup for cold winter days or the raw spring weather."

1 large can tomato juice
1 teaspoon basil
½ bay leaf
½ teaspoon oregano
Juice of 1 lemon
4 beef bouillon cubes
1 cup hot water

Combine ingredients and heat to boiling point. Set on back of stove to simmer. Remove bay leaf and serve as bouillon in cups, or as a hearty pickup in pottery mugs. —CAPRILANDS HERB FARM

1 MEASURE OF DRIED HERB = 3 MEASURES OF FRESH

CHEDDAR SOUP

Parsley • Basil

MAKES 1 QUART SOUP.

¼ cup butter
¼ cup diced onion
¼ cup diced celery
2 tablespoons flour
2 teaspoons chicken flavor base or 2 bouillon cubes
1 ½ cups hot water
1 ½ cups milk
8 ounces cheddar cheese, grated
¼ teaspoon dried parsley
¼ teaspoon dried basil

Melt butter in 2-quart saucepan, add onion and celery, and saute until tender. Stir in flour. Cook 3 minutes, stirring constantly. Combine chicken flavor base with water. Slowly add broth and milk to saucepan. Heat to boiling, stirring constantly. Lower heat and stir in remaining ingredients. Stir with wire whisk until cheese is melted. Simmer 5 minutes at low heat. Serve hot with herbed croutons (see below); garnish with fresh herb of your choice.

HERBED CROUTONS

MAKES 1½ CUPS CROUTONS.

Slice one-half loaf Italian bread in ½-inch slices. Trim crusts from bread. Cut slices in ½-by-1-inch pieces. Set aside. Melt ½ cup butter in skillet. Add ⅛ teaspoon instant garlic powder, ⅛ teaspoon instant onion powder, ½ teaspoon dried basil leaves, and ½ teaspoon dried marjoram leaves. Saute bread cubes in hot butter mixture, turning to brown on all sides. Drain on paper towels. Serve on soup or salad.

1 MEASURE OF DRIED HERB = 3 MEASURES OF FRESH

To vary crouton recipe, substitute ⅛ teaspoon each dried chopped chives, dried tarragon leaves, and dried thyme leaves in place of other herbs.

—ADAPTED FROM McCORMICK/SCHILLING

DILL SWIRL BREAD

Dill • Chives • Parsley

MAKES ONE 8-BY-4-INCH LOAF.

One 13¾-oz. package hot roll mix
1 stick (4 ounces) butter
¼ cup dried dill weed
¼ cup dried chopped chives
¼ cup dried parsley flakes
¼ teaspoon salt
¼ teaspoon ground black pepper
½ teaspoon onion powder

Prepare hot roll mix following package directions. Let rise until double in size. Roll out in a rectangle 8 by 14 inches. Melt butter, then stir in remaining ingredients. Spread herb mixture over dough. Roll tightly from short side to make a loaf 3 by 8 inches. Place, seam side down, in greased 8½-by-4-by-2½-inch loaf pan. Lightly grease top of loaf. Cover with damp towel and let stand in warm place until double in size. Bake in 375°F oven 40 to 45 minutes. Serve warm.

—McCORMICK/SCHILLING

1 MEASURE OF DRIED HERB = 3 MEASURES OF FRESH

HERB BISCUITS

Marjoram • Oregano • Thyme

These quick drop biscuits also make good dumplings for beef stew or chicken fricassee.

MAKES 10 BISCUITS.

2 cups biscuit mix
¼ teaspoon dried marjoram leaves
¼ teaspoon dried oregano leaves
½ teaspoon dried thyme leaves
¼ teaspoon onion powder
1 cup milk

Combine biscuit mix with herbs. Stir in milk. Drop from spoon to make 10 equal biscuits, on lightly greased baking sheet. Bake in 425°F oven 12 to 15 minutes or until lightly browned. Serve hot.

—McCormick/Schilling

HOT HERB BREAD

Oregano • Garlic

MAKES 4 SERVINGS.

2 tablespoons margarine
1 teaspoon lemon juice
1 teaspoon dried oregano
¼ teaspoon garlic powder
⅛ teaspoon black pepper
2 French rolls (5- to 6-inch), split lengthwise

Beat margarine, lemon juice, oregano, garlic, and pepper in bowl until softened and smooth. Spread on French rolls, wrap in foil, and bake in 400°F oven for 15 to 20 minutes or until hot. Cut each roll into 4 slices and serve. —Spice Islands

1 MEASURE OF DRIED HERB = 3 MEASURES OF FRESH

CHAPTER TEN

Salads and Salad Dressings

- If you have an herb garden, gather up a handful of fresh herbs just before you make a green salad; chop them and scatter over the greens before adding the dressing.
- Make your salads extra special by adding edible flowers of herbs: nasturtiums (yellow and orange), borage (blue), bergamot (red), chives (pink). For garnish, leave flowers whole; if you want people to actually eat them, tear the larger ones into separate petals.
- Cut a clove of garlic in half lengthwise and rub it all over the inside of your wooden salad bowl. That way you get the garlic flavor throughout the salad but you don't have to worry about anyone biting into a chunk of garlic.
- Herb-flavored vinegars (see chapter 14) all by themselves make a nice dressing for tomato salads.
- Check the Soup chapter for herb-flavored croutons that are also great on salads.

BASIC HERB DRESSING

Add your favorite herbs, either singly or in combination, fresh or dried, for your personal version of classic oil and vinegar dressing.

1/3 cup vinegar (herb-flavored, if desired)
2/3 cup salad oil or olive oil
1 teaspoon Dijon mustard
½ teaspoon salt
¼ teaspoon pepper
¼ cup fresh herbs, chopped fine

Whisk together all ingredients till well blended.

HONEY HERB DRESSING

Garlic • Mixed herbs

Especially good with tomatoes.

1 cup honey
½ cup oil
5 tablespoons basil vinegar
1 clove garlic
1 tablespoon celery seed
1 tablespoon salt
1 cup assorted chopped fresh herbs, such as chives, chervil, parsley, burnet, tarragon, basil

—CAPRILANDS HERB FARMS

1 MEASURE OF DRIED HERB = 3 MEASURES OF FRESH

FRESH SORREL DRESSING

Sorrel • Basil • Parsley • Garlic

This combination of lemony sorrel with basil and orange juice makes a scrumptious light herbal dressing that is good on any tossed green salad.

1 large bunch sorrel leaves, stems removed (about 12–15)
5 sprigs fresh basil leaves
½ cup fresh parsley leaves
½ cup olive oil
1 clove garlic
Fresh juice of 2 oranges
Salt and pepper to taste

Combine all the ingredients and whirl together in blender until liquefied. Add salt and pepper to taste and toss with any fresh lettuce salad.

—SHEPHERD'S GARDEN SEEDS

GREEN GODDESS SALAD

Parsley • Chives • Garlic • Tarragon

1 ½ quarts rinsed salad greens (spinach, endive, assorted lettuces)
2 cups cut fresh vegetables (cucumber, green pepper, celery, tomato and/or carrots)
½ cup slivered almonds, toasted

Toss salad greens, vegetables, and nuts with dressing and serve.

1 MEASURE OF DRIED HERB = 3 MEASURES OF FRESH

GREEN GODDESS DRESSING

MAKES 4 SERVINGS.

¼ cup dried parsley leaves, packed
1 tablespoon white wine vinegar
2 teaspoons dried chives
1 teaspoon minced garlic
1 teaspoon dried tarragon
½ teaspoon sugar
1 cup plain yogurt

Combine ingredients, except yogurt, in blender or food processor. Whirl until finely chopped. Stir in yogurt (do not use blender, it thins too much).

—SPICE ISLANDS

LAYERED SALAD

In straight-sided bowl, alternate layers of shredded lettuce, broccoli flowerets, cauliflowerets, radishes, cucumber slices, cherry tomatoes, and green pepper rings or pieces. Serve with Creamy Dill Dressing.

1 MEASURE OF DRIED HERB = 3 MEASURES OF FRESH

CREAMY DILL DRESSING

Chives • Dill • Garlic

MAKES 1¼ CUPS.

½ cup sour cream
½ cup mayonnaise
2 tablespoons milk
1 teaspoon dried chives
¼ teaspoon dried dill weed
1 teaspoon lemon juice
Dash ground white pepper
Dash garlic powder

In medium bowl combine all ingredients. Mix thoroughly. Chill 24 hours to allow flavors to blend. If a thinner dressing is desired, add additional milk. —McCormick/Schilling

1 MEASURE OF DRIED HERB = 3 MEASURES OF FRESH

TUSCAN POTATO SALAD

Garlic • Parsley • Chives

Celebrate your home-grown potatoes with this simple, rustic dish that sings with good earthy flavors.

SERVES 6.

6 medium potatoes, cooked, peeled, and sliced into thick slices
2 tablespoons olive oil
1 large or 2 small cloves of garlic, very finely chopped
1 tablespoon balsamic vinegar
2 tablespoons finely chopped fresh parsley
2 tablespoons finely chopped fresh chives
¼ teaspoon salt
¼ teaspoon freshly ground pepper

Combine all the ingredients and toss lightly. Allow to stand about ½ hour to blend flavors before serving at room temperature.

—SHEPHERD'S GARDEN SEEDS

1 MEASURE OF DRIED HERB = 3 MEASURES OF FRESH

LAYERED TOMATO SALAD, VINAIGRETTE

Basil • Garlic • Parsley

SERVES 12.

12 ripe tomatoes, thickly sliced
¼ cup chopped green onions
½ cup olive oil
⅓ cup wine vinegar
8 fresh basil leaves or 2 teaspoons dry
1 teaspoon salt
½ teaspoon dry mustard
2 cloves crushed garlic
1 tablespoon fresh parsley, minced
1 teaspoon sugar
Mozzarella cheese (optional)
Onion (optional)

Combine all but optional ingredients in a bowl and marinate at least 4 hours. Serve on lettuce. Good with mozzarella cheese coarsely grated and sweet onions (such as Walla Walla or Vidalia) in rings.

—ALBERTINA'S I

1 MEASURE OF DRIED HERB = 3 MEASURES OF FRESH

MINTED MELON AND GRAPE SALAD

Mint

SERVES 10–12.

DRESSING

1 cup plain yogurt
2 tablespoons honey
½ teaspoon grated fresh ginger (or ¼ teaspoon powdered ginger)

Mix dressing in the blender. Refrigerate.

SALAD INGREDIENTS

4 cups seedless grapes (see note)
1 tablespoon minced fresh mint
2 medium melons, peeled, seeded, and cut into chunks
Lettuce leaves
Whole mint leaves for garnish

Toss grapes with mint and chill. Cut melon into chunks. Chill. Combine melon chunks and grapes and place on lettuce leaves. Drizzle dressing over the top and garnish with mint leaves.

Note: Use red grapes with honeydew melon and green grapes with cantaloupe. This is also pretty served in a stemmed glass with no lettuce.

—ALBERTINA'S II

1 MEASURE OF DRIED HERB = 3 MEASURES OF FRESH

CHAPTER ELEVEN

Main Dishes

- When baking whole chickens, put fresh herbs in the cavity, along with a lemon into which you have cut a few short slits.

- Next time you make shish kebab, thread whole bay leaves next to the meat pieces.

- A flavorful way to cook fish: steam it using celery instead of a metal steamer. Put sprigs of fresh herbs (fennel is a good one) in the hollows of several ribs of celery. Lay the fish on top of the celery, and add water up to the level of the celery. Cover the pan and simmer till fish is done. The fish, which is held up out of the water by the celery, absorbs the herb flavors while it steams.

- If you're making fish and chips, or any kind of batter-fried fish, dip a few pieces of fresh parsley into the batter and fry; serve at end of meal as a breath freshener.

CRISPY HERB-TOPPED CHICKEN

Sage • Savory • Parsley

SERVES 8.

8 boned and skinned chicken breast halves
8 ounces Swiss cheese, grated
One 10-oz. can cream of chicken soup
¼ cup white wine (or milk)
2 cups seasoned bread crumbs (see note)
⅓ cup melted butter
3 tablespoons almond slivers

Preheat oven to 350°F. Place chicken breasts in ovenproof casserole and sprinkle cheese evenly over all. Mix soup and wine and distribute evenly over chicken, spreading to cover chicken completely. Sprinkle crumbs over chicken, and drizzle melted butter over the top. Scatter almonds over all. Bake for 30 to 35 minutes.

SEASONED BREAD CRUMBS

2 cups fine dry bread crumbs
½ teaspoon dried sage
¼ teaspoon dried savory
¼ teaspoon onion powder
1 teaspoon dried parsley flakes

Note: As a shortcut, purchase bread crumbs already seasoned, and add herbs of your choice. —ALBERTINA'S II

1 MEASURE OF DRIED HERB = 3 MEASURES OF FRESH

SICILIAN PIZZA

Basil • Oregano

A thick, soft-crust pizza loaded with goodies.

One 16-oz. package hot roll mix
One 6-oz. can tomato paste
1 ½ cups water
½ teaspoon dried basil
½ teaspoon dried oregano
¼ teaspoon cracked black pepper

TOPPINGS

Italian sausage, mild or hot, sliced and cooked
Mushrooms, sliced
Green pepper, seeded and chopped
Red pepper, seeded and chopped
Onion, peeled and chopped
Bacon, cooked and crumbled
Mozzarella cheese, shredded

Prepare hot roll mix, following package directions. Put dough in lightly oiled 15-by-11-by-1-inch jelly roll pan. Press dough to line bottom and sides of pan. In saucepan, combine tomato paste with next 4 ingredients. Heat to a boil, reduce heat, and simmer for 30 minutes. Pour over crust, spreading to coat evenly. Sprinkle your choice of toppings over the sauce. Top with shredded cheese. Bake in 375°F oven 30 minutes. —MCCORMICK/SCHILLING

1 MEASURE OF DRIED HERB = 3 MEASURES OF FRESH

BAKED FISH

Dill · Tarragon

MAKES 4 SERVINGS.

3 tablespoons margarine
1 teaspoon dried dill weed
1 teaspoon dried tarragon
2 teaspoons olive oil
4 salmon, bass, or halibut steaks or fillets (1 ½ to 2 lbs.)
¼ cup thinly sliced shallots or green onion
1 lemon, thinly sliced

Combine margarine, dill weed, and tarragon in a small bowl. Cut 4 sheets of foil, each 4 times wider and 6 inches longer than the fish fillets. Rub center portion of foil with ½ teaspoon olive oil and center fish on oiled area. Spread ¼ of the margarine mixture on each fish fillet. Sprinkle shallots or green onion over fish and carefully arrange lemon slices on top. For each packet, wrap foil up and around fish and seal seam by making several small folds. Roll up ends of foil and tuck underneath fish to completely seal fish inside. Lay packets in baking pan and bake at 450°F for 8 to 10 minutes or until fish is just cooked through (do not overcook). Cut a small slit through foil into the fish to check. —SPICE ISLANDS

1 MEASURE OF DRIED HERB = 3 MEASURES OF FRESH

MEAT LOAF

Fennel • Parsley • Oregano • Basil • Garlic

¼ cup chopped onion
1 clove garlic, minced
2 tablespoons olive oil
1 pound hamburger meat
1 egg, lightly beaten
½ teaspoon fennel seeds
½ teaspoon dried oregano
½ teaspoon dried basil
¼ cup fresh parsley, chopped
1 teaspoon salt
½ teaspoon pepper
Beef bouillon, as needed

Saute onion and garlic in oil till soft. In mixing bowl, combine ground meat, egg, herbs, and spices. Add onion and garlic, and mix thoroughly (it's easier if you use your hands). If mixture seems too dry, add a bit of liquid beef bouillon. Shape into loaf, put in loaf pan, and bake 1 hour at 350°F.

BROCCOLI BASIL FETTUCINE

Basil • Parsley • Garlic

Nutrient-rich broccoli is the base for a creamy pasta sauce. Garnish with lots of toasted pine nuts and grated Parmesan cheese.

MAKES 4 SERVINGS.

One 10-oz. package frozen chopped broccoli or 1 ½ cups chopped fresh broccoli
1 cup half and half
¼ cup fresh parsley leaves
½ cup toasted pine nuts
2 cloves garlic
1½ tablespoons dried basil
Salt and pepper to taste
½ pound fettucine, cooked and drained

Lightly steam broccoli. Place in blender or food processor with remaining ingredients; whirl until blended. Toss broccoli mixture with cooked fettucine. —SPICE ISLANDS

1 MEASURE OF DRIED HERB = 3 MEASURES OF FRESH

CHAPTER TWELVE

Side Dishes: Vegetables, Pasta, and Rice

- Herbed rice is delicious and easy: cook rice your favorite way; while hot, quickly mix in chopped fresh herbs. Try parsley, marjoram, dill, lovage, or mint.

- To make herbed rice with dried herbs, melt some butter and let herbs "soak" in it while you cook rice as usual; when rice is done, quickly stir in herb butter.

- For easy rice pilaf, melt butter in saucepan, saute herbs and dry rice for a few minutes, then add appropriate amount of chicken stock, cover, and cook till rice is done and liquid is absorbed. Lemon thyme is especially good for this.

- Add chopped herbs when you make mashed potatoes.

- For herbed new potatoes, first boil potatoes till done; separately, melt butter and saute herbs, then roll the potatoes in the butter before serving.

MEDITERRANEAN RICE

Thyme • Savory • Marjoram • Garlic

SERVES 4 TO 6.

1 onion, minced
1 clove garlic, minced
1 tablespoon olive oil
1 cup uncooked long-grain rice
1 teaspoon minced fresh thyme
1 teaspoon minced fresh oregano
1 teaspoon minced fresh summer savory
½ teaspoon minced fresh marjoram
1½ cups chicken or beef stock
1½ cups peeled and chopped tomatoes

Saute the onion and garlic in oil over low heat until soft. Add the rice, thyme, oregano, savory, and marjoram, and cook for a few minutes more, stirring constantly.

Add the stock and the tomatoes; cover and bring to a boil. Lower the heat and simmer for approximately 50 minutes, or until the liquid has been absorbed and the rice is tender.

SAVORY GREEN BEANS

Savory

SERVES 4.

1 pound green beans
1 tablespoon butter
2 teaspoons minced savory

Steam beans until they are just tender; do not overcook. Toss with butter and savory.

1 MEASURE OF DRIED HERB = 3 MEASURES OF FRESH

DILL-BRAISED BRUSSELS SPROUTS

Dill

A new favorite for enjoying sprouts' sweet crispness.

SERVES 4.

1 pound fresh brussels sprouts
2 tablespoons olive oil
½ teaspoon salt
¼ teaspoon fresh ground pepper
3 tablespoons chopped fresh dill leaf
⅓ cup water
2 tablespoons fresh lemon juice
1-2 teaspoons butter
3 tablespoons grated Parmesan cheese

Slice off ends of brussels sprouts. Cut into 3 or 4 slices, or if small, cut in half. Heat oil in a skillet, add sprouts, and stir-fry until coated with oil and bright green. Add salt, pepper, dill, water, and lemon juice; cover and cook 2 minutes or until tender but still crunchy. Toss with butter and Parmesan cheese.

—SHEPHERD'S GARDEN SEEDS

1 MEASURE OF DRIED HERB = 3 MEASURES OF FRESH

HERBED CORN-ON-THE-COB

Basil • Marjoram

This corn is a special treat, whether prepared outdoors on the grill or served, year-round, piping hot from the microwave.

6 ears of corn, in husks
½ cup butter, softened
1 teaspoon instant minced onion
½ teaspoon dried basil
½ teaspoon dried marjoram
¼ teaspoon seasoning salt
½ teaspoon paprika
Dash ground red pepper

Loosen husks of corn enough to remove silk. Soak corn in cold water 30 minutes or longer. When ready to roast, drain well. Combine remaining ingredients and spread generously over corn. Rewrap husks, then wrap in aluminum foil. Place on grill about 5 inches from coals. Cook 25 minutes, turning several times. Remove foil and husks. Serve hot.

Microwave directions: In a microwavable bowl or measuring cup, melt butter and add herbs and spices; cook on low power for 2 minutes, and set aside. Prepare corn as above (remove silk, spread butter on corn, rewrap husk) and wrap in waxed paper, twisting the ends. Place corn on microwavable plate or shallow casserole. Cook 10 to 12 minutes, turning corn and rotating once. Let stand 5 minutes.

—McCormick/Schilling

1 MEASURE OF DRIED HERB = 3 MEASURES OF FRESH

HERB-SAUTEED CHERRY TOMATOES

Rosemary

A splash of tangy vinegar and a dash of rosemary bring out the best in these cherry tomatoes. This may become one of your favorite dishes for entertaining.

MAKES 4 SERVINGS.

1 tablespoon butter
1 pint cherry tomatoes, washed (about 36 tomatoes)
2 teaspoons dried rosemary, crushed
2 teaspoons red wine vinegar, plain or herb-flavored
Black pepper to taste

Heat butter in large skillet over medium-high heat. Add tomatoes, rosemary, vinegar and pepper; gently stir and cook for 2 to 3 minutes until heated through.

—SPICE ISLANDS

1 MEASURE OF DRIED HERB = 3 MEASURES OF FRESH

VEGETABLE MEDLEY IN FOIL

Garlic • Thyme • Tarragon

Cooking vegetables in foil packets on the grill makes it easy to prepare, serve, and clean up at outdoor parties. Children and adults enjoy opening individual packets to discover a fragrant and colorful vegetable surprise.

MAKES 4 SERVINGS.

Heavy-duty aluminum foil
1½ cups julienned (cut into thin strips) carrots
1½ cups julienned zucchini
1 cup sliced fresh button mushrooms
2 tablespoons butter
2 tablespoons lemon juice (about ½ lemon)
2 teaspoons garlic salt (or equivalent amount salt plus minced garlic)
1 teaspoon dried tarragon
½ teaspoon dried thyme

Cut 4 pieces of heavy-duty aluminum foil, approximately 8 by 10 inches. Divide carrots, zucchini, and mushrooms into 4 portions; center each portion on lower half of each foil piece. Top each portion with ½ tablespoon butter, ½ tablespoon lemon juice, ½ teaspoon garlic salt, ¼ teaspoon tarragon, and a pinch of thyme. Fold upper half of foil over vegetables and seal all edges to form a packet. Place packets on barbecue grill, 4 inches above medium coals, for 10 minutes or until vegetables are hot. To serve, cut an "X" in top of packet and fold foil back.

To bake in oven: Place packets on baking sheet; bake at 450°F for 15 minutes or until vegetables are tender-crisp. Serve as directed above. —ADAPTED FROM SPICE ISLANDS

1 MEASURE OF DRIED HERB = 3 MEASURES OF FRESH

BAKED SQUASH WITH ROSEMARY AND HONEY

Rosemary

SERVES 6.

2 pounds butternut squash, cleaned and cut into 6 serving pieces

2 tablespoons softened butter

2 tablespoons honey

1 teaspoon fresh rosemary, finely chopped

Preheat oven to 375°F. Place squash pieces cut side down in a greased baking pan. Bake 35 minutes or until softened. Turn squash over. Combine butter, honey, and rosemary and spread a spoonful of the mixture over each squash piece. Bake for 20 minutes longer until bubbly and tender. —SHEPHERD'S GARDEN SEEDS

1 MEASURE OF DRIED HERB = 3 MEASURES OF FRESH

CHAPTER THIRTEEN

Desserts and Beverages

- A very easy and very delicious summertime punch is two parts herb tea (your choice) to one part fruit juice (your choice). The art, of course, is in the combinations.
- On a blustery winter night, treat yourself to a hot herbal toddy. Start with hot herb tea [your favorite blend]; fill cup ⅔ full, then add 1 or 2 tablespoons rum, and lemon and honey to taste.
- Just a simple sprig of fresh mint makes canned lemonade seem special.
- Spicy-tasting herbs add a delicious note to fruit desserts; you can't quite put your finger on that subtle taste, but it's very good. Try bay with peaches (remove bay leaf before serving); cinnamon basil with apples; nutmeg thyme or lemon thyme with pears; and rose geranium with strawberries.
- For an old-fashioned treat, put rose-scented geranium leaves into the bottom of the cake pan before you pour in the batter.

- For very special occasions, decorate your cake or fruit tray with crystallized mint leaves. Start with fresh leaves that are thoroughly dry and perfectly shaped. Paint both sides with beaten egg white, dip leaves in sugar to cover completely, shake off excess, and lay on waxed paper to dry.

TOMATO JUICE PUNCH

Basil • Lemon basil

1 large can tomato juice

2 cups orange juice

1 can limeade (concentrate) mixed with 1 can water

2 tablespoons fresh basil or 1 tablespoon dried basil

Lemon basil for garnish

If dried basil is used, soak in the liquid to soften the leaves. Combine ingredients and garnish each cup with a sprig of lemon basil.

—CAPRILANDS HERB FARM

1 MEASURE OF DRIED HERB = 3 MEASURES OF FRESH

HERB TEA PUNCH

Cinnamon basil • Lemon balm • Peppermint

This is a basic recipe; try other combinations based on your favorite tea herbs.

1 cup cinnamon basil
1 cup lemon balm
½ cup peppermint
Honey to taste
1 liter club soda, lemon-lime soda, or grapefruit soda
Fresh mint for garnish

Use the three herbs and about a quart of boiling water to brew a strong batch of tea. Add honey to taste, keeping in mind the sweetness of the soda you will be using. Refrigerate the herb tea base till serving time, then mix with cold soda and serve over ice. Garnish each glass with sprig of fresh mint.

1 MEASURE OF DRIED HERB = 3 MEASURES OF FRESH

LEMON BASIL SNAPS

Lemon basil

MAKES ABOUT 5 DOZEN.

2 cups flour
½ teaspoon baking soda
¼ teaspoon salt
¾ cup butter or margarine, at room temperature
¾ cup sugar
1 egg
1 tablespoon grated lemon rind
1 tablespoon lemon juice
⅓ cup chopped fresh lemon basil

TOPPING

⅓ cup finely chopped pistachio nuts
3 tablespoons sugar

Sift together the flour, baking soda, and salt. Set aside. In a bowl cream the butter and sugar until light and fluffy. Beat in the egg, mixing until combined. Add lemon rind, lemon juice, and lemon basil. Stir in the dry ingredients, blending thoroughly. Wrap and chill the dough for 1 hour or until firm.

Preheat oven to 350°F. Shape the dough into 1-inch balls. Combine pistachio nuts with 3 tablespoons sugar. Roll the balls of dough in the mixture until coated. Place 2 inches apart on ungreased baking sheets. Press cookies down with the palm of hand to flatten them slightly. Bake 10 to 12 minutes or until golden. Transfer to racks to cool.

—SHEPHERD'S GARDEN SEEDS

1 MEASURE OF DRIED HERB = 3 MEASURES OF FRESH

SCENTED GERANIUM WITH APPLES

Scented geranium

SERVES 4.

4 large cooking apples, washed and cored
¼ cup butter
⅔ cup raisins
4 fresh scented geranium leaves
Pancake or maple syrup to taste

Wash and core 1 apple for each serving. In a baking dish place a dab of butter or margarine under each apple. Fill the holes in the apples with raisins. Top each with a scented geranium leaf. Spoon syrup around the apples and bake in a moderate oven for 40 minutes, or until the apples are soft. The geranium leaves will become crisp.

VARIATIONS

Other possibilities for filling the apple hole: combination of raisins and nuts, candied citrus peel, raisins plus a bit of candied ginger, or apple jelly.

1 MEASURE OF DRIED HERB = 3 MEASURES OF FRESH

CHAPTER FOURTEEN

Condiments

This is the "miscellaneous" chapter, with a little bit of a lot of things: herbal vinegar, jelly, sauces, relishes, and butter spreads—all ways to add the special flavor of herbs to your table.

Sauces

GREEN SAUCE NO. 1 (COOKED)

Mixed herbs

For vegetables, fish, or light soup. Vary this basic sauce by choosing herbs that complement the dish you're serving.

1 tablespoon butter or oil
1 tablespoon flour
½ cup chicken stock
½ cup milk
2 tablespoons chopped fresh mixed herbs, such as parsley, salad burnet, sage, tarragon, or oregano
1 teaspoon lemon juice
2 tablespoons sour cream or yogurt

Melt butter or oil in saucepan, then add flour and cook without allowing it to brown. Add the stock and milk and blend well. Add herbs and lemon juice and simmer for 2 to 3 minutes. Stir in sour cream or yogurt just before serving.

GREEN SAUCE NO. 2 (UNCOOKED)

MAKES ABOUT 3 CUPS.

1½ cups mixed greens and herbs, your choice (suggestion: spinach, nasturtium leaves, tarragon, chives)
4 shallots, peeled (or 1 tablespoon minced onion)
½ cup mayonnaise
1 cup plain yogurt
½ cup sour cream
½ cup lemon juice

Combine all ingredients in blender or food processor and mix thoroughly.

—THE COOK'S GARDEN

1 MEASURE OF DRIED HERB = 3 MEASURES OF FRESH

SORREL SAUCE

Sorrel has a tangy, tart flavor that will remind you of lemons. The sauce is good on baked chicken, poached fish, or steamed vegetables.

1 tablespoon butter
1 shallot, finely chopped (or substitute 1 teaspoon minced onion)
2 cups chopped sorrel leaves
½ cup cream
⅛ teaspoon nutmeg

Saute shallots or onion in butter till translucent. Add sorrel and cook till it wilts, about 2 minutes. Add cream and nutmeg. Cook for 2 minutes more, stirring. —THE COOK'S GARDEN

1 MEASURE OF DRIED HERB = 3 MEASURES OF FRESH

PESTO SAUCE

Basil • Garlic

Add to hot cooked spaghetti, to vegetables, to poached fish, or to minestrone.

MAKES ABOUT 1 CUP.

2 cups fresh basil leaves
2 cloves of garlic
½ cup parmesan cheese
½ cup olive oil (approximately)

Put first 3 ingredients into blender container; use on/off switch to chop and blend. Then, a little at a time, add olive oil until you get a thick paste. To keep pesto from turning black, store in small jar and pour a thin layer of oil on top.

VARIATIONS

Add ⅓ cup pine nuts or walnuts to blender and puree along with the basil. Classic pesto is made with basil, but there's no reason you cannot use other green herbs.

1 MEASURE OF DRIED HERB = 3 MEASURES OF FRESH

BARBECUE GLAZE

Oregano • Basil

If you decide on the spur of the moment to have a cookout, and have no time to marinate the meat, use this tangy sweet glaze instead. It's delicious with chicken, pork, or ribs. Start the meat cooking and then make the glaze. When the meat is almost done, brush on the glaze.

MAKES 1 CUP GLAZE.

¼ cup powdered mustard
⅔ cup vinegar
½ cup brown sugar, firmly packed
¼ cup honey
2 teaspoons dried oregano
2 teaspoons dried basil

In a small saucepan, mix mustard and vinegar into a paste. Add sugar, honey, and herbs and blend well. Heat to boiling and then simmer until thickened, about 2 minutes. —SPICE ISLANDS

1 MEASURE OF DRIED HERB = 3 MEASURES OF FRESH

LEMON/ONION RELISH

Thyme

Good with baked chicken, ham, or lamb; on Thanksgiving, serve it alongside cranberry sauce.

MAKES 1¾ CUPS.

2 tablespoons olive oil
2 medium onions, cut into thin strips
2 medium lemons
2 tablespoons lemon juice
¼ cup water
5 tablespoons sugar
Pinch of salt
1 tablespoon chopped fresh thyme leaves

Heat oil in a medium skillet, add onions, cover. Cook on very low heat until soft but not brown, about 15 minutes.

Meanwhile, prepare lemons. Squeeze out juice and save 2 tablespoons. Cut rinds into strips ¼ inch wide and put them into a saucepan. Cover with water, bring to boil, then drain off water; do this three times. Add to onions along with reserved lemon juice and remaining ingredients. Cook uncovered at low heat for about 20 minutes, stirring occasionally, until most of the liquid is evaporated and onions and lemons are glazed.

Put up in glass jars; store in refrigerator.

—SHEPHERD'S GARDEN SEEDS

1 MEASURE OF DRIED HERB = 3 MEASURES OF FRESH

HERB JELLY

Herb jellies, with their savory-sweet flavor, are good with meats, or with cold cuts in a sandwich; try them spread on crackers with cream cheese for a party snack.

Here's a general approach. Use your favorite apple jelly recipe, but substitute an herbal infusion for the water called for. Make the infusion by steeping the herbs in boiling water for 30 minutes, then strain. Herbs to try this way: lemon thyme, sage, tarragon, rosemary, and of course mint.

CINNAMON BASIL JELLY

A dark pink clear jelly, good for glazing a baked chicken or for a sweet bread with afternoon tea.

MAKES APPROXIMATELY 3 HALF PINTS.

1½ cups cinnamon basil leaves
2¼ cups cold water
3 tablespoons lemon juice
3½ cups sugar
1 3-ounce pouch liquid pectin

With a wooden spoon, bruise the basil or coarsely chop, and place in a saucepan with cold water. Bring to a full boil, cover, and remove from heat. Allow to steep for 15 minutes. Strain "tea" into a large saucepan; you should have about 1¾ cups. Add lemon juice and sugar, bring to a full roiling boil that can't be stirred down. Remove from heat, add pectin, stir. Quickly ladle into hot sterilized jars. Seal with two-part canning lids or with paraffin. —THE COOK'S GARDEN

1 MEASURE OF DRIED HERB = 3 MEASURES OF FRESH

HERB-FLAVORED BUTTER

If you have a container of premixed herb butter waiting in your refrigerator, you will find many, many ways to use it:

- vegetables
- baked potatoes
- grilled meat or fish
- sauces
- and, of course, bread

Any time you would want to add both butter and an herb to a dish, just pull out your herb butter and dip out a spoonful.

BASIC HERB BUTTER

½ cup butter or margarine

1 to 3 tablespoons chopped fresh herbs, or half that amount of dried herbs

Let the butter or margarine soften till you can easily mix in the herbs. Let sit at room temperature for an hour or so for the flavors to blend, then store in refrigerator.

VARIATIONS

- Add 1 teaspoon lemon juice. Lemon juice accentuates the flavor of many herbs.
- Gradually beat in small amounts of water until mixture is light and fluffy; you now have a delicious version of the whipped butter served in elegant restaurants.

1 MEASURE OF DRIED HERB = 3 MEASURES OF FRESH

- Instead of just one herb, use a combination; here are a few suggestions:

  chives and garlic
  marjoram, thyme, and chives
  parsley, tarragon, and thyme
  basil and chives
  dill and parsley
  tarragon, dill, and chives
  mint and lemon balm (delicious on blueberry muffins)

HERBAL VINEGAR

Vinegar richly flavored with one or more herbs is a marvel; once you try it, you'll never make salad dressing with ordinary vinegar again. Once you discover how easy it is to make, you'll soon need a whole shelf for your vinegar collection.

Here's the basic process: put bruised or chopped fresh herbs, or crumbled dried herbs, in a clear glass jar.

Most herbs, fresh:	4 tablespoons of herbs per cup of vinegar
Fresh basil and tarragon:	½ cup herbs per cup of vinegar
Dried herbs:	1 tablespoon of herbs per cup of vinegar

Pour in vinegar. Let sit on a sunny windowsill for about one week or in a dark cupboard for three to four weeks. Taste after a week; when you like the flavor, it's ready. Strain out the herbs.

Pretty easy, right?

1 MEASURE OF DRIED HERB = 3 MEASURES OF FRESH

The vinegar draws out the oils from the herbs, a process which is accelerated with some heat. The sun will do it nicely, but you can also heat the vinegar on the stove or microwave before adding the herbs. *Do NOT let it come to a boil.*

A few of the fine points:

- Use good-quality vinegar. The best choices are white wine and red wine vinegar. White distilled vinegar is satisfactory, and so is cider vinegar as long as it's not "cider flavored." For an Oriental blend, start with rice wine vinegar.
- If your container has a metal lid, don't let the vinegar touch it. If you want to fill the jar full, use a liner of plastic wrap or waxed paper.
- Whenever you think of it, give the jar a shake while it's "brewing."
- To tell if it's ready, be sure to taste it; don't go by smell. Easy way: dip a piece of white bread into the vinegar.

The most familiar herb vinegar is tarragon, but you can use any herb, or a combination. **Caution:** if you use whole garlic or shallots, remove after 48 hours.

Herbs for White Vinegar

tarragon
marjoram
borage
salad burnet (for a cucumber taste in the middle of winter)
lemon thyme
lemon verbena
thyme
rosemary

Herbs for Red Vinegar

sweet basil
garlic
thyme
bay

1 MEASURE OF DRIED HERB = 3 MEASURES OF FRESH

rosemary
oregano
sage
savory
cilantro

Add to White Vinegar for Color

Chive flowers (turns vinegar pink)
Sage flowers (rosy pink)
Borage flowers (blue)
Purple basil leaves (rich red)

A Few Combinations

Garlic and basil
Garlic, oregano, basil, parsley
Garlic and chives
Sage and chives (good with chicken)
Basil, savory, garlic (good with beef)
Sage and lovage (for poultry)
Tarragon and lemon balm
Salad burnet and chives
Dill and lemon balm (for fish)

Remember: take garlic cloves out after 48 hours.

Herbal vinegars have a double place in our lives: not only are they excellent condiments for salads and other uses, but this is a very effective and very easy way to preserve the flavor of fresh herbs, especially those that do not dry well. If you have a bumper crop of basil and have made all the pesto you can use, make a few jars of vinegar out of the rest.

These beautiful herbal vinegars also make wonderful gifts. Here, where appearance counts almost as much as taste, you may want to strain the vinegar twice, using a coffee filter the second time, to remove all the flotsam. Some people like to put one sprig of the herb

1 MEASURE OF DRIED HERB = 3 MEASURES OF FRESH

in the jar, but it does tend to create a certain amount of sediment after a while.

For more information on herb vinegars, Shepherd's Garden Seeds (see Appendix) has a very helpful brochure.

A Note About Herbal Oils

Since we're talking about vinegar, this is a good place to make special mention of homemade herbal oils—salad oil in which you infuse fresh herbs or garlic for several days or weeks. In a word, **don't.**

The U.S. Department of Agriculture has recently concluded that this is dangerous. Herbs and garlic do not have enough acid in them to counteract the organisms that can cause botulism. Commercially manufactured garlic and herbal oils are safe because they have been processed, but homemade products are just too risky.

CHAPTER FIFTEEN

Herb Tea

Most people are introduced to herb tea when they buy a box of packaged tea in the supermarket; many delicious flavors are avail able, and the specialty blends are definitely worth exploring. If you've never made iced tea from a fruity herbal tea blend, you're missing a bet.

But if you have access to fresh herbs, you need not be limited to the commercial products. You can brew a cup of fresh mint tea any time. You can add some of your home-dried herbs to commercial packaged tea, for a unique taste. Or you can dry your herbs and create your own special blend from scratch, to enjoy on a cool winter's night or to give to friends.

MAKING HERB TEA

Although many people talk about herb tea as if it had magical properties, there's nothing mysterious or esoteric about the process of making it. Herb tea is made just the same as regular tea: by steeping the leaves in hot water. The herbs can be either fresh or dried, either a single variety or a combination.

Herb tea in general has a lighter, more delicate taste than regular black tea, and it is lighter in color. It takes a larger quantity of herbs for a cup than China tea, and it takes longer to brew, but it will never get the color of Lipton's, no matter how long you leave it to steep.

To Make a Perfect Cup of Tea

1. Put cold tap water into a kettle; bring to a boil.
2. Measure the herbs into a china or crockery teapot (or anything that is not metal): one teaspoon of dried—or two to three teaspoons of fresh—per cup of water. If using fresh herbs, chop finely. You can either use a tea ball or put them directly into the pot, in which case you'll have to strain the tea before drinking.
3. Pour boiling water onto the herbs. Cover and let steep for 5 to 10 minutes. Strain into cup.
4. Sweeten with sugar or honey, if you wish.

Iced tea is made the same way, except it should be stronger to accommodate the dilution of melting ice cubes. Iced herbal tea is a real treat in the summertime. Add a fresh mint leaf for color and pizazz.

Herbs to Use for Tea

Through the years many different plants have been used for tea; many of them still are, although like everything else certain flavors go in and out of style. In theory, you can make herb tea out of any herb that you cook with, and many others besides. Whether it tastes good is a matter of, well, taste.

If you have herbs growing in your garden, you have lots of opportunities to try many kinds of herb teas. But even if you don't, you can still experiment with some of the herbs you already have on hand in your kitchen.

Herb Tea from Your Spice Rack

Anise Tea made from anise seed has a mild licorice flavor, and is soothing to an upset stomach. For one cup of tea, lightly crush one teaspoon of seed lightly, then add to boiling water. Simmer for about 10 minutes, then strain and sweeten to taste.

Basil Let dried leaves steep in hot water for about 5 minutes. Because we are so accustomed to associating basil with tomatoes, your taste buds may perceive this as a broth rather than a tea.

Caraway Crush caraway seeds lightly and simmer in boiling water for 10 minutes or so. Caraway tea feels warm in the stomach and thus has long been used for babies with colic.

Cumin If you have whole seeds, crush them lightly and simmer in boiling water for about 15 minutes. This tea is said to have a calming effect on stressed-out people.

Fennel Fennel tea is an old remedy for babies with colic; it gives a warm feeling in the tummy. For the same reason, many adults enjoy it before bedtime. Crush fennel seeds lightly, simmer in boiling water for 10 to 15 minutes, strain and sweeten if desired.

Parsley You probably already know that parsley is full of vitamin C, so here's another way to take your vitamins: drink it. Parsley tea is light and refreshing; if the color green had a taste, this would be it. One teaspoon of dried parsley per cup of boiling water; let steep for 10 minutes.

Rosemary A pleasant-flavored tea that is said to be good for headaches and colds. Dried rosemary leaves are hard, like fir needles; crumble them with your fingers before pouring on the boiling water, then strain carefully.

Thyme Dried thyme makes an aromatic tea with a subtle taste. Some believe it helps ease a hangover.

TEA FROM YOUR GARDEN

If you have an herb garden, or a friend who will let you browse through hers, you can make tea from fresh herbs. The process is the same as for dried herbs, except that you use more herbs. The general rule of thumb is, 2 to 3 teaspoons of the herb, chopped fine, per cup of water, and steep in hot water for 5 to 10 minutes.

From a home garden, you can enjoy familiar herbs in fresh form, as well as some of the less common ones that you will never find in the supermarket.

Angelica Tea made from the leaves of this dramatic plant has a light, sweet licorice taste, and some say it helps digestion. Not recommended for daily use.

Anise Tea can be made from the feathery leaves as well as the seeds; has the same licorice flavor.

Bergamot This plant is sometimes called Oswego tea, after the beverage brewed by Native Americans in New York State. This citrusy beverage was one of the "protest" teas during the American Revolution. Simmer the chopped leaves about 10 minutes.

Catnip This mint relative is high in vitamin C. Makes cats crazy, but very soothing to humans. This was a favorite early remedy for babies with colic. Drinking the tea before meals stimulates appetite; drinking it afterward helps digestion.

Chamomile The delicate and fruity taste of chamomile tea is so popular that it is widely available as a commercial herb tea. But if you grow chamomile you can make your own. In either case, the part that is used for tea is the flower heads. A very soothing tea that is popular as a nightcap.

Costmary Tea made from costmary should be steeped just a few minutes, or the minty taste will become bitter.

Geranium The leaves of scented geraniums can be used to make tea, and the flavor will echo the fragrance: rose geranium tea tastes faintly like roses, lemon geranium like lemon, peppermint geranium like peppermint, and so on. In most cases, there is a truer source of the flavor, and so probably you would make geranium tea for the novelty of it.

Horehound Horehound syrup and candy are classic remedies for coughs, and the tea has some of the same qualities, although it is of course much more dilute. It tastes like menthol, and therefore if you are making it purely as a beverage you will probably find it more pleasing as part of a blend with other herbs.

Lemon balm You can occasionally find lemon balm tea in the store, but if you have it growing in your yard you have a never-ending supply. The leaves (fresh or dried) make a delicious tea that is both lemony and minty, and it is very nice in combinations with other teas.

Lemon verbena Use the leaves to make a rich lemony tea; add to regular China tea in place of lemon slice. Blends nicely with spearmint.

Lovage Want to try a tea that tastes like celery? Use any part of the lovage plant: leaves, stem, or seeds, or all three. Add a bit of garlic or salt, some other culinary herbs like marjoram, and you have a savory broth. Think of it as nature's bouillon.

Mint	Of course you can buy mint tea in the store, and it's delicious. But if you grow it in your garden, you can have flavors you'll never see on the supermarket shelves: orange mint, apple mint, pineapple mint, chocolate mint, to name a few. And you can create your own special blend.
Salad burnet	This salad herb has small leaves that taste like cucumber. A tea made from them has the same fresh flavor and, some say, a pick-me-up effect.
Sweet cicely	Leaves or seeds produce a sweet tea that tastes like licorice and is reputed to help us digest heavy foods.
Thyme	Thyme tea from fresh herbs is fun because there are so many delicious varieties of thyme. If you grow lemon thyme, for instance, you can have a tea that is both lemony and savory.

Herbal Tea Combinations

Once you have brewed a cup of tea from an herb and made note of what it tastes like, you're ready to move to mixing herbs together into your own blend. The combinations are very much a matter of taste and experimentation. Try two that you think would taste good together (a few combinations are suggested here, to get you going), then maybe add a third or a fourth. When you get a combination you really like, write down the formula so you can make it again later.

Try These Together

Marjoram and mint
Thyme and rosemary
Ginger and mint
Costmary and orange mint
Ginger and chamomile
Lemon verbena and mint
Rose geranium and mint
Lovage and salad burnet
Bergamot and sweet cicely

If you're lucky enough to know someone who has a large herb garden, or have one yourself, you can dry quantities of lots of herbs in the summer and spend the winter experimenting. It's something like the Mad Scientist in the kitchen: add a handful of this, a pinch of that, a touch of this other. To get your creativity going, here are a few recipes.

EMMA'S BLEND

3 parts apple mint
1 part spearmint
1 part orange mint
1 part peppermint

—Willamette Valley Herb Society,
Aurora, Oregon

SWEET MEADOW TEA

This delicious blend is made from dried herbs. Mix thoroughly; store in glass jars. Use 1 teaspoon to make one cup of tea.

¼ cup orange mint
2 tablespoons rosemary
1 tablespoon sage
2 tablespoons lemon thyme
1 tablespoon calendula petals
3 tablespoons chamomile
1 tablespoon fennel leaves

—Joyce Laitinen, Canby, Oregon

And one more suggestion, which isn't really a recipe, from Adelma Simmons of Caprilands, the grande dame of herb growers. Honoring the legendary virtues attributed to various herbs, she has created this whole-souled blend.

CAPRILANDS TEA

1 part calendula, for cheerfulness and a clear complexion
1 part chamomile, for a calm spirit and a good night's sleep
1 part marjoram, for happiness
1 part mint, for wisdom
1 part rosemary, for remembrance
1 part sage, for long life and domestic happiness
1 part thyme, for bravery

Herb Tea/China Tea Combinations

Another way to have fun with tea herbs is to add them to regular black tea. (I use the term *black tea* in a general way—to distinguish from herb tea. In other words, it's the tea you have been buying all your life, usually in tea bags, to make a cup of hot tea or iced tea. In this book *China tea*, *black tea*, and *regular tea* all mean the same thing.)

Once again, let your taste buds guide you. Think about the taste of the individual herb, then mentally add it to the taste of your regular tea. Then try it out, and make note of the combinations you really like.

When you make a pot of tea, or a cup, add any of these herbs (dried or fresh) for an unusual taste.

Basil
Lemon balm
Bergamot (make your own Earl Grey blend)
Chamomile
Costmary
Lemon thyme
Lemon verbena
Mints
Sweet cicely

There is really no limit on the number of ingredients that can be blended together into a tasty tea. Go ahead—play Mad Scientist. Even if the results are awful, you haven't wasted much.

Here are a few spicy blends to try.

ROSE SPICE TEA

2 tea bags of black tea
2 tablespoons of dried rose geranium leaves (or 4 fresh)
1 cinnamon stick

ORANGE SPICE TEA

2 tea bags black tea
2 tablespoons dried orange mint *or* grated rind of one orange
3 cloves

LEMON SPICE TEA

2 tea bags black tea
1 tablespoon dried lemon verbena or lemon balm
1 tablespoon dried rose geranium leaves
1 pinch ground allspice

TEA AND POLITICS

Can you imagine, as you settle down in the evening to enjoy a quiet cup of herb tea, that you are committing an act of political protest? Two hundred years ago, that's exactly what the American colonists did.

These settlers from England loved their tea, but the Crown added taxes to tea sent to the colonies, making it too expensive for many colonists. As the force of revolution began to build, this tax took on greater significance: it became a symbol of the dominance from afar.

From the Native Americans the colonists learned to enjoy teas brewed from New World plants such as Oswego tea (bergamot), and soon they were blending their own concoctions from their back-door gardens: raspberry leaves, hyssop and chamomile, thyme and red clover. These teas became known as Liberty teas, and colonists defiantly drank them in place of the imported black tea.

Then in December 1773 a group of colonists disguised as Indians climbed aboard three British ships lying in Boston Harbor and threw 342 chests of tea into the water. The Boston Tea Party was the most flagrant protest yet against the hated tax, and served to accelerate the movement toward independence.

Tea Tips

* The method for preparing herb tea depends on what part of the plant is involved. If the herb was originally leaves (most of our common kitchen herbs), make tea as you do regular tea: boil water, add herbs, remove from heat, let steep. If the herb is in the form of seeds or roots, either whole or powdered, you'll need to simmer it on the stove for 10 minutes or more.

* General proportions are: 1 teaspoon of dried herb per cup of water, or 2 to 3 teaspoons of fresh herb.

* Steeping time is longer than regular tea.

* To tell if your tea is ready, go by taste or aroma, not color. Herb tea is very pale (usually yellow or green), not brick red.

* Herb tea is caffeine free.

* To fully enjoy herb tea, don't compare it to regular tea that comes in tea bags; try to think of it as something completely different.

PART FIVE

Herbal Crafts and Household Products

Introduction

This section will introduce you to some of the many ways herbs can be used in your daily life. The first time you soak in a tub filled with lavender-scented water, or replace smelly mothballs with a pretty little wormwood-filled sachet, or present a bride-to-be with a special nosegay built around the symbolism of herbs, you will realize you have stepped through a door into a new world.

You have joined the line of those who consider herbs as much more than something to cook with, people who cherish herbs for all their utilitarian and symbolic values. It is a line that stretches back through the centuries and forward to the future, and into which you are warmly welcomed.

Some assumptions of the chapters in this section are:

- You do not have to have an herb garden. All the materials can be purchased at a craft supply store or mail-order company.
- On the other hand, if you do have herbs growing, you will learn how to work with them.
- You do not have to be an experienced craftsperson; full instructions are included, in beginning-level terms.

CHAPTER SIXTEEN

Potpourri

In the Middle Ages bundles of dried herbs were hung throughout the house or tied to the furniture, to sweeten the air and make the room smell fresh. In those days, when windows were kept tightly closed and baths were not everyday occurrences, these natural room fresheners were important for hygiene and emotional sanity.

Today we have air conditioners and showers, and we don't worry so much about stuffy rooms and pungent odors, but the gentle, sweet smell of dried herbs and flowers still adds a touch of grace to any home.

Potpourri (pronounced poh-poor-EE) is a mixture of dried flower petals, herbs, and other plant materials, blended with spices and oils for fragrance and set into a pretty container that permits us to enjoy its visual beauty and sweet aroma.

In almost every kind of retail store—supermarket, department store, variety store—you can buy premade potpourri in plastic bags. The cost is modest but the quality can be disappointing; the aroma doesn't last and the ingredients are chosen for economy. Most traditional potpourri makers shudder at the very high proportion of wood chips in those cellophane bags. It's a bit like hot dogs: once you know what's in them, they don't seem so appealing.

In gift shops and home decor shops you can also buy high-quality potpourri products that are lovely to look at and smell heavenly, but they are not cheap.

There's a third option: you can make it yourself. It's easy, it's fun, it's very satisfying, and when you're all done you have lots of nifty stuff to give as special little presents.

Two Kinds of Potpourri

There are two basic types of potpourri: wet and dry. Wet potpourri is made from partially dried flower petals that are packed in salt, where they ferment, then mixed with spices and allowed to "cure" for weeks or sometimes months. The process is tedious and time-consuming, and many people who have tried it have given up in frustration because the mixture has a distressing tendency to mold before it is finished curing.

One other drawback is that the finished product, while it smells wonderful, is not pleasant to look at. The word *potpourri* is French for "rotten pot"; that should give you a clue! However, it does have a deep, rich aroma that lasts for years, literally. Wet potpourri is usually kept in pretty ceramic containers that have a top with holes to let the scent through.

Dry potpourri is made from materials that were dried first. The flowers and flower petals retain some of their original color, and so the final product is pretty to look at as well as sweet smelling. It doesn't have to be hidden away in a covered jar.

In this chapter we are going to concentrate on dry potpourri, for the simple reason that you can hardly go wrong. Just about any combination of dried materials will work, and you can add any kind of fragrance. You can mix and blend colors, textures, and spicy undertones to your heart's content. So let's get started. First, a review of the various categories of ingredients.

What Goes in a Potpourri Mixture

Making potpourri is not unlike making meat loaf: there are hundreds of recipes, and some of the best preparers don't use a recipe at all. In broad terms, potpourri is made of four categories of materials:

1. *Dried flowers, leaves, and other plant material.* In other words, all the "stuff" in a potpourri mixture.
2. *Spices.* To add richness to the aroma.
3. *Oils.* This is where the primary fragrance comes from.
4. *Fixative.* To keep the fragrance from evaporating.

The Dried Material

This is the part you see—all the dried flowers, herbs, flower petals, berries, leaves, seed pods, cones. Sometimes this is all collectively referred to as *the botanicals*, since they were once part of a living plant.

Some of the flowers, and all the herbs, are included for the fragrance they add. In this group you will find, for instance:

For Fragrance: Flowers

roses
sweet pea
lilac
lavender
carnation (the variety called clove pink)
violet
honeysuckle
jasmine

For Fragrance: Leaves

mints
tarragon
sweet woodruff
rosemary
marjoram
angelica
lemon balm
lemon verbena
scented geraniums (leaves)
sage
costmary
hyssop

- bay
- thyme (especially lemon or nutmeg thyme)
- basil

Unscented flowers, or those that don't have much fragrance after drying, are added for color. Any kind of flower will work here; it's a matter of finding colors that blend nicely. A few examples:

For Color

- calendula
- cornflower
- carnation
- nasturtium
- primrose
- daisy
- zinnia
- bachelor's button
- peony
- larkspur
- delphinium
- tulip
- poppy

If you have flowers in your yard, or access to wildflowers, or a generous neighbor, you can dry your own; later on in this chapter you'll learn how. If you don't have any of these things, you can buy dried flowers and other botanical materials from a number of mail-order sources; check the Appendix, under the category Crafts Supplies.

Traditional potpourri is made from flowers, primarily roses; in fact, the finished product used to be called a rose bowl. But there is no reason it has to be limited to flower petals. In the plant kingdom are a number of other things that make nice contributions to a potpourri: berries, unusual seed heads, small cones, snips of evergreen foliage, pieces of bark, anything that looks interesting. The mixtures that feature this kind of material often evoke autumn and winter landscapes, and so are popular in the Thanksgiving-Christmas holiday season.

A lot of what many folks call weeds look wonderful in a wintertime potpourri. Think "potpourri" as you walk through any field or forested area and you will see many interesting things you never noticed before. As soon as you take on this perspective, you will find dozens of beautiful items. If you're sure you're in a place where it is appropriate to do so, start collecting these dried seed heads, cones, dried moss, for a truly unique potpourri.

Spices

In both ground and whole form, many of the world's spices are added to potpourri to add depth to the fragrance blend. Usually you don't see them, or at least they aren't a prominent element. Possibilities include:

lemon peel	orange peel	allspice
aniseseed	cloves	cinnamon sticks
star anise	coriander	vanilla bean
ginger	juniper berries	nutmeg

Oils

Here's a surprise: in modern potpourri the main fragrance comes not from the botanicals but from a bottle—in the form of concentrated oil. In earlier times, flowers used to make potpourri were highly aromatic; today's hybrids have been bred for other qualities and the fragrance is not so strong. So, we compensate by adding a few drops of scented oil.

The oils can be purchased in gift and craft stores, retail herb shops, and some natural foods stores; and several mail-order sources have an amazing selection (check the Appendix, under Craft Supplies). Just to give you an idea: coconut, pine, magnolia, peach, apple blossom, wisteria, jasmine, lime, tangerine, honey-suckle, rose geranium . . . there are hundreds.

As you start exploring this fascinating world, first you should know about the different types of oil.

- *Essential oil* has been distilled from the plant. It is thus pure essence of, say, peppermint or lavender (not "essential" in the sense of being mandatory). Some essential oils are also what is termed *food quality*, meaning approved for use in cooking.

- *Synthetic oil* has been created in a laboratory, from ingredients that chemically duplicate the aroma of natural oils.

- *Fragrance oil* can be either a blend of synthetic oil and an essential, or an essential oil diluted with alcohol.

Not all suppliers distinguish between synthetics and fragrance oils. They lump everything into two groups: (1) essential oils and (2) everything else, and often they call this second group simply fragrance oils.

Essential oils are, as you might imagine, more expensive, but still quite reasonable, especially since you need just a small amount. Remember that all these oils are *highly* concentrated, and you should not apply them directly to your skin.

Fixatives

Over time, the aromas of the fragrance oils fade. Think about it: the reason we can smell them at all is that they have evaporated into the air, and once there, they're no longer in the potpourri bowl. But it is possible to slow down the evaporation rate, by adding to the mixture certain substances that chemically bond with the oils and then release them slowly.

These substances are collectively called fixatives, and there are several kinds. They can be bought in craft shops that have supplies for floral crafts, or from most of the same mail-order sources that sell craft supplies.

Originally, fixatives were taken from animals: ambergris, from the sperm whale; civet, from the glands of an African cat; and musk, from the musk deer found in central Asia. Today environmental concerns, not to mention economics, have diminished the use of these animal fixatives; if you see musk or ambergris listed in a catalog, those are almost certainly synthetic.

Fixatives derived from plants are used nowadays; the most common are these:

- *Orris root,* the most popular fixative, is the root of a particular species of iris, called Florentine iris. It comes in powder form and in granules about the size of ice cream salt. Some people are allergic to the powder but can usually tolerate the granular form. Don't get curious and nibble a piece; it can cause vomiting. Orris root has its own fragrance, a faint violet scent, and so is best used in floral potpourris.
- *Oakmoss,* which is actually a lichen, looks like a tangled mass of grayish green thread. It goes well with lavender and citrusy blends.
- *Calamus root,* the dried roots of the marsh plant known as sweet flag, has a light spicy aroma that is compatible with woodsy or spicy mixes.
- *Gum benzoin,* the gum of an Asian tree, is an excellent fixative as well as an ingredient in Oriental incense.

Recently, as potpourri manufacture has become big business, enterprising people have searched for new and more economical products that have fixative properties. One is ground-up corn cobs, euphemistically listed as "natural cellulose"; word is that it works reasonably well.

Gathering and Drying Material

The potpourri that you produce is a way to capture the beauty of the garden or woodland, preserve it, and set it close by for indoor memories. All year long, you will want to keep an eye out for things that would go well in a potpourri, starting with the very earliest spring flowers, on through the lush blooms of summer and the berries and cones of winter.

Flowers bloom at different times; as each comes into its season, take a few and dry them for potpourri. Store them in airtight containers out of the sun. When you have a good supply of various colors and fragrances, you're ready.

Flowers

Generally, flower petals (rather than whole flowers) are used in potpourri, and most of the time it's easier and faster to dry them as individual petals. Very small flowers and buds can be dried whole.

Start with flowers that are dry (that is, not covered with dew or raindrops). To air-dry, pull the petals apart and spread them on something flat that lets air through (check the section on drying in chapter 6 for suggestions). Keep the drying tray in a place that is dry, well ventilated, and away from direct sun. (Sunlight will fade the colors.) You can overlap most types of flowers (one that has to be in a single layer is peony), but if you do you should stir them around once a day. The petals are ready when they are crisp-dry; that takes anywhere from a few days to a week, depending on their size.

Another technique for air drying is hanging bunches upside down. This works best with plants that have small flowers in a tight cluster, such as:

lavender	tansy
larkspur	heather
hydrangea	bachelor buttons
blue salvia	yarrow

Everlastings (see chapter 18) are also dried this way, and they make terrific additions to potpourri—great color but no scent.

Because lavender is such a popular ingredient in potpourri, we'll take a moment to talk about drying it. You want to dry the flower buds just before they open, for that's when the fragrance is highest. So when the first buds open up into flowers, cut off entire flower stalks, bundle them together, and hang to dry. (They also dry on their own if you just stand them in a vase with no water; while they're drying, you have a pretty bouquet to enjoy.) When completely dry, strip the flower buds off the stem; they are quite small, like grains of purple rice.

You can also dry flower petals in the microwave. Spread in a single layer on a paper towel, cover with a second paper towel, and microwave for 30 to 40 seconds. Two disadvantages: they burn easily, and it's a time-consuming way to do a large batch of petals.

And let us not forget the flowers of herbs:

chives (pink flowers)	sage (blue flowers)
bergamot (red)	feverfew (white)
borage (blue)	santolina (yellow)
hyssop (pink, blue)	calendula (yellow)

One of the prettiest ways to display potpourri is to add a single whole dried flower right on top, for a color accent and visual focal point. The herb flowers listed just above work nicely this way; because they are relatively small, their contribution is subtle. Larger flowers, such as one deep red rose or a bright yellow tulip, make a stronger accent. Chapter 18 contains information about drying whole flowers.

Herbs

Herbs for potpourri are dried just the same as if you were drying them to make tea or to cook with. Check the drying instructions in chapter 6. When they are thoroughly dry, strip the leaves from the stem but try to keep the leaves as whole as possible. Now they are ready to be stored away in airtight jars until you're ready to make your potpourri.

Other Materials

If you collect berries, cones, or bark in outdoor spaces, they may be very damp, especially if they were lying in the rich spongy ground of the forest floor. Spread them out on your drying racks, or on cookie sheets in a very low oven, until all the moisture is gone. With cones, you'll know when that is because they open up.

You never want to add anything to a potpourri mixture that is not completely dry; if even one item is damp, its moisture will be reabsorbed by the dry petals, and then you have danger of mold.

Making the Potpourri

Potpourri, like meat loaf, has a mix of ingredients in fairly standard proportions. Meat loaf is mostly meat, with breadcrumbs or eggs for extra volume and herbs and spices for flavoring. Potpourri is mostly the botanicals, with herbs and spices for extra richness and oils for aroma.

As with meat loaf, there are precise recipes for potpourri, and several are included in this chapter by way of example; but part of the joy of the process is letting your creativity free. The art lies in the details—putting together colors that enrich each other and a fragrance that enhances rather than conflicts. When this is achieved, the whole is greater than the sum of the parts.

How do you get started?

1. *First, choose a theme.* If you have been building up an inventory of things for potpourri, start by evaluating what you have. Line up all your containers of "stuff" so you can see the entire collection at once. What do you have the most of? Does one color family predominate? Do you have just one type of flower, or a mixture? Do you have more woodsy items than flowers? Try dividing the collection into two batches, by color range or type of botanical. Shift the jars around until you are pleased with the combinations.

   Now, what do those combinations suggest to you? If you have lots of gold, orange, yellow, maybe your theme is "Autumn Meadow." A grouping of small cones with cinnamon sticks and red berries says "Old-fashioned Christmas." A combination of pink rose petals, blue and purple statice, and dark red tulip petals has a Victorian look, so your theme is "Victorian Garden."

On the other hand, if you do not have your own dried materials but plan to buy everything from a catalog, you can decide on a theme ahead of time and order plant materials that contribute to that theme.

2. *Select a compatible fragrance.* Unless you have a local source you will have to order the oils, so allow a few weeks for this part of the process. The catalog will tell you whether the bottles come with medicine dropper tops; if not, order a few separately. You need a very small amount of oil per batch of potpourri, and a dropper is the easiest way to control this. Also, most potpourri recipes specify a certain number of drops.

   And while you're at it, order fixative too. (Of course, if you're ordering the dried materials from a catalog you'll order everything all together.)There's nothing to prevent you from using more than one oil; careful blends are often better than a single fragrance. For instance, a blend of lime and lemon is richer than either one alone.

   Which fragrances go well with your theme? This is the creative part. In your imagination, try out various combinations. For the Christmas batch, how about pine, clove, and tangerine? If you have dried lavender flowers, you can deepen the aroma with lavender oil and sharpen it with orange or lime. Rose oil is a natural for your Victorian blend, with a touch of lemon or lime so it's not overly sweet. And so on. (See additional tip on blending in chapter 17.)

   Shortcut: Several mail-order sources sell their own blended formulas, as well as individual oils.

3. *Choose herbs and spices to complement your blend.* Now that you know the theme and the main fragrance, think about herbs and spices that will enhance the mixture. Try to imagine the layers of fragrance. For example:

   - Cloves and cinnamon are nice undertones to rose.
   - The sweetness of lavender is highlighted with rosemary.

- Bay seems to go naturally with pine or fir.
- Lemon or peppermint geraniums go well with most floral blends.
- Sweet woodruff adds a light vanilla layer.
- And mint is delicious with almost everything.

If you don't have your own herb garden, you can order dried herbs in bulk from mail-order companies too. In a pinch, you can use commercial herbs and spices from the supermarket, but in the quantity you need it's not cost effective.

4. *Gather your containers.* This can be done while you're waiting for your ordered materials to arrive. You'll need large jars to keep the potpourri in while it is aging, and possibly others to store it in until gift-giving time. Get in the habit of saving all the glass jars with airtight lids that pass through your household. Avoid plastic, which adds its own smell. And start collecting unusual small containers for your gift potpourris.

5. *Make the potpourri.* When you have all your materials on hand, time to start mixing. At this point there are several ways to go, but the one described here seems the most surefire.

   - Prepare the fixative base. In a small glass jar with a tight lid, put a small amount of fixative, then add your oils. Shake and let stand for at least a day; two days is better. This way the fragrance of the oil will be fully dispersed into the fixative.
   - In a large bowl (glass, pottery, or stainless steel), put the flowers and herbs. Sprinkle with the spices, then the oil-infused fixative. With a wooden spoon, gently mix all together.

6. *Set it aside for aging.* Put the finished potpourri into a covered container (not plastic) away from sunlight for approximately six weeks; gently stir every few days. During this period of

aging, the oils will blend and "set" into the mixture. The fragrance of the final product will be mellower and softer than the original aroma you had in Step 5.

BASIC POTPOURRI PROPORTIONS

6 cups dried flowers or other botanicals
1 cup dried herbs
3 tablespoons spices
¼ cup fixative (but use 1 cup of oakmoss)
10 drops oil (approximately 1 teaspoon)

Remember, this is a rough guideline only. Make up your own mix, using these relative proportions. Here are a few recipes to get you started.

OLD-FASHIONED ROSE POTPOURRI

4 cups dried rose petals
1 cup dried lavender flowers
¼ cup dried spearmint leaves
¼ cup dried lemon verbena leaves
1 tablespoon cloves
2 tablespoons orris root
4 drops rose oil
2 drops lavender oil

HINT-OF-MINT LAVENDER POTPOURRI

2 cups dried lavender buds
1 cup dried mint leaves
¼ cup dried rosemary
1 tablespoon orris root
3 drops lavender oil
1 drop spearmint oil

LEMON POTPOURRI

1 cup lemon balm
1 cup lemon thyme
1 cup lemon verbena
1 lemon rind, grated and dried
1 tablespoon orris root
4 drops lemon oil

MOUNTAIN MEADOW POTPOURRI

2 cups dried flowers in yellow/orange range: calendula, santolina, zinnia, strawflowers
1 cup dried herbs: rosemary, marjoram, basil
1 handful seed heads such as teasel or poppy
½ cup hop flowers
1 tablespoon cloves
1 tablespoon allspice
2 tablespoons orris root
3 drops bergamot oil
2 drops spearmint oil

CHRISTMAS POTPOURRI

3 cups small cones, such as hemlock or alder, or sweetgum balls
1 cup star anise pods
6–8 cinnamon sticks, broken into 1-inch lengths
1 cup dried orange peel cut into narrow strips
½ cup bay leaves
¼ cup whole cloves
2 drops pine oil
2 drops bergamot oil

Optional but pretty: lightly spray the star anise with gold glitter.

Displaying Potpourri

A big part of the charm of potpourri is that it is pretty to look at. So when your batch is finished with the aging process and ready to be put out on display, take some time to think about the container.

Clear glass works beautifully with all types of potpourri; it allows all the pretty things to be seen from all angles. Any type of glass bowl makes a perfect container, but you don't have to limit yourself to bowls. Here are some ideas:

- Sugar bowl
- Wineglass
- Champagne goblet (the kind with the broad top)
- Small rounded vase
- Brandy snifter

Other glass in all types of colors can also be used. Solid black is a dramatic background for floral potpourri. Colored glass is nice if the colors are compatible.

Other containers offer an unlimited range of possibilities for matching the theme of the potpourri to its container.

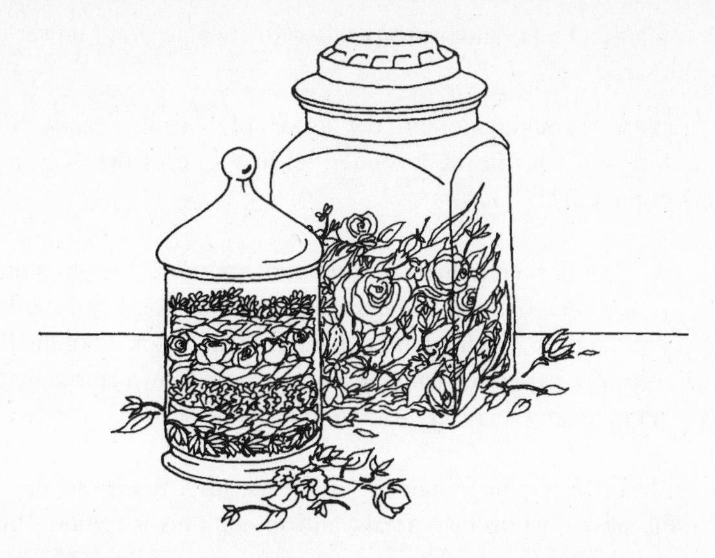

Clear glass apothecary jars are ideal for storing and displaying potpourri. Separate layers of flowers and petals (***left***) are especially pretty.

- A small brass bowl is pretty for woodland mixtures that feature cones and other brown tones.
- A small basket holds potpourri based on wildflowers (set a clear glass bowl inside so the small pieces don't fall through).
- An old cream pitcher painted with roses holds rose potpourri.
- That silver candy dish you got as a wedding present is a perfect background for lavender potpourri.

Next time you're in a secondhand shop or antique store, look around with new eyes. Think "potpourri" and you'll come up with many creative ideas.

And while you're at it, look for ways to add a decorative flourish to your container. For instance:

- Put one or two miniature Christmas balls, silver or bright red, in your holiday mix.

- Top a floral mix made with petals with a whole dried flower of the same type.
- Fit a lacy handkerchief into the bottom of that silver candy dish before you pour in the lavender; let just a bit of the lace spill over the edge.

Some of the best containers for potpourri are those straight-sided glass jars with glass lids, called apothecary jars. If you keep the lid on most of the time, the fragrance will last much longer. Take the lid off when you're expecting company, or when your own spirits need a lift. And here are two pretty ways to fill them:

- Build up layers of individual elements: pink rosebuds, green mint leaves, white rose petals, and so on. This is tedious, but the end result is gorgeous.
- Fill the jar as usual, with a mixture, then add a few whole flowers. Slide a plastic knife (the picnic kind) down next to the edge, pushing the mix aside; carefully fit a whole flower, face out, into the empty space.

Keeping Potpourri Fresh

Eventually potpourri will lose its fragrance. You cannot avoid that, but you can delay it.

1. Don't put your container in direct sunlight; it fades the colors and dissipates the oils.
2. Keep a lid on the container; remove it for special occasions. (Bonus: this will also keep dust out.)

And when the aroma is gone, you can add more. Mix up a batch of fixative-plus-oil, remove the potpourri mix from its container, and fold in the new fixative.

In some gift and craft shops you can find mixed fragrance blends in aerosol form—just spray it on. It doesn't last as long, but it's certainly a convenient way to refresh potpourri, especially when you're in a hurry.

Eventually, however, you will want to replace old potpourri with a new batch. The colors fade, household dust does its usual damage, and there doesn't seem much point in trying to revive it. If you have a fireplace, burn the old batch; it sends a wonderful aroma into the room, like incense. Or add new oil to old potpourri and sew it into a sachet (see chapter 17), where the faded colors won't matter.

Potpourri Tips

* Absolutely *anything* can be used in a potpourri mixture, as long as it harmonizes with the theme. I know someone who puts small pieces of old lace ribbon in a Victorian-style rose potpourri; it's exquisite. But don't mix too many things of different character, or you'll end up with sweet-smelling clutter.

* Keep all the botanicals away from direct sun throughout the process—while they are drying, while the mixture is in the aging jar, and while it is out on display. Bright sun fades the colors.

* Experiment with color and fragrance combinations—that's the fun of it all—but keep notes as you go along so that when you get something you really like you'll be able to make it again.

* Make your own simmering potpourri from spices you already have in the cupboard: all-spice, cloves, cinnamon, ginger, or any combination. Train your kids to save orange peels, and dry them. Add a few drops of vanilla or some of those flavored extracts you've had on the shelf forever: orange, lemon, mint, almond. Proportions: 2 cups water, ½ cup spices. Simmer on stove or bake in very slow oven with the door open.

* No flowers of your own? Volunteer to maintain the rosebushes in your neighborhood park or your church's garden; the blossoms need to be trimmed off constantly to keep the bushes blooming, so you might as well make use of the trimmings.

CHAPTER SEVENTEEN

Potpourri Crafts and Similar Items

A crystal bowl filled with rose petals and lavender flowers is a thing of beauty unto itself. But that is not the only way to enjoy and make use of your potpourri blend. Once you have the potpourri made up, you have the basis of some very nice craft items, for yourself or for gifts.

In this chapter we are going to look at a few of the many things you can do with potpourri, plus some other assorted ideas based on similar principles.

SACHETS

A sachet, which is nothing more than potpourri in a small fabric bag, allows you to put the clean smell of potpourri in places where an open container would not work—a dresser drawer, for instance.

One nice thing about sachets is that the ingredients are hidden from sight. So if you have some dried flowers that didn't turn out as

Sachets are small fabric bags filled with sweet-smelling potpourri; they can be made in many shapes.

you hoped, or have become faded, they can be turned into sachet bags quite satisfactorily.

Sachets can be any shape—round, rectangular, heart-shaped, even in the form of an animal or bird, if you're very good with needle and thread. One traditional shape is a rectangle about three inches wide and six inches long, tied at the top. Choose light-weight fabric that breathes (cotton, linen, or silk are best) in delicate prints or solid colors, and select harmonizing ribbon. Cut and sew following the general directions on page 356. And while you're at it, make *lots,* because as soon as they see them, your friends will want one too.

For a quick no-sew sachet, start with a square of fabric and trim the edges with pinking shears. Even faster, use a lacy handkerchief; the edges are already hemmed. Put a small pile of potpourri into the center, pull the sides up, and tie with a ribbon.

A pretty combination: one square in bright colored satin or silk, covered with an outer layer of filmy lace that lets the colored fabric show through. For a delicate all-lace look, use an inner layer of thin fabric the same color as your lace. (If you use just lace, some of the finer particles of potpourri will dribble through.)

Use sachets in lingerie drawers, linen closets, shoe bags, any closets or clothes storage areas. Hang one from the bedpost or doorknob and give it a gentle squeeze to release the fragrance. Slip one behind

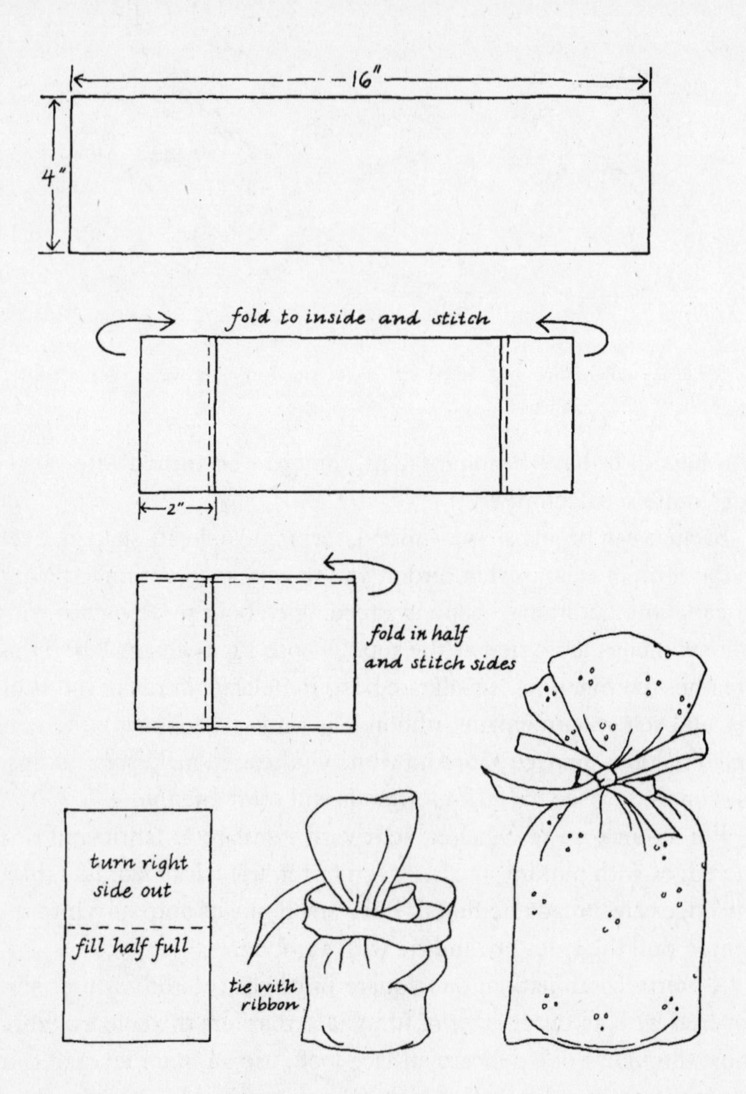

Basic sachet construction. Fill small bags with prepared potpourri, tied closed with a ribbon, and you have sachet in an instant.

the sofa cushions. Put one on the coat rack by the front door. Or on that shelf behind the backseat in your car. Or in the baby's stroller. Or any other part of your world that could use a little sweetening.

Mini-sachets

Some natural food stores and mail-order sources sell small bags made of special porous paper for homemade herb tea: you fill them with dried herbs and heat-seal them with an iron. The same little bags can be used to make a batch of miniature sachets. Use them in out-of-sight spots where their unadorned appearance won't matter, such as your purse or the glove box of the car, or where a normal-sized sachet wouldn't fit, such as a box of stationery. To order the bags, check Nichols Garden Nursery, Harvest Health, or Dabney Herbs in the Appendix.

SACHET NO. 1

1 part lemon geranium leaves
1 part rose geranium leaves
1 part lavender flowers

To a quart of mixture, add 2 tablespoons orris root blended with 1 drop lemon oil, 1 drop rose oil, 1 drop lavender oil.

SACHET NO. 2

1 part lemon verbena
1 part lemon balm
1 part spearmint
1 part orange *or* apple mint

To 1 quart of dried leaves, add 2 tablespoons of orris root that has been preblended with 3 drops lemon oil and 1 drop mint oil.

Here, as in most other herb recipes, you can freely substitute if you don't have a particular item. For instance, all the lemon-scented herbs can be used interchangeably: lemon verbena, lemon balm, lemon thyme, lemon basil.

SACHET NO. 3

2 parts lemon balm
1 part rosemary
1 part lavender leaves

To 1 quart of mixture, add 2 tablespoons orris root preblended with 2 drops lemon oil and 1 drop lavender oil.

Note the use of lavender leaves in this recipe. Generally, "lavender" in a potpourri recipe means dried flower buds; but the leaves have aroma too, and are particularly appropriate in sachets, where the visual is not important.

SCENTED PILLOWS

At one time all young ladies (and some insomniac men) had a "sweet pillow," a small bed pillow filled with the herbs that were thought to calm the spirit and encourage a good night's sleep. Frankly, I don't know how they slept through all the crunching noise, but that tradition, with some modification, is worth reviving.

The modern version is smaller than a bed pillow but larger than a sachet. It is covered in pretty fabric that matches or harmonizes with the bed covering, to adorn the bed and send out a subtle fragrance during the day. Then, as she climbs into bed, milady can give it a squeeze, breathe in the fragrance, and have sweet dreams.

This small pillow is also a convenient size to carry with you for car trips or airline travel. It also makes a nice addition to the throw pillows on a sofa, releasing its aroma whenever someone leans against it. And it is a thoughtful gift for someone in the hospital.

To make a sweet pillow, stitch a fabric bag into a finished size about 6 by 12 inches, following the sachet directions above. Of course you can't wash this, so you may want to make an inner bag of plain muslin and an outer case of more decorative fabric.

SCENTED PILLOW NO. 1 (TRADITIONAL)

1 part hop flowers
1 part chamomile flowers
1 part mint

Both hops and chamomile have the reputation of soothing frazzled nerves. It is said that King George III of England was never without his hop pillow.

SCENTED PILLOW NO. 2 (MODERN)

1 part chamomile flowers
1 part lemon balm *or* lemon verbena
1 part sweet woodruff

To 1 quart of dried herbs add ½ cup oakmoss blended with 2 drops lemon verbena oil and 2 drops bergamot oil. You can also use orris root if you're sure no one is allergic.

HOT PAD

Here's a nice gift for your favorite cook (or yourself): a thick herb-filled pad to protect your dining table from hot dishes. When a hot

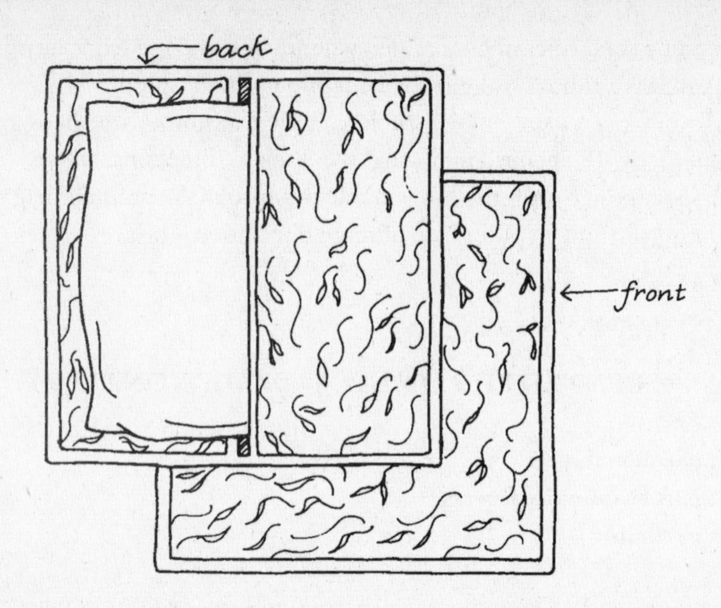

Hot pad made of thick fabric encases a plain cotton bag filled with dried herbs. When hot dishes are set on it, the aroma of the herbs is released.

casserole is set on it, the heat releases the aroma. Makes even ordinary macaroni and cheese taste special.

To make the pad, first stitch a bag about 8 inches square out of plain cotton (see sachet directions). Leave one edge open, fill with herb or spice mixture (suggestions below), then stitch closed.

Now cut two pieces of padding material just a bit larger. Quilt batting makes good padding, or an old mattress pad; if you have a bath towel that has seen better days, cut squares out of the still-thick sections. Assemble a sandwich: padding, spice insert, padding.

To finish the pad, make an outer bag of pretty fabric. If you like, you can make this outer bag openable, so that you can slip it off to launder it. Slide the "sandwich" inside, and you're done.

Here's an alternate method, even simpler: forget the inner bag and the padding; just make one bag out of thick quilting material. You won't be able to throw it in the laundry, but if you choose a dark pattern it will hide spills.

HOT PAD MIXTURE NO. 1

½ cup whole cloves
½ cup orange peel (tiny pieces)
1 cup sweet woodruff
1 teaspoon orris root
1 teaspoon ground cinnamon
2 drops cinnamon oil
2 drops sweet orange oil

First mix the orris root with the ground cinnamon and the oils; blend in other spices and herbs.

All the ingredients in a hot pad mixture should be quite small; you don't want any bumps that might create an uneven surface.

HOT PAD MIXTURE NO. 2

1 cup rosemary
1 cup thyme
1 cup sage
10 bay leaves
1 tablespoon orris root
5 drops rosemary oil

HOT PAD MIXTURE NO. 3

1 cup tarragon
1 cup mint
1 cup basil
¼ cup lemon peel, grated then dried
1 teaspoon coriander seed
1 teaspoon ground allspice
1 tablespoon orris root

Of course you can also use this same idea—and these same recipes—to make special potholders for yourself, for gifts, or for your church bazaar. Add a tablespoon or so of a spicy blend to your basic padded potholder, and every time you use it the heat will send the aroma into the kitchen.

Moth Bags

A special kind of sachets for your closet are bags filled with a mixture of herbs that repel moths. These really do work, and they are far more pleasant than commercial mothballs.

Make a sachet bag as usual, and use a very long string or ribbon so you'll be able to tie the bag onto clothes hangers or a hook on the closet wall.

These are the primary moth-repellent herbs:

southernwood
wormwood
tansy
santolina

As far as I know, the only source of these herbs is your own garden (or a friend's). But several other, more common herbs work almost as well; it seems that the moths just don't like the smell:

lavender	rosemary
thyme	mint
sage	marjoram
rue	costmary

Add a bit of whole cloves to your mixture, approximately 1 tablespoon per cup of dried herbs.

Another ingredient that we know works well as protection against moths is cedar, and there is an easy way to add it to moth bags. In pet stores you can find small bags of cedar chips; they are intended to be added to the dog's bed to keep fleas away, but they're a perfect size for moth potpourri. When you use cedar shavings, you don't need fixative; the cedar itself will absorb the oils.

MOTH SACHET NO. 1

2 cups dried lavender
1 cup dried southernwood
½ cup dried mint
½ cup dried sage
½ cup dried rosemary
4 tablespoons cloves
1 tablespoon orris root
10 drops rosemary oil

MOTH SACHET NO. 2

1 cup santolina
1 cup lavender
½ cup rosemary
2 tablespoons cloves
1 tablespoon orris root
10 drops clove oil (or half clove oil and half lavender)

MOTH SACHET NO. 3

2 cups cedar shavings
½ cup mint
¼ cup whole cloves
5 cinnamon sticks, crushed
5 drops clove oil
5 drops pine oil

MOTH SACHET NO. 4

2 cups tansy (flowers and leaves)
2 cups cedar shavings
1 cup thyme
2 cinnamon sticks, in small pieces
5 drops lemon oil
5 drops pine oil

Catnip Mouse

If you have catnip growing in your garden, dry some and make your cat ecstatically happy with this toy.

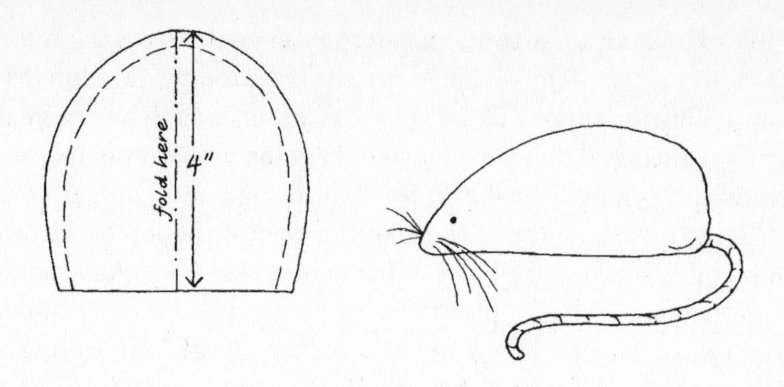

Catnip mouse is easily made from a small piece of heavy fabric

Cut a half-oval piece of fabric (see above); use something sturdy like denim. Sew together, leaving a small opening; turn seams inside, and stuff with a mixture of dried catnip and foam or fiberfill scraps, or catnip alone. Switch the hole closed.

Sew on a tail of braided yarn, whiskers of yarn or embroidery thread, and ears of felt. Paint eyes with a permanent marking pen. Add ribbon or a lace collar if your cat seems the type.

Pomanders

Pomanders are not new. Like much else in the world of herbs, this particular item that we enjoy today for its beauty and sweet smell was developed centuries ago for a very practical reason.

During the Middle Ages, when infectious diseases were commonplace, carrying a small metal ball with holes in the top was the primary defense against plague. Into the ball was put a mixture of the herbs thought to keep a person from contracting an illness, or cure him if he did. Because the balls were about the size of apples, they came to be known as *pomme d'ambre* (apple of ambergris, because that was the fixative used then).

Pomanders were hung in homes, and people wore one around their neck or waist when they had to go outside. Today this tradition remains: in some gift shops you can find decorated ceramic balls with holes, designed to be filled with potpourri.

But most of us know the pomander as that orange we stuck full of cloves when we were in kindergarten and proudly presented to Mom at Christmastime. These last for years, making the room smell like Christmas and doing a fine job of keeping moths away too. You already know how to make it: Take an orange and cover it completely with whole cloves. To make this part of the job easier, use something sharp to poke holes in the orange skin first, like a nail or a knitting needle. If you plan to tie a ribbon around the pomander, leave a small track for it; otherwise, cover the orange completely but don't jam the cloves into each other. The orange will shrink as it dries, drawing the cloves tighter.

This next step may be new to you: after the orange is completely covered with cloves, put it in a bowl filled with a mixture of ground spices and powdered orris root in equal proportions. The spices can be cinnamon, allspice, nutmeg, or cloves, or a combination. Roll the orange in the mixture until all surfaces are dusted. Leave it in the bowl, turning it every day, until the orange has hardened, which may take several weeks. Add a ribbon with a long loop for hanging. Once hardened, the orange will last forever. It keeps getting smaller, but it does not rot.

The orange is the fruit we usually associate with pomander, but apples, lemons, and limes can be used too.

Working with Fragrance Oils

It's a dead-level certainty that once you acquire a few bottles of oil, you will want more. They are not expensive, and the wide range of "flavors" is irresistible. It's also a good bet that the first year you make potpourri you will have oils left over. So when it comes time to make potpourri next year, you have a good collection to start with, plus whatever new ones you get.

Custom Blends

Use leftovers to advantage by combining custom blends. Here's a nifty suggestion for trying out combinations, from Grace Wakefield of Tom Thumb Workshops:

Cut a plain piece of cardboard into strips.

On one strip, put one drop each of two different oils, one on top of the other.

Smell, and then consider adding a third drop—either one of the original two or a third fragrance.

On the cardboard, write down what you did.

Try other combinations on other strips.

Turn the strips over so you can't see the notes, then walk outside for a few minutes.

With a fresh nose, sniff the cardboard strips; which ones do you like best? Ask others to give you their opinions too.

On the same cardboard strips, write down the results: "too sweet"; "bland"; "smells like blueberry jam"; "Dan's favorite"; and so on.

What to Do with Leftover Oils

- Put a few drops into the bathwater before you climb into the tub. You'll be bathing in a cloud of lavender, or roses, or whatever; it's very relaxing.

Sachet Tips

* To release the scent, give your sachet a squeeze.

* Whole spices work better in sachets than powdered forms, which tend to work their way through most fabrics. If very large, they can be broken into pieces.

* For the same reason, granular orris root works better than powdered; also, people who are allergic to powered orris can usually tolerate the granular form.

* Moth sachets need to be strong; use about twice as much fixative/spices/oils as you would with potpourri.

* For the doggie bed, make up sachets filled with dried *pennyroyal,* which has been used for centuries to repel fleas. Pennyroyal is also said to discourage mosquitoes. Use dried leaves of this mint relative; oil of pennyroyal is toxic.

* *Mint* is known for its ability to keep mice away; add either dried leaves or oil to sachet and moth bags if you have this problem.

- Make massage oil: a couple of drops of essential oil in ¼ cup of baby oil, almond oil, or even salad oil, if it has no scent of its own. Remember, don't put straight, undiluted essential oil on your skin; it causes rashes for some people.
- Apply oil to cardboard, cut into small pieces, and put them wherever you'd like to put a sachet but have room only for something really flat. For instance, along the sides of your lingerie drawers, or in your wallet. Or use a piece of your kids' construction paper and slide a colorful scented insert into a birthday card. (Blotter paper works even better than cardboard, but who has blotter paper lying around these days?)
- Make soap (see chapter 19).
- Take one box of baking soda, add 5 or 6 drops of oil (lemon or pine is nice, but whatever you like), and mix well. Sprinkle on your carpet, let sit for an hour, then vacuum up. Good-smelling room and clean carpets!
- If you've used up all your flowers, you can still make small sachets. Drop oil onto cotton balls, put several into a gingham bag, tie with ribbon.

- Add to lamp oil.
- Burned smell in your kitchen? Simmer a pan of water to which you have added a few drops of clove oil.
- If you make candles, add essential oil to the paraffin mixture for herb-scented candles.

CHAPTER EIGHTEEN

Wreaths and Floral Arrangements

In this chapter we look at some of the many ways herbs can be used to decorate the home. You can use many of the ideas in this chapter even if you don't have an herb garden, but if you do, you'll have more options and more room for creativity.

Drying Whole Flowers

All the projects in this chapter can be done completely with herbs. But every one of them will be enhanced with the addition of a few accent flowers.

Certain dried flowers can be purchased from mail-order sources (see Appendix) and from large craft shops. But if you have access to fresh flowers, you can dry your own, which is more fun. And while your mail-order selection is limited, you yourself can dry practically anything.

Let's look at two ways of drying flowers to maintain their color and shape.

Drying Agents

The standard technique used by florists and other craftspeople involves some kind of material that draws moisture out of flower petals. One such substance is called silica gel, which has been used commercially for years and recently has become available to individual crafters. It looks like white sand with little blue flecks in it.

Flowers dried in silica gel keep their color well and, if you are careful in your technique, their original shape too.

Here is a brief description of the process; for more detailed instructions, check the bibliography at the back of this book for books on crafts, and Roberta Moffitt's books on flower drying (see Appendix).

1. Fill a wide, shallow container that has a lid (like a shoebox) with about an inch of silica gel.

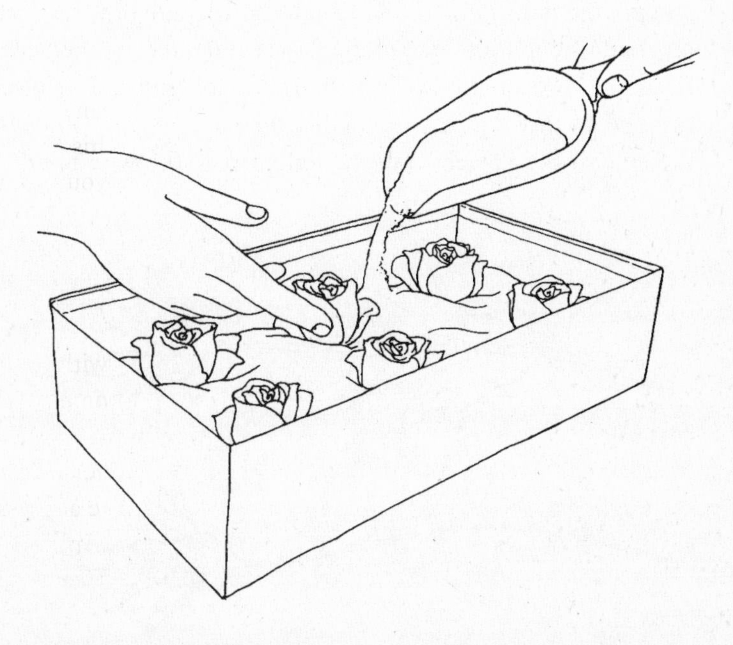

Drying whole flowers with a drying agent such as silica gel preserves their shape and color for special crafts projects.

2. Set the flowers into the silica gel; they should not be touching each other. Flat flowers like daisies and zinnias go face down. Others go face up; make a little dimple in the silica gel and set the base of the flower in it. Slide the fingers of one hand underneath the flower to support the petals in their natural position while with the other you carefully cover the flower with more silica gel, working it under and around the petals.

3. Cover the box. Check after two days. If not dry, re-cover the flower and leave for another day. Really dense flowers can take a week to dry thoroughly. It's counterproductive to leave longer than necessary.

4. If you plan to use the flowers in a vase, you will have to provide a "stem" of thin wire, which you can get in any craft shop or hardware store. And because you won't be able to add the wire after the flower is dry (too fragile), you'll have to do it before you put the flower into the silica gel. Cut a length of wire, push one end through the base of the flower and out the other side, bend the top completely over in a U shape and pull it back through so that you have a double thickness of wire through the core of the flower. Turn the long part of the wire to a 90-

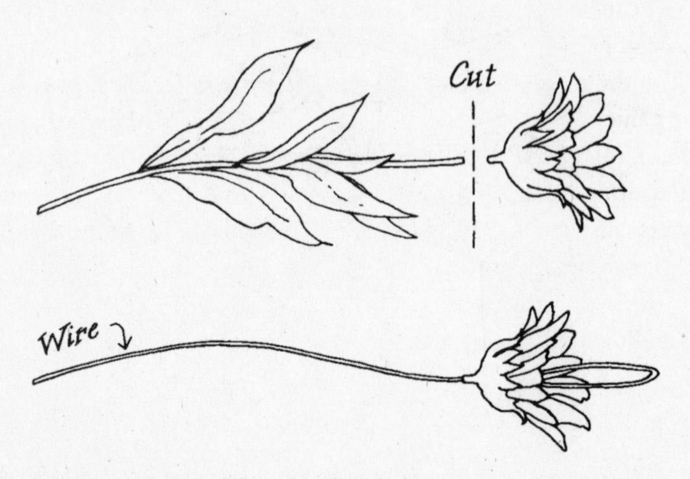

Wire stems must be added to the flower head before drying.

degree angle just below the flower head so the wire will lie flat in the box but the flower can sit face up.

Once you get the hang of working with this material, you will be amazed at what you can do. Tulips, lilies, irises, daffodils, large roses—all these can be preserved intact. Little flowers with a single layer of petals, like pansies or petunias, dry very easily.

Silica gel can be purchased from mail-order craft suppliers or from craft shops. It is not inexpensive, but it can be used over and over again indefinitely.

Long before silica gel was invented, people were drying flowers using ordinary sand. If you want to try this, you can buy small bags of sand in your local garden center, where it is sold as a soil amendment, or very large bags at the building supply store, where it is sold for making cement. The technique is exactly the same as described above for silica gel.

Even easier, you can use something you may very well already have around the house—kitty litter. The type with the very fine particles works best. This is the ideal way to get started, if you just want to experiment with drying a few flowers. Fair warning, though: it's so much fun you'll soon be doing more than a few.

You can speed up the process by combining a drying agent and a source of heat. The box with the silica gel (or sand or kitty litter) can go into the oven, where the flowers will dry in a matter of hours, or in the microwave, where they will dry in a matter of minutes. Note, though, that you can't put prewired flowers into the microwave.

Experimenting with drying flowers is the best way to learn. All flowers can be dried this way; some colors hold up better than others. In general terms:

- Yellows and oranges retain their natural color best
- Pink and blue flowers turn softer and mellower
- White flowers become a slightly dusty shade of ivory
- Red and purple turn darker, almost black

After your flowers are dry, take note of these tips:

- Put a few drops of white household glue down inside the base of large flowers with prominent individual petals such as tulips or lilies, whose shape would be ruined if one petal fell off.
- If you're not going to use them right away, store away from sunlight so the colors don't fade.
- Spray the flower all over with hair spray (yes, hair spray); it will make the color more intense.

Air Drying

Some kinds of flowers can be dried hanging in bundles, the same way you dry your herbs (see chapter 6). Roses can be dried this way, if they are still buds. The ones that work best are flower heads that are clusters of small blossoms, like salvia or delphiniums. If the flower heads are large—for example, hydrangea or yarrow—hang them individually so the full shape is maintained.

Most of these same flowers can also be dried standing upright, in a jar or vase. Make sure each one has lots of room; if they are pressed together, they'll dry with one flat side.

Air drying is the ideal way to handle *everlastings*—the flowers that dry naturally and keep their original color and shape all on their own. Baby's breath is an everlasting. Have you ever noticed when you get a bouquet from the florist that after all the other flowers have died the baby's breath looks just the same as on the first day? That's what "everlasting" means.

Another very popular everlasting, used quite a lot in florist arrangements, is statice, which comes in many shades of pink and purple, as well as white and yellow. Other everlastings are globe amaranth, German statice, and strawflowers. All of these can be grown in your garden, and if you get serious about dried arrangements you may want to order seeds for next year. They will dry right on the plant if you leave them there.

Crafts with Dried Herbs and Flowers

With a selection of herbs and dried flowers, you have the materials for an unlimited number of decorative items. Everything that can be done with fresh flowers can also be done with dried flowers and herbs—and then some.

In this section we look in detail at two sample projects: wreaths and tussy-mussies. Some of the many other possibilities include:

- Door swags
- Garlands for hanging over the bed, mantel, or doorway
- Miniature nosegays for individual table decorations
- Tiny wreaths for Christmas tree ornaments
- Flower-decorated straw hats
- And, of course, all types of floral arrangements

Wreaths

Dried wreaths are among the loveliest of all floral crafts. Using floral materials (flowers, herbs, pretty leaves or seed heads) that you dried yourself or ordered from a supplier, and your own good taste, you can create exquisite works of art to grace your front door. You can also plan to display your wreath on an interior wall, selecting colors that harmonize with your color scheme.

Grapevine Herb Wreath

The decorated grapevine wreath is quite popular in "country-look" decorating styles. A beautiful variation is an all-herb wreath. The basic idea is wonderfully simple: fresh herbs are entwined into the wreath in an attractive pattern and left to dry in place, right on the wreath.

Start by considering where the finished wreath will go; that will help you decide which herbs to use. For a kitchen wreath, you

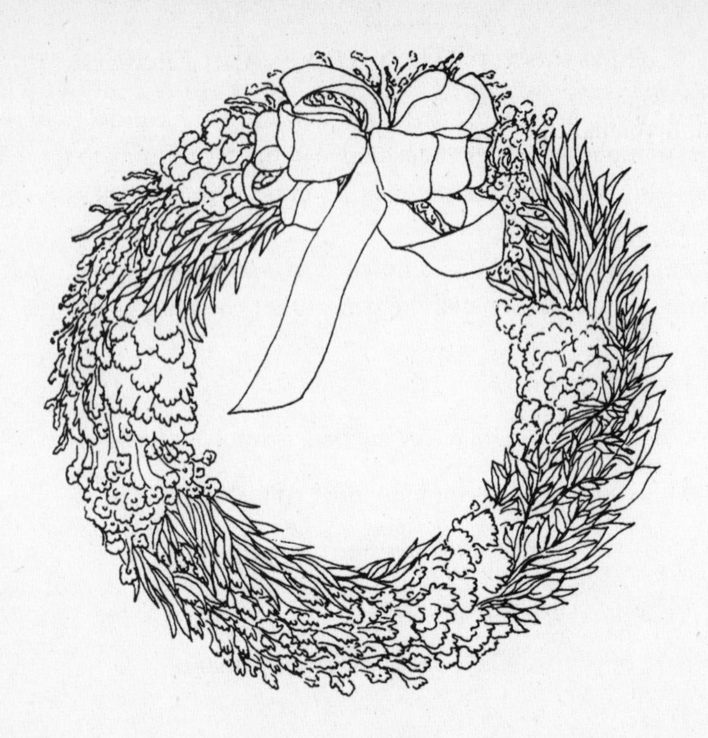

Herb wreaths can be made from any combination of dried herbs. All-herb wreaths have subtle colors; add ribbon or dried flowers for color accents.

would probably choose cooking herbs; for other parts of the house, the range of possibilities is unlimited.

On your work table, spread out piles of the various materials you will use. Then arrange them—still on the table—in a circular pattern until you get a combination you like. Think about color, texture, and fragrance. What colors go well together? For instance, try silvery santolina with dark green sage. Use contrasting textures: the soft feathery leaves of sweet cicely with the strong spiky stems of rosemary. And don't overlook the possibility of using just one plant: a big wreath of nothing but bay leaves, for example, is striking.

Once you are satisfied with your basic pattern, start putting the herbs into place. It's a simple process, but it needs a steady hand. First, strip off the bottommost leaves so you have bare stem for an inch or so. That stem goes down into the wreath; try to twist it around one grapevine branch to secure it. Then add another herb right next to the first one, overlapping slightly so it covers any bare stem. If you have planned one dark herb for the base layer (which is attractive), complete this layer all the way around and then go back and add the contrasting herbs on top.

You may choose to fill in the complete wreath with herbs, or to leave part of the bare grapevine showing. Wherever you put herbs, be generous. Remember that as they dry they will shrink somewhat. Also, if you're creating a kitchen masterpiece, the cook may want to snip off some of the herbs for the stewpot.

An all-herb wreath has a rustic, earthy look and feel that is especially appropriate in informal rooms; it would make a nice housewarming gift for a friend's mountain cabin. Of course there's nothing to prevent you from adding in dried flowers and seed stalks to your herb wreath. This increases the range of colors and textures available.

Over time, dried herbs lose their pungency and color. For this reason, you should think of herb wreaths as temporary decorations. After a couple of years, they can take on a dingy, dusty look. There's

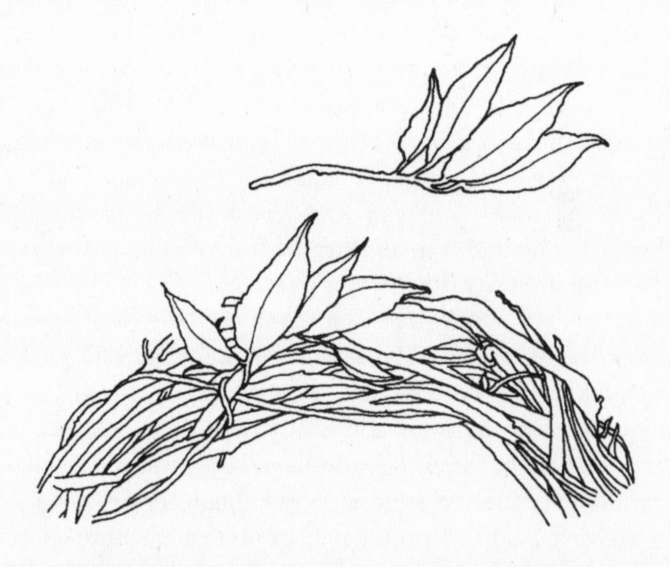

Grapevine herb wreaths start with fresh (not dried) herbs. Strip off lower leaves, wind herb stem around grapevine, and leave to dry in place.

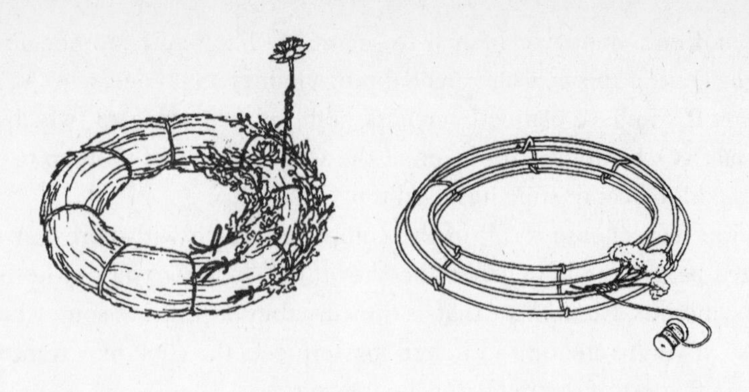

Wreath forms of wire or straw from a crafts shop can be used for herb wreaths. Tie dried herbs or flowers on with fine-gauge wire, or use toothpick-shaped florist pins.

no way to refresh the herbs themselves, so they should be discarded, but you can use the wreath form again.

Other Styles

The grapevine wreath is lovely, but it is not the only way to make an herb wreath. You can use other bases: dried straw forms, woven birch stems, metal wire frames. To use the wire frames, tie the plant materials on with very fine wire (from craft shops or hardware stores). To work with the straw bases, attach plants with florist pins purchased at the craft shop, or make your own pins by bending wire into a U shape or breaking paper clips into two U-shaped halves.

Still another approach: you can weave the herbs themselves together, using no frame at all. Wreaths that you make this way will be smaller than those made using a form.

Choose herbs with flexible stems, and cut long pieces. Strip off the lower leaves, leaving about half the stem bare. Overlap two stems together, staggered so that the leaves of one stem cover the bare part of the second stem, and gently twist them together so you have one long stem. Then add a third, and a fourth, and so on.

When your combined stem is long enough, bring it around to form a circle shape. Keep adding new stems to anchor the old twists, and soon it holds together by itself.

You may want to add a little security in the form of fine-gauge wire

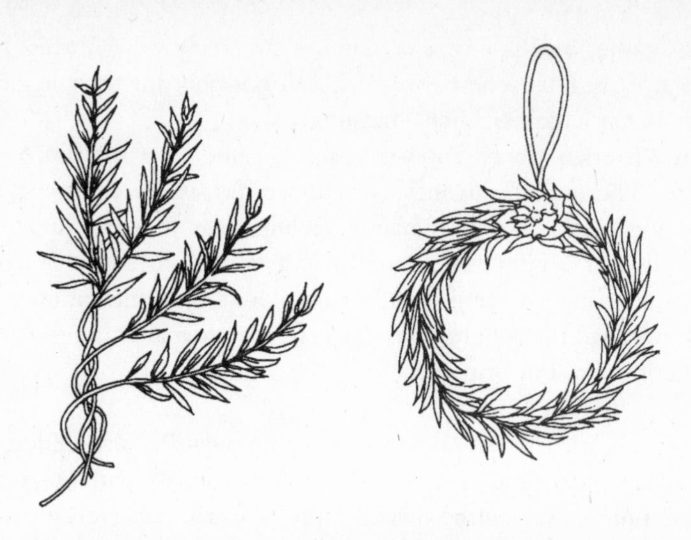

Twisted herb wreath uses only herbs, without extra support. Remove lower leaves, then twist stems together *(left)* until you have a long rope. Then bring the ends together to make a circle and fasten with wire or ribbon, leaving enough extra ribbon for a hanger.

or fishing line, but this is not really necessary. Once the stems dry, they will be permanently entangled. If you wish, you can decorate this small wreath with ribbon or glued-on flowers.

Tussy-Mussies

The name *tussy-mussy* is a modern spelling of a very early English term for "flower." It is used in this book to mean a small nosegay because the term is so closely identified with the world of herbs.

Originally these bouquets had a medical purpose. They were made from the herbs that had astringent qualities; sixteenth- and seventeenth-century Europeans carried them around and sniffed at them (hence the term *nosegay*) whenever they were in places where the air was unhealthy or simply stale-smelling.

Later another tradition was added: the symbolic language of herbs and flowers. This idea of using plants to communicate messages had been brought to Europe from the Middle East by the Crusaders centuries earlier, and now was applied to the nosegays. With this new aspect, tussy-mussy herbs were chosen not only for their hygienic value but also their symbolic meaning.

In Victorian times, tussy-mussies became very elaborate creations. The social conventions in those days were complex, and speaking frankly about romantic feelings was frowned upon. By carefully combining several herbs and flowers in a single tussy-mussy, a young man could send a very precise communication to his lady love, and thus get his message across while maintaining acceptable etiquette. For instance:

- A red carnation ("alas for my poor heart") surrounded by chamomile flowers and leaves ("I will be as patient as you require") and southernwood ("my love will persevere through your neglect").

She, of course, could respond in the same fashion, and did.

- Lavender ("I cannot trust your intentions") mixed with white daisies ("I am but an innocent child").

And this message in turn would be answered with another tussy-mussy:

- Rosemary ("I shall never forget you"), basil ("good wishes always"), and bay ("I change but in death").

We can only wonder whose job it was to replace all the flowers and herbs that got used up in the name of true love.

In those days young men and women had to be on their toes, for some plants had several meanings. Chamomile could be interpreted more than one way. Basil was used to symbolize both love and hatred; tansy meant either "our love is immortal" or "I declare war against you." Then as now, communication about matters of the heart was fraught with potential for misunderstanding.

Today, most people construct tussy-mussies with an eye toward how the herbs and flowers look together rather than what they mean. But it's still fun to work a message into your bouquet. Here, for example, is a flower and herbal tussy-mussy for Mother's Day:

> We thank you (agrimony for gratitude) for the many things you do (thyme for activity), for the festive meals (parsley for festivity) and all the things you taught us (cherry leaves for education). Your love (rose for love) is a constant (bluebells for constancy) inspiration (angelica means inspiration). We will remember you (rosemary for remembrance) in our thoughts (pansies mean thinking of you).
>
> —BARBARA REMINGTON, DUTCH MILL HERB FARM

For a very memorable gift, you might make a special tussy-mussy for these occasions:

- happy birthday
- best wishes for the bride and groom
- welcome to a new baby
- get-well wishes
- congratulations on a promotion

Make up a special card, explaining the symbolism of all the ingredients.

As a practical matter, you have to work with whatever flowers and herbs you have. And not every "message" is in bloom at the same time. But by making use of dried flowers and herbs—and by interpreting the language of flowers broadly, just as the Victorians did—you can send your sentiments in this sweet, old-fashioned way.

How to Make a Tussy-Mussy

A tussy-mussy can be made from fresh materials or dried, or a combination of the two. If you make your tussy-mussy from dried herbs and flowers, you don't have to worry about it wilting, nor are you limited to whatever is blooming at the time. You can concentrate on your message and the visual blend of ingredients.

The standard, classic design has one prominent flower in the center, surrounded by one or more circles of smaller flowers intermixed with foliage accents, all on a background bed of greenery. To make the tussy-mussy, follow these steps:

1. Gather your materials and arrange them loosely on the work surface until you are pleased with the combinations.

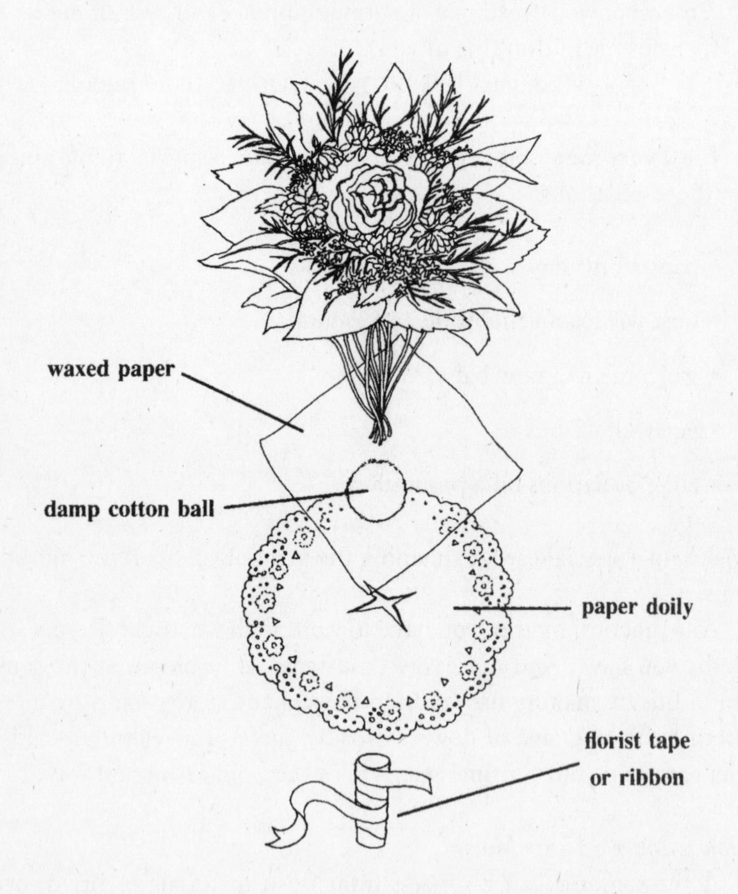

A tussy-mussy is an old-fashioned nosegay of flowers and herbs, rich with meaning. A damp cotton ball keeps fresh herbs from wilting; a square of waxed paper keeps dampness away from the paper doily.

2. Use a small glass or a narrow-necked vase to hold the materials as you work.

3. Put enough of your background leaves in the vase to create a circle. Insert the main, central flower. Fill in around it with the smaller flowers, variegated leaves, and special accents. Usually, the center is higher than the outer edges.

4. Holding the entire creation carefully in one hand, tie the stems together so that the shape is maintained.

5. At this point you can wrap the stems together into one combined stem, using stretchy green florist tape. Or you can add ribbon and a frilly collar made from a paper doily, for an even more romantic look.

6. To add the doily, first cut a large X in its center; this is easier if you choose a kind that has a solid center. Bend the four points backward and slide the bundled stems through. Now wrap the stems with ribbon or florist's tape, and add the prettiest ribbon you can find.

To work with fresh materials, you would follow these same steps but make some provision for keeping the stems damp so your gift doesn't wilt too soon. One way to do that is to add a layer of damp sphagnum moss at the base of the bouquet; to keep the doily from getting soggy, add an inner liner made of waxed paper or plastic wrap. As an alternative, some people run the bundled stems through a wet cotton ball (see drawing).

Another way to keep fresh flowers fresh is to purchase a special nosegay holder at craft shops, the type florists use for bridesmaids' bouquets. These holders come in two parts: a lace collar made of either fabric or plastic, and a round center filled with florist foam. The foam holds several times its own weight in water, and will keep flowers fresh for several days.

The Symbolic Language of Flowers and Herbs

Agrimony	Thankfulness
Angelica	Inspiration
Anise	Something is about to change
Basil	Hatred; love; good wishes
Bay leaf	I change but in death; I admire you but cannot love you
Borage	Courage; bluntness; please don't persist, you embarrass me
Buttercup	Childish behavior
Calendula	Happiness; joy; grief; cruelty in love
Caraway	Faithfulness; someone has betrayed our secret
Red carnation	Alas for my heart
Striped carnation	Refusal
Chamomile	Humility; patience; may your wishes come true; energy in adversity; don't despair; I admire your courage
Chervil	Sincerity
Chives	Why are you crying?
Coriander	Hidden merit; your closeness is welcome
Daisy	Innocence
Dandelion	Oracle

Fennel	Praiseworthy; heroic; I do not believe your promises; flattery
Ferns	Sincerity
Forget-me-not	True love; don't forget me
Garlic	Go away, you evil one
Nutmeg geranium	An unexpected meeting
Rose geranium	Preference
Globe amaranth	Unfading love
Honeysuckle	Generosity; devotion; bonds of love
Hops	Injustice
Hyssop	Cleanliness; sacrifice
Iris	Message
Ivy	Fidelity
Jonquil	Desiring a return of affection
Lavender	Distrust; I cannot understand you; silence; cleanliness; devotion; luck
Lemon balm	Sympathy
Lilac	Innocence; first stirrings of young love
Marjoram	Happiness; blushing innocence; charm against witchcraft
Mint	Love; passion; humble virtue; find someone your own age; you are overreacting about a small thing
Nasturtium	Patriotism

Pansy	Happy thoughts; thinking of you
Parsley	Festivity; the lady of the house is in charge here
Pennyroyal	Go away
Peppermint	Warm feelings
Petunia	Never despair
Rose	Love
Cabbage rose	Ambassador of love
Rose de la France	Meet me by moonlight
Yellow rose	Jealousy
White rose	I am worthy of you
Red and white roses together	Unity
Damask rose	Brilliant complexion
Rosebud	Pure; innocent of love; I confess my love
Rosemary	Remembrance
Rue	Disdain; sorrow; repentance; virtue
Sage	Domestic virtue; long life; wisdom; good health; esteem; I would suffer anything for your love
Salvia (blue)	I think of you
Savory	The truth is bitter
Sorrel	Affection
Southernwood	Jest; perseverance; constancy
Spearmint	Warm sentiments

Sweet woodruff	Be cheerful, rejoice
Tansy	Immortality; I declare war against you
Tarragon	Unselfish sharing
Thyme	Activity; courage; strength; happiness
Tulip	Declaration of love
Violet	Modesty; faithfulness
Wisteria	I cling to you
Wormwood	Bitterness; absence; displeasure
Yarrow	War
Zinnia	Thinking of one who is absent

CHAPTER NINETEEN

Bath and Personal Products

Want to try an experiment? Go into your bathroom or wherever you keep shampoos, body lotions, that sort of thing, close your eyes, and pick one at random. Then read the list of ingredients. When I tried it, here's what I got:

> Water, stearalkonium chloride, monosodium citrate, ceteth-2, citric acid, dimethyl stearamine, stearyl alcohol, phenoxyethanol, glyceryl stearate, fragrance, methylparaben, panthenol, fd&c yellow no. 6, fd&c blue no. 1, d&c red no. 19.

What is it? Conditioner, for your hair. It's a fairly well known brand, made by a company whose name is a household word. The only ingredient I'm confident I understand is the first one—water.

Not that there's anything wrong with any of those other ingredients. In fact unless you decide to drink them nothing in any of those jars in your bathroom will cause you harm; they've all been tested and approved by the federal government. But wouldn't it be nice, at least once in a while, to use a product that had ingredients you could pronounce?

That's just one of the many reasons that people find homemade bath and beauty preparations so appealing: they know what's in them.

Another reason, important to many, is the desire to refrain from using products whose manufacturers relied on animal testing. And many people who are allergic to certain commercial ingredients can avoid a reaction by using their own products that avoid those ingredients.

In earlier centuries, beauty and personal care products were made from available household materials and garden herbs, taking advantage of the natural qualities in certain plants. Some herbs are astringent. Some have antiseptic qualities. Some will brighten hair color. Others will improve skin problems.

All these beneficial effects of herbs have been scientifically verified. Today's products are, in some respects, a laboratory duplication of those old formulas. In cosmetics, as in medicine, we have developed synthetic versions of old herbal remedies, and we smugly call them "modern."

So why not use the original versions? Maybe you don't want to throw away all your drugstore conveniences—I certainly don't—but you will find much pleasure in occasionally using these old-fashioned herbal products. They are gentle on the body and on the soul.

THE COSMETICS FACTORY AT YOUR DOORSTEP

Basil	Hair rinse
Bergamot	Hair rinse
Borage	Skin softener
Calendula	Hair lightener; skin healer (flowers)
Chamomile	Skin softener; hair lightener; antiseptic; mild antiseptic (flowers)
Chervil	Skin cleanser

Comfrey	Smooths rough or abraded skin; conditions dry hair
Costmary	Hair rinse
Fennel	Skin softener (leaves)
Feverfew	Skin cream
Garlic	Dandruff control
Hyssop	Skin cream
Lavender	Astringent for skin
Lemon balm	Skin astringent
Lemon verbena	Skin freshener
Marjoram	Antiseptic; encourages hair growth
Marsh mallow	Heals rough skin
Mint	Astringent; antiseptic
Parsley	Skin whitener; hair rinse; dandruff control
Rosemary	Hair care: makes hair glossy, adds body, darkens color, prevents dandruff
Sage	Darkens and conditions hair; astringent
Salad burnet	Skin softener
Southernwood	Helps hair grow, brightens hair, prevents dandruff
Thyme	Deodorant
Yarrow	Astringent for oily skin

What About Allergies?

One of the reasons people like herbal products is they tend to contain fewer of the chemical ingredients that create allergic reactions.

And if you make your own things, and already know what you're allergic to, you can simply leave out the problem ingredients.

But we can't say across the board that herbs are "safe" in this respect, for no doubt someone, somewhere, is allergic. What we can say is that people who use products with natural ingredients seem to have less trouble with allergic reactions.

If you're thinking of making some of these products, and especially if you tend to have sensitive skin, it's a good idea to check for reactions. Make up a small batch and put a couple of drops on the gauze pad of a bandage; wear it on your inner arm for a day. (Be careful with essential oils. They are so concentrated that they can easily irritate *anyone's* skin; dilute them in water before doing the test.)

Herbal Baths

There is no better cure for the daily stresses of a complicated life than a long soak in a hot tub. The restorative value of being immersed in hot water is so well documented that modern science has given it a name: *hydrotherapy.* But even better than plain water is a leisurely soak in an herbal bath.

It is pure heaven to step into a bath scented with lavender. (Or mint, lemon verbena, rosemary, or any other personal favorite.) For a short time the whole room is turned into a magical cloud of fragrance, and your only task is to enjoy it. That fragrance alone is worth the price of admission, but that is not the only benefit.

Which Herbs to Use

We know that certain herbs have beneficial effects on the body, and when they are added to your bathwater you get the double effect of the healing herb and the soothing warm water. Here is a summary of the helpful effects you can create.

Soothing and Relaxing

- Catnip
- Chamomile
- Hops
- Hyssop
- Marsh mallow

Invigorating (Stimulates Blood Circulation)

Basil	Mint
Bay	Rosemary
Fennel	Sage
Lavender	Tansy
Lemon balm	Thyme

Good for Rough or Damaged Skin

Calendula
Comfrey
Spearmint
Yarrow

For Sore Muscles

Bay
Oregano
Sage

Astringents (Tighten Skin Pores)

Bay	Sage
Comfrey	Salad burnet
Nasturtium (flowers)	Southernwood
Rosemary	Yarrow (flowers)

And, of course, combinations of herbs can be individually blended for bath therapy. You can experiment to your heart's content, for you're in no danger of hurting yourself with an herb by merely soaking in it (assuming, of course, that you've already checked for an allergic reaction).

To make your herbal bath—in fact, for all the products in this chapter—you can use fresh herbs from your garden, or dried herbs that you dried yourself or purchased in bulk from a mail-order supplier (see Appendix).

HERBAL BATH NO. 1

1 part lavender
1 part rosemary
1 part sage

HERBAL BATH NO. 2

1 part peppermint
1 part sage
1 part rosemary
1 part thyme
2 parts chamomile flowers

HERBAL BATH NO. 3

1 cup lavender
1 cup uncooked oatmeal
½ cup dried orange peel
½ cup rosemary
10 bay leaves, broken

Preparing an Herbal Bath

How do you get the herbs into the bathwater? Well, you could just throw a handful in while the water's running. That would work fine as far as getting the qualities of the herb into the water, but then you'd have all those little green flecks all over your body when you get out.

There are easier ways.

Herbal Water. The basic idea here is to make a strong "tea" of the herb and then add some to the bathwater. This is technically called an *infusion,* but you make it just like tea: boil water, pour it over the herbs, let it steep, then strain.

You can use either fresh or dried herbs; if fresh, chop the herbs first. Use a lot of herbs, much more than for tea, because it is going to be diluted in the bathtub. General proportions are 3 to 4 tablespoons of dried herb per cup of water; twice that much for fresh. Steep for fifteen minutes to an hour; the longer you let it steep, the stronger concentration you will have.

If you happen to be using an herb for which the active part is the root (as in ginger) or seeds (as in fennel), the process is a little different. Here you make what is known as a *decoction.* Chop or crush the material, place in a pan of cold water, bring to a boil, simmer for about half an hour, then strain.

Use about one cup of herbal water in your bath. The rest will keep in the refrigerator for a few days; if you leave it too long, you'll know when it has gone bad: it smells awful.

Bath Vinegar. Vinegar has the ability to draw the essential oils out of an herb. So, after an herb is left to soak in vinegar for a day or so, all the good stuff that was originally in the herb is now in the vinegar, and the herbs are a lifeless blob that's ready for the compost pile. The vinegar smell is now an undertone to the aroma of the herb you used.

And did you know that vinegar is good for your skin? It cleanses the pores and restores the natural acid balance that healthy skin has. So you get double benefit: the vinegar softens your skin, the herbs do their magic.

There is one more benefit, less tangible but no less valuable. If you use flowers of herbs, the vinegar draws out the color as well as the oils, so the finished product is beautiful to look at. A particular favorite of mine is lavender vinegar. The purple blossoms produce a rich magenta vinegar that glistens in the sunshine.

Because vinegar itself is a preservative, your herbal vinegars do not have to be stored in the refrigerator. To enjoy the visual treat, put your vinegar in a glass jar or bottle and keep it on the windowsill. A salad cruet, the kind with a stopper, is both pretty and easy to pour from. Another possibility is to keep it in a narrow-necked vase. Because the top is open, the scent will lightly fill the room all the time.

To make the vinegar from fresh herbs, start with a glass jar of any size. Fill it with the herbs, which you have chopped or crushed slightly. Then pour in enough white vinegar to cover the herbs, and let it sit overnight or longer; a longer time will make a stronger solution. Strain out the herbs, and strain again through a coffee filter to remove any little flecks. Store in your prettiest bottle.

This is stronger than herb-flavored vinegar for salads, because it will be diluted by the bathwater. Add about half a cup to a tubful. This vinegar can also be used to make a wonderful rinse for your hair; see Hair Care section below.

Essential Oils. The easiest way to create an herbal bath is to add a few drops of essential oil or fragrance oil to the tub. If you have been making potpourri (see chapter 16), you probably have some oil left over. Even if you have not, you may want to buy a bottle or two just for the bath; they are relatively inexpensive, and nothing could be simpler: while the tub is filling, add a few drops of oil.

Bath Bags. A bath bag is a sachet—a bundle of herbs in a small fabric bag—that is added to the bathtub for a few minutes, long enough for the herbs to steep into the water. (See chapter 17 for general instructions on making sachets.) There are two ways to use it: throw the bag into the tub after it has filled, or tie the bag to the faucet so that it hangs down and the water runs through it. In either case, the bags can be reused several times.

Bath sachets should be made of colorfast fabric and tied with plain string instead of ribbon, so the color doesn't leach into the water.

A nice way to take full advantage of these sachets is to store several in a basket on the counter. That way you can enjoy their subtle fragrance in between bath times. This is especially nice for a guest bathroom; welcome your travel-weary visitors with a soothing herbal bath.

Shortcuts

- If you don't sew, or don't want to, you can buy small muslin drawstring bags to use for your bath bags. Several mail-order sources carry them; check listings in the Appendix for Meadowbrook, Dabney Herbs, Rasland Farms, Sandy Mush Herb Nursery, and Tom Thumb Workshop.

- Another ready-made option is the small porous bags intended for use with herbal teas. You fill them with your own dried tea herbs and seal closed with an iron. There's no reason you can't use them to make small bath bags. In the Appendix, check Nichols Garden Nursery, Dabney Herbs, and Harvest Health.

- Easier still: use a real tea bag from the grocery store—herbal tea, that is. Chamomile, for instance, is a wonderful herb for baths, and commercial chamomile tea is just plain chamomile flowers. This is a very good way to sample the experience of an herbal bath: just throw a couple of tea bags into the tub.

- One final shortcut: a metal tea ball filled with herbs can dangle from the faucet or be tossed into the tub for a few minutes. The larger size, intended to make a pitcherful of tea, works better than the individual teacup size.

Hair Care

Using herbal products for beautiful, shiny hair is not a new idea. Women in ancient Rome used herbs to give their hair body and luster, and to heighten its color. You can too—either by purchasing those fancy herbal shampoos in the store or by making your own version.

Herbs for Hair Care

To lighten the color
- Calendula
- Chamomile

To darken the color
- Sage

To condition dry hair
- Comfrey
- Marsh mallow
- Parsley
- Sage

To add shine and body
- Calendula
- Nasturtium
- Parsley
- Rosemary
- Sage
- Southernwood

To make hair grow faster
- Catnip
- Marjoram
- Nasturtium leaves
- Rosemary

To condition oily hair
- Calendula
- Lavender
- Lemon balm
- Mint
- Rosemary
- Southernwood
- Yarrow

To help prevent dandruff
- Chamomile
- Parsley
- Rosemary
- Southernwood

To make hair softer
- Chamomile

You can use fresh or dried herbs, and you can use them in either shampoo or rinses, or both. You will get the specific benefits of the herbs, plus your hair will smell absolutely wonderful.

Herbal Shampoo

Start with a very mild shampoo, unscented if you can find it. Baby shampoo works well. Pour a little bit into a cup, enough for one shampoo, and then add the herb or herbs of your choice, either in the form of a strong herbal water or an essential oil.

- Make a small amount of very strong herbal water, following the directions in the section on herbal baths (page 393). Add about 2 tablespoons to the shampoo.

Or:

- Add 3–4 drops of essential oil to shampoo; blend very thoroughly before using.

The main herb for blonds is chamomile; for brunettes, sage and rosemary.

Herbal Hair Rinse

After you shampoo and rinse out all the soap, treat yourself and your hair to an herbal rinse. You can enrich the color, add shine and softness, soothe the scalp, and give your hair a wonderful fresh scent.

To make the rinse, first choose the herb or herbs for your hair color and condition.

For light hair	Chamomile
For dark hair	Sage, or rosemary, or both
For hair or scalp problems	Add other herbs from the list in this chapter (page 397).

Then, using any of the three methods below, add the herbs to warm water. Pour through your hair. If it's convenient, catch the rinse in a bowl or basin and pour through a second or third time.

To 1 pint of water add:

- 5–6 drops essential oil

  Or
- ½ cup herbal bath vinegar

  Or
- ½ cup strong herbal water

Directions for bath vinegar and herbal water are in the Herbal Baths section of this chapter (page 394). Hair rinse made from herbal vinegar has extra benefits: the vinegar helps correct the natural acid balance of the scalp, controls dandruff, and will get rid of any soap film.

If you want to try a hair rinse, you already have all the ingredients in your kitchen.

HERBAL RINSE FOR LIGHT HAIR

1 cup white vinegar
1 tea bag of chamomile tea
Grated peel of one lemon

Combine the tea with vinegar and lemon peel. Heat to a simmer, but do not boil. Remove from heat and let steep for 20 minutes. Strain.

To use: mix ½ cup of vinegar rinse with 2 cups water. Pour through hair; catch into a basin and pour again.

HERBAL RINSE FOR DARK HAIR

1 cup cider vinegar
1 tablespoon dried sage
1 teaspoon dried rosemary

Heat till simmering, but do not boil. Remove from heat and let steep 20 minutes. Strain.

To use: mix ½ cup vinegar rinse with 2 cups water; pour through hair as final rinse.

Skin Care

There is almost no end to the variety of herbal skin care products you can make. In the rest of this chapter we will look at just a few.

Herbs for Skin Care

For all skin types
- Fennel
- Lavender
- Rosemary

For dry skin
- Borage
- Chamomile
- Comfrey
- Marsh mallow
- Parsley

For oily skin
- Lavender
- Lemon balm
- Mint
- Rosemary
- Sage
- Salad burnet
- Yarrow

For rough or irritated skin
- Borage
- Calendula
- Chamomile
- Comfrey
- Marsh mallow
- Parsley

Herbal Soap

The basic procedure involves melting down a bar of soap and adding chopped herbs or essential oil.

Start with the purest soap you can find: glycerine soap or castile soap from the drugstore, if you can find it, plain white soap like Ivory if you can't. You want something with the least amount of scents or extra ingredients.

Then decide which herbs you want to add—either for their beneficial effect on the skin, or for their fragrance, or both. You can add the herbs themselves, either fresh or dried, chopped up very fine; or essential oils; or a combination of the two forms. The herbs give an added texture to the soap that is helpful for removing dry skin cells, but this is purely a matter of personal choice.

Craft stores sell special soap molds in fancy shapes, which are fun if you really get into soap making. But if you just want to try it, you can use any small heatproof container. Pour the prepared soap into soap molds or containers that you have lightly coated with vegetable oil. Set aside to cool and harden. The finished product will be a little softer than the soap you started with.

By the way, if you use Ivory soap all the time, you end up with lots of little pieces that are too small to use but too good to throw away. This is a good way to use them up.

First, two general recipes; then a sampling of special combinations.

HERBAL SOAP NO. 1 (SMOOTH TEXTURE)

1 bar soap, in small pieces
¼ cup herbal water (see page 394)
3–4 drops essential oil

Melt soap with herbal water in top of double boiler. Stir in essential oil. Pour into oiled containers.

HERBAL SOAP NO. 2 (ROUGH TEXTURE)

½ cup water
3 tablespoons dried herb, crumbled fine
1 bar soap, cut into small pieces

In top of double boiler, heat water to simmering and add herb; remove from heat and let steep 15 minutes. Return to heat, add soap, and melt. Pour into oiled containers.

OATMEAL HERB SOAP

This soap is good for acne and other similar skin problems. The rough texture helps rub off the dead skin cells; the lemon balm and lavender add astringency for oily skin.

¼ cup dried lemon balm
1 cup water
1 bar soap, in small pieces
½ cup rolled oats, uncooked
4 drops essential lavender oil

Crumble the lemon balm leaves through your hands into the water in top of double boiler. Bring to simmer and let steep about 10 minutes. Add soap, heat till melted. Remove from heat; stir in oatmeal and essential oil till well blended. Pour into oiled containers.

VARIATIONS

Substitute oils of other astringent herbs such as rosemary or sage.

LEMON LAVENDER SOAP

2 tablespoons dried lavender flowers
Grated rind of one lemon
½ cup water
1 bar soap
2 drops lemon or lime oil
2 drops lavender oil

Run the lavender and lemon rind through a blender to pulverize them; this is easier if you first allow the rind to dry partially. In top of double boiler, bring water to simmer and add the lavender/lemon mixture. Add the soap, heat till melted. Remove from heat and mix in the oils. Pour into oiled containers.

Moisturizers

All those fancy moisturizing creams and lotions at the cosmetic counter, in the elegant bottles with the elegant prices, are essentially alike. They have some kind of waxy substance as a base, oils for the creamy texture, and water; cosmetics manufacturers add various scents (usually synthetic), coloring agents, and other mysterious polysyllabic ingredients.

Homemade facial creams use a base of either beeswax or paraffin, an oil such as safflower, and an infusion of one or more herbs. Lotions, with their more liquid texture, have a foundation of either lanolin or glycerine. To make an herbal preparation, first choose the herbs, based on your skin condition, and make a strong infusion (like making herb tea; see Herbal Water on page 394).

You might enjoy experimenting with face creams and lotions. Two generic recipes are suggested below. Lanolin and glycerine can be purchased from your pharmacist. Buy paraffin at the grocery store, where the canning supplies are. Beeswax is at some craft shops and a few mail-order suppliers (check Herbally Yours, Penn Herb Company, and Dabney Herbs in the Appendix).

For dry skin: calendula, chamomile, comfrey, parsley

For oily skin: lavender, mint, sage, rosemary, yarrow

To soften skin: chamomile, salad burnet, fennel

MOISTURIZING CREAM

½ ounce beeswax or paraffin
½ cup mild vegetable oil
3 tablespoons herbal water (see page 394)

Heat the wax and the vegetable oil together in top of a double boiler. Separately, heat the herbal water (microwave works well for this). Stir the two hot liquids together. Pour into jar or other wide-mouthed container and cool.

MOISTURIZING LOTION

2 parts herbal water (see page 394)
1 part lanolin or glycerine

Mix thoroughly.

An even simpler way to experiment with using herbs for skin care is this quick version of herbal face cream:

Shortcut: To half a cup of unscented cold cream, add 1 tablespoon of herbal water.

Skin Freshener/After-Shave

Another group of skin care products uses an alcohol-herb base. Alcohol has the effect of tightening pores and removing oil from the skin, and the herbs contribute their special properties.

When herbs are steeped in alcohol, the qualities of the herb are dissolved out of the leaves. The process is called *extraction*, and the resulting liquid is technically known as a *tincture*. Many herbal medications are alcohol extractions, and in fact the term *tincture* usually carries the sense that it is some kind of medicine. But *any* alcohol extraction is a tincture. In fact, that's what perfumes and colognes are: blends of flowers, herbs, and spices distilled into fragrant alcohol.

The tincture base can be made into toilet water, after-shave lotion, or any kind of skin freshener. Water is added to dilute the mixture to the appropriate strength, and sometimes essential oils are added for extra fragrance. Distilled water is preferred to tap water, which often has impurities; distilled water can be purchased at most supermarkets and drugstores.

To make any of these skin fresheners, first make the tincture. Pure grain alcohol, which is colorless and odorless, is best, if you can find it. If you can't, ordinary vodka works fine too. Don't use rubbing alcohol for this, because its medicinal smell will fight the fragrance you're trying to achieve.

Decide what herbs you want to use, or try some of the recipes below. Fill a glass jar with the herbs, add alcohol to cover, and let sit for several weeks. Strain out the herbs; filter a second time if needed. Once you have the tincture, you can:

- Add distilled water for a lightly scented floral water. These waters were used as a light perfume in our grandmothers' day, and they are just as lovely today. Also, keep them in an open bottle to refresh stale-smelling rooms.
- Add a few drops of glycerine to make a smooth, lotion-textured freshener for dry skin.
- Add essential oils for your own personal cologne.
- Add spices and oils of astringent herbs for after-shave.

SKIN FRESHENER

An all-purpose skin toner for men or women

1 part sage
1 part lavender
1 part lemon balm
Alcohol or vodka

Fill glass jar with herbs. Cover with alcohol. Let stand for two weeks or more, then strain.

LAVENDER WATER

A fragrant floral water

Fresh or dried lavender flowers
Alcohol or vodka
Distilled water

Fill a glass jar with lavender; pack down tight. Cover with alcohol, let stand 2 to 3 weeks, then strain. Dilute with distilled water, approximately half and half.

VARIATIONS

Any fragrant flowers or combination of flowers and herbs can be used to make floral water.

Shortcut: For floral water in any fragrance, add essential oils to alcohol; dilute with distilled water as needed.

AFTER-SHAVE LOTION

1 cup rosemary
1 cup sage
½ cup peppermint
10 bay leaves, broken
1 tablespoon whole cloves, crushed lightly
Alcohol
Distilled water
Glycerine (optional)

Put herbs and spices into glass jar, cover with alcohol. Let stand 2 to 3 weeks, then strain. Dilute with distilled water to desired strength. For dry skin, add 1 teaspoon of glycerine per cup of lotion.

Rubbing Lotion

Athletes know about the wonderful restorative effects of an alcohol rubdown; you can make it even more special by adding aromatic herbs. The medicinal smell is softened by the sweet, clean scent of your favorite herb. Use this lotion after exercising, after a bath, or any time you feel hot and sweaty.

To make the lotion, put a handful of either fresh or dried herbs into a clean glass jar. Then add a cup of plain rubbing alcohol from the drugstore. Leave for about two weeks (longer wouldn't hurt), shaking the jar once in a while. Strain off the herbs and pour alcohol into a clean bottle.

You can choose herbs for their healing powers or their fragrance, or both. Here are a few suggestions; also see the list of skin-care herbs on page 400.

Calendula
Chamomile
Comfrey
Scented geraniums
Lavender
Lemon verbena
Marjoram
Mint
Rosemary
Thyme

You can, of course, mix several herbs together. You could also mix comparable essential oils, or use a combination of oils and dried herbs. To give you an idea of the range of possibilities, here are two old recipes.

RUBBING LOTION NO. 1

½ cup dried lemon balm
¼ cup lemon peel
1 teaspoon ground nutmeg
1 teaspoon ground cinnamon
1 teaspoon ground cloves
2 cups (16 ounces) rubbing alcohol

Mix all the herbs and spices in a blender, then add to the alcohol. Let stand for a week, shaking the jar occasionally. Strain out herbs; to remove all sediment from the ground spices, you may want to run through a coffee filter after straining. Store in a clean bottle.

RUBBING LOTION NO. 2

2 parts dried sage
2 parts dried rosemary
2 parts dried lemon balm
2 parts peppermint (*or* any mint)
1 part lavender
1 part fennel seed
Rubbing alcohol

Mix all herbs together in a large bowl. Fill a clean glass jar with the mixture, then add rubbing alcohol to cover. Leave in jar for two weeks; then strain and filter.

Shortcut: Add a few drops of essential oil to a bottle of rubbing alcohol.

Massage Oil

In recent years a new aspect of herbal medicine has become popular. *Aromatherapy* is a way of administering the healing qualities of certain herbs through massage. The theory is that with the massaging, the essential oils work their way through the skin and into the bloodstream, spreading their beneficial qualities throughout the body. Aromatherapy practitioners carefully blend massage oils with essential oils of herbs selected for specific conditions: muscle aches, colds, arthritis, and so on.

Whether or not you accept the theory, you will certainly enjoy a massage with oil scented with your favorite herbal fragrance. Nothing could be simpler: any mild vegetable oil can be turned into massage oil, simply by adding the essential oils of your choice.

Start with an oil that doesn't have a strong scent of its own; massage therapists prefer almond oil, but you can also use others such as corn, safflower, canola, or sunflower. Add any essential oil or combination of oils. The usual proportions are 20 to 25 drops of essential oil to ¼ cup of vegetable oil. Just remember two things:

- Don't use essential oils directly on your skin. Always dilute in vegetable oil first.
- Use only true essential oils. Synthetic oils won't hurt you, but all they have is fragrance. Only essential oils contain the therapeutic properties that were originally present in the herb.

Trading massages with a friend is best, but you can give yourself one very special treat: a foot massage with scented oil.

Bath and Cosmetic Tips

* Herbal concentrations made with either vinegar, alcohol, or water are versatile. Any one of them can be used in the bathtub, as a skin tonic, as a hair rinse, or as an air freshener.

* Alcohol and vinegar bases last indefinitely; water-based infusions should be used the same day you make them, or refrigerated for no more than three days.

* Any of the products in this chapter can be made with essential oils as well as with the herbs themselves.

* In the summertime, keep a jar of herbal vinegar or floral water in the refrigerator. For a quick refresher, dip a handkerchief or washcloth in the cool liquid and wipe your face and hands.

* Label all cosmetics and lotion formulas NOT FOR DRINKING.

PART SIX

Healing with Herbs

CHAPTER TWENTY

Home Remedies

For at least five thousand years, people have been using the plants that grew around them as cures for illness and disease. Herbal remedies were used in ancient Greece and Rome a thousand years before Christ, and noted in the writings of famous poets like Homer and Virgil. The Hippocratic Oath, which all modern doctors honor, is named for Hippocrates, a physician who kept records on the medicinal uses of some four hundred herbs in the fourth century B.C. In China, herbalists have been treating sick people for many thousands of years, prescribing herbal preparations still in use today in Chinese medicine.

Modern medicine, with its high-tech surgery and miracle drugs, tends to frown on the old remedies, often with complete justification. Many of the "cures" in the old herbals are bizarre, even dangerous. For instance, Nicholas Culpeper, a seventeenth-century herbalist who is often quoted in contemporary books about herbs, said that the way to prevent miscarriages was to hold a sprig of tansy near a pregnant woman's navel.

In the days before science made chemical analysis possible,

herbal doctors tried to decipher the hidden meaning of herbs. If a plant had a tangled root system that looked like a bed of young snakes, it was presumed to be good for snakebite. If a certain flower seemed to resemble the human eye with red streaks in it, it was used to make a treatment for eye diseases and blindness. A plant with yellow flowers was said to be effective against jaundice, which turns the skin yellow. This is known as the *doctrine of signatures* (each plant has its own "signature"), a theory that still has its proponents among contemporary herbalists.

Modern medical research has confirmed that in some cases these old remedies have a basis in science—and many do not. Just because something appears in an old herbal as a prescription for a certain illness, that doesn't mean it's medically valid. Tansy won't keep you from miscarrying, and no herb is going to restore your sight.

If you're sick, go to a doctor.

However, many minor ailments can be treated at home, and this is where some of the old herbal remedies come in. Many of the herbs you already have in your garden, even on your spice shelf, can be used as home remedies for commonplace conditions such as indigestion, colds, sore throats, nausea, and more. That is the focus of this chapter.

Making Herbal Remedies

How do you go about making these homey treatments? First, let's learn a few of the terms.

Infusion When the part of the herb that you're using is the leaf, you make an infusion, which is made the same way as herb tea. Heat water to boiling, pour it over the herb leaves, let steep for a while, strain. What makes an infusion, as medicine, different from tea, as beverage, is the strength. Infusions are more concentrated: one ounce of dried herb (and you'd be surprised how much it takes to equal an ounce) to one pint of water. Because it is stronger, you don't gulp down several cups as you would tea. Usually you make a batch and store it in the refrigerator, pouring out a little bit to sip on several times a day.

Decoction If the part of the plant you're using is something hard, like the root, seeds, or a woody stem, you make a decoction. Rather than steeping, the herb is actually cooked in simmering water for half an hour, then strained and stored. Same proportions: one ounce of herb to one pint of water. Sip it, a tablespoon at a time.

Tincture A very concentrated form of herbal preparation, a tincture has a base of alcohol such as vodka or grain alcohol. Dried or chopped fresh herbs are steeped in the alcohol for several weeks, then strained. Use 4 ounces of herb to one pint of alcohol. The resulting tincture is strong; one dose is a few drops, diluted in juice, water, or tea.

Poultice Infusions, decoctions, and tinctures are all taken internally. A poultice is for external use—sore muscles, bruises, rashes, burns, and so on. In a poultice, herbs are put directly on the skin; sometimes they are chopped and mixed with water and perhaps oatmeal to make a paste that's easier to spread. A cloth or bandage is added to hold the poultice in place. As every Boy Scout and Girl Scout knows, this is a common first-aid treatment for minor injuries or insect bites.

One thing to keep in mind: there is no such thing as an herb that is absolutely, positively 100 percent safe—because someone, somewhere, is allergic to it. Before you begin any treatment program, take a sample first, and watch for negative reactions. If your rash gets worse instead of better, stop using the herb.

Home Remedies

For Skin Problems

Irritated or rough skin

- *Calendula*—make a poultice or lotion from flower petals. (To make lotion, steep petals in warm salad oil for half an hour, strain.)
- *Thyme*—make an infusion from leaves. Use as a face wash for oily skin and as a lotion for mild athlete's foot (the thymol in thyme is antiseptic).
- *Comfrey*—make a poultice from the leaves.

For Bruises, Swelling, Cuts and Scrapes

Ordinary cuts and scrapes; minor burns

- *Comfrey*—make a poultice from the leaves.
- *Hyssop*—make a poultice from the leaves; helps reduce black-and-blue marks.

For Indigestion or Intestinal Gas

- *Dill*—make infusion from seeds or leaves.
- *Fennel*—make infusion from seeds or leaves.
- *Lemon verbena*—make infusion from leaves.
- *Catnip*—make infusion from leaves. Extra bonus: catnip has lots of vitamin C.
- *Chamomile*—make infusion from flowers; especially good for gas.
- *Peppermint*—make infusion from leaves. Don't give to babies; the menthol can make them choke.

For Babies' Colic

- *Anise*—make a weak tea.
- *Dill*—make a weak tea.

- *Fennel*—make a weak tea.
- *Chamomile*—add to any of the first three, because it calms fretful babies.

For Sore Muscles

- *Comfrey plus chamomile*—make infusion, add to bathwater for a long soak.
- *Thyme, calendula, and lemon verbena*—another combination for soothing bath.
- *Rosemary*—make a strong infusion of leaves and flowers, massage into tired muscles.

For Colds and Flu

- *Hyssop*—make an infusion of leaves and flowers; mix with honey because the infusion itself is rather bitter tasting; especially good if your chest is congested.
- *Horehound*—make infusion from leaves. Try this special blend: 1 handful horehound leaves, 1 teaspoon crushed anise seed, 2 tablespoons honey or sugar, juice of 1 lemon. Simmer leaves and seed in boiling water for 20 minutes, strain, add lemon and sweetener. Horehound is excellent for all symptoms of a cold.
- *Mint*—make infusion.
- *Lemon balm*—make infusion.
- *Chamomile*—make infusion.
- *Sage*—make infusion.

For Coughs

- *Horehound*—make infusion, candy, or syrup. For syrup, add sugar or honey to infusion. For candy, add sugar to infusion and boil till it gets thick; pour into oiled shallow pan and cut into small pieces when cool.

For Sore Throat

- *Horehound*—make infusion; it contains mucilage, which is soothing to a raw throat.
- *Sage*—make infusion, use as a gargle.
- *Sage plus thyme*—make an infusion.
- *Hyssop*—make infusion, sweeten with honey.

For Nausea

- *Mint*—make infusion.
- *Lemon balm*—make infusion.

For a Mild Sedative

To calm children who are not feeling well, frightened by nightmares, or fretful; or adults who are restless, anxious, or having trouble falling asleep. If treating children, make the infusion weak.

- *Chamomile*—make infusion from the flowers.
- *Catnip*—make infusion from the leaves.
- *Lemon balm*—make infusion from leaves.
- *Fennel*—make infusion from leaves or seeds.

For Headaches

- *Feverfew*—make infusion from leaves; some report it eases migraines.
- *Rosemary*—make a mild infusion from leaves.

For Menstrual Cramps

- *Peppermint*—make infusion.

For Bee Stings

- *Lemon balm, hyssop, or savory*—crush the leaves and rub on the sting.

If you're interested in learning more about herbal treatments, check the references suggested in the Bibliography.

APPENDIX

Mail-order Resources

If you do not live in a large city, you may find it easier—perhaps necessary—to use some of these mail-order sources for herbs and herb-related products. Even if you do live in a city that offers varied shopping opportunities, looking through these catalogs is a heck of a lot of fun.

The list here doesn't pretend to include every mail-order company that has something to do with herbs; it was not feasible to find them all, and some did not respond to requests for information. The ones listed here are those from whom I received firsthand information.

Two other excellent access guides, both of which include more categories, are recommended: *Northwind Farms Herb Resource Guide* (see Northwind Farms entry in this chapter) and *The Herb Companion Wishbook and Resource Guide* (see Bibliography).

The listings are accurate as of publication time, but alas, things change. For more up-to-the-minute information, look through the ads in herb magazines and newsletters; this is a good way to find brand-new companies.

This chapter is divided into two sections. The first, which contains full information on each company, including the main categories of product lines, is organized alphabetically. The second, which lists company names only, is divided by product categories. The categories are:

Craft supplies. Materials for making potpourri, dried wreaths, and other craft projects: the plant materials, the fragrances, and other assorted accessories.

Gardening supplies. Garden hardware (in the high-tech sense of the word): tools, gadgets, fertilizers, seed-starting supplies—everything but the seeds and the dirt.

Herbal products. A catch-all category including all sorts of home and personal products with herbs as an ingredient: shampoo, skin cream, scented candles, flea collars for your pet, things like that.

Kitchen supplies/recipes. Cooking gadgets, gourmet food items, tea-making accessories, sources of recipes.

Medicinal herbs and herbal supplies. Herbs sold for their medicinal properties, in various forms and formulations; also related accessories.

Packaged herbs. Regardless of the type of container, these are just plain herbs, dried and ready for use in cooking, crafts, or tea.

Publications/associations. Publications (newsletters and magazines, plus specialized books) about herbs; and herb associations. Some associations are also publishers.

Seeds/plants. Businesses that sell plants, seeds, or both by mail order.

Albertina's
The Old Kerr Nursery
424 NE 22nd Ave.
Portland, OR 97232
cookbooks

Albertina's is a volunteer-run restaurant housed in a historic building that once served as an orphanage. All its proceeds, including the servers' tips, go to support social service programs for children and families. Recipes from the popular restaurant have been compiled into two cookbooks known as *Albertina's I* and *Albertina's II;* $14 each, including postage and handling.

American Botanical Council
P.O. Box 201660
Austin, TX 78720
512/331-8868
publications/association

This organization is concerned with herbal medicine and has an educational focus. It publishes a quarterly magazine, *HerbalGram* (subscription $25 per year), and a series of booklets on individual herbs.

American Spice Trade Assoc.
P.O. Box 1267
Englewood Cliffs, NJ 07632
publications list, free • publications/association • recipes/cooking

This is the professional association for commercial herb and spice producers, and many of its publications are quite technical. However, inexpensive booklets, spice charts, and brochures are available for the general consumer.

Berkshire Botanical Garden
5 W. Stockbridge Rd.
P.O. Box 826
Stockbridge, MA 01262
413/298-3926

This enterprise, formerly known as Berkshire Garden Center, is not a nursery but a botanical garden, with a fifty-year-old display herb garden open to the public.

Dorothy Biddle Service, Herb Dept.
HC01 Box 900
Greeley, PA 18425-9799
717/226-3239
catalog 50 cents • craft supplies • gardening supplies

A long-established business now run by Dorothy Biddle's granddaughter, this company sells flower-arranging supplies, including many items useful in herbal craft projects.

Bluestone Perennials
7211 Middle Ridge Rd.
Madison, OH 44057
catalog free • plants

As the name suggests, this company specializes in flowering perennials; they have a small collection of herbs.

W. Atlee Burpee & Co.
300 Park Ave.
Warminster, PA 18974
215/674-4900
catalog free • seeds/plants • gardening supplies

The granddaddy of seed catalogs (at least one of them, anyway). The comment of their friendly customer service person says it well: "We are primarily and most happily a home gardener's catalog." Vegetables, flowers, herbs, gardening tools, and their own books. The photos will make you hungry.

Caprilands Herb Farm
534 Silver St.
Coventry, CT 06238
203/742-7244
catalog free; SASE requested • seeds/plants • craft supplies • publications

Caprilands is the well-known enterprise of Adelma Grenier Simmons, author and herb enthusiast for some forty years. Herb tours and lectures in the display gardens. Herbal products and gifts, books (including those by Mrs. Simmons), potpourri supplies, etc. by mail order.

Carroll Gardens Inc.
P.O. Box 310
Westminster, MD 21158
410/848-5422
catalog $2.00, credited to first • order • seeds/plants

Perennial flowers, scented geraniums, and herb plants. Catalog has very detailed information and excellent instructions. Greenhouses open to visitors.

Cherchez, Ltd.
P.O. Box 550
Millbrook, NY 12545
914/677-8271
catalog free • packaged herbs • craft supplies • herbal products

Dried herbs for potpourri, essential oils, and scented gift items, from the company of Barbara Ohrbach, author of *The Scented Room.*

Common Scents
3920-A 24th St.
San Francisco, CA 94114
415/826-1019
catalog free • herbal products

An intriguing line of beauty products; their focus is products with natural ingredients that do not use animal testing. Among the herb-related items are herbal bath gels, shampoos, and lavender hair conditioner.

Companion Plants
7247 N. Coolville Ridge Rd.
Athens, OH 45701
614/592-4643
catalog $2 • seeds/plants

The company's slogan is "common and exotic herbs," and they have certainly succeeded. The catalog, deceptively small, is loaded with interesting varieties: 27 kinds of sage, 18 varieties of rosemary, and 42 thymes! Display gardens open to the public from March to Thanksgiving.

Comstock, Ferre & Co.
Box 125
Wethersfield, CT 06109
203/529-6255
catalog $3.00 • seeds

This company, now in its 172nd year, sells seeds for herbs, vegetables, and flowers—and they list the herbs first.

Cook's Garden
P.O. Box 535
Londonderry, VT 05148
802/824-3400
catalog $1.00 • seeds/plants • gardening supplies • kitchen supplies/recipes • books/gift items

This is a small, family-run organization that takes pride in environmentally responsible practices in all aspects of the business. Their specialty is salad greens, with more kinds of lettuce than you knew existed. The herb seeds, like everything else, are organically grown. The excellent catalog is filled with detailed information and sprinkled throughout with owner Ellen Ogden's recipes. They also sell a few select gardening and kitchen tools, as well as books, including two written by the Ogdens.

Curtis Woodward
4150 Boulevard Pl.
Mercer Island, WA 98040
206/343-9296
price list free • craft supplies

Natural-dried flowers, cones, and seed pods from all over the world. Mrs. Eunice Curtis, an amateur botanist who collected plant materials in Australia and Africa, started the business in the 1940s to create interest in the world's flora. Their focus is unusual, quality items for crafters and floral designers.

Dabney Herbs
P.O. Box 22061
Louisville, KY 40252
502/893-5198
catalog $2 • seeds/plants • packaged herbs • herbal products • craft supplies • kitchen supplies • gardening supplies • books

A very comprehensive selection of all sorts of products having to do with herbs: a very wide range of books, each one described in detail; cosmetics and beauty products; dried herbs in bulk, for tea or cooking; herbs, spices, and fixatives for potpourri; fragrance and essential oils; and assorted gift items. Also, a full range of herb plants, and herb and flower seeds.

Dutch Mill Herb Farm
6640 NW Marsh Rd.
Forest Grove, OR 97116
503/357-0924
plant list free with SASE • plants

Barbara Remington has assembled the largest collection of lavenders on the West Coast—close to 100 varieties. Demonstration gardens and local sale of hundreds of herbs; mail order sales limited to lavender. Send SASE (self-addressed stamped envelope) for list of available species and shipping costs. Dutch Mill is a certified organic farm.

Elixir Farm Botanicals
General Delivery
Brixley, MS 65618
417/261-2393
catalog free • medicinal herbs/herbal supplies • seeds/plants

The emphasis here is on herbs as medicine; they sell a few plants, books, and a flower press—but primarily seeds. The catalog is in the form of a poster, with drawings and descriptions of about 30 medicinal herbs.

Essential Oil Co.
P.O. Box 206
Lake Oswego, OR 97034
503/697-5992
catalog free • medicinal herbs/herbal supplies • craft supplies

This company sells materials for massage therapists and other holistic health practitioners. It also offers a nice range of oils (both essential and synthetic) for individual consumers interested in making potpourri or homemade bath and beauty products. Also related items such as bottles and medicine droppers, and a small line of books.

The Flora-Line
7336 Berry Hill (MS)
Rancho Palos Verdes, CA 90274-4404
310/377-7040
quarterly, $16.95 a year • sample copy, $3.95

Dody Lyness, teacher and floral designer, is editor of this quarterly newsletter for professional crafters, formerly titled *Potpourri Party Line.* Ms. Lyness is also the author of a book on potpourri, available from the same address.

Fragrant Fields
129 Front St.
Dongola, IL 62926
catalog $1.00 • seeds/plants

Herb plants (including some unusual ones) and perennial flowers. Display garden and greenhouse open to visitors.

Frontier Cooperative Herbs
The Herb and Spice Collection
P.O. Box 299
Norway, IA 52318
319/227-7991
catalog $5.00, credited to first order • packaged herbs • kitchen supplies • herbal products

This cooperatively owned company sells more than 5,000 items to wholesale distributors and retailers: dried herbs, herb and spice blends, teas, essential oils, natural skin care products, and so on. Individuals should ask for the retail catalog.

Garden Spot Distributors
438 White Oak Rd.
New Holland, PA 17557
717/354-4936
catalog free • herbal products • medicinal herbs

This company is a wholesale distributor for several manufacturers of natural foods products, including two herbal lines that you might not be able to find locally: Nature's Way, with herbal products meant to be taken as medicine (in capsules), and Solid Gold, billed as "America's only natural herbal dog food." They also sell to individuals; write for retail catalog.

Garden Way Publishing
Storey Communications Inc.
Schoolhouse Rd.
Pownal, VT 05261
catalog free • publications

Publisher of excellent herb craft books and the "Country Wisdom" series of booklets. (See Bibliography.)

Gardener's Supply Co.
128 Intervale Rd.
Burlington, VT 05401
802/863-1700
catalog free • gardening supplies • kitchen supplies • herbal products • seeds/plants

Primarily a supplier of quality tools and serious equipment for gardeners, this company offers a small selection of herb plants as well as natural pesticides and flea repellents.

Goodwin Creek Gardens
P.O. Box 83
Williams, OR 97544
503/846-7357

retail shop: The Secret Garden
154-1/2 Oak St.
Ashland, OR 97520
503/488-3308
catalog $1.00, credited to first order • seeds/plants

Goodwin Creek, in business since 1977, is a small family operation specializing in herbs and everlastings. Catalog does not show what the plants look like but has good written descriptions of the various species; also instructions on starting seeds and preserving flowers. The company also carries a line of books, including the definitive book on growing everlastings, written by owners Jim and Dotti Becker.

Gourmet Gardener
4000 W. 126th St.
Leawood, KS 66209
913/345-0490
catalog $2.00 • seeds • kitchen supplies • herbal products • craft supplies • books

Seeds for herbs, gourmet vegetables, and flowers—including edible flowers and flowers to grow for drying and using in craft projects. Specialty is imported seeds for unusual varieties. Also books and a few gift items. This company was formerly known as The Herb Gathering.

Gurney's Seed & Nursery Co.
110 Capital St.
Yankton, SD 57079
605/665-1671
catalog free • seeds/plants

A major home gardener's catalog, with seeds for herbs, vegetables, and flowers, plus gardening supplies and kitchen items. Ask for their free bulletin about growing herbs.

Harvest Health, Inc.
1944 Eastern Ave. SE
Grand Rapids, MI 49507
616/245-6268
catalog free • packaged herbs • medicinal herbs • craft supplies • kitchen supplies

A very wide range of dried herbs, some for medicinal purposes and some for cooking. Also a nice selection of essential oils for potpourri, and useful items like bottles with medicine droppers and heat-sealable tea bags. Company has been in business since 1952.

Heirloom Garden Seeds
P.O. Box 138
Guerneville, CA 95446
catalog $2.50 • seeds

Seeds for more than 400 plants—herbs in the broad sense of the word, for cooking, healing, and ornamentals. Catalog is wonderful reading (they call it the "storybook catalog," and that's a good description): full of herb lore and nice old drawings, as well as cultivation information. If you already know what the plants are like, just ask for the free (and very well organized) order form.

The Herb Companion
Interweave Press
201 E. Fourth St.
Loveland, CO 80537
303/669-7672
$21 a year, six issues • publications/associations

A truly wonderful magazine for people who love herbs. Lovely photos, attractive layout, and full of good information: major feature articles plus calendar, plant profiles, growers' tips, and much more. The many small ads are a good way to find up-to-the-minute access to suppliers of everything under the herbal sun. This same company also publishes books, including *The Herb Companion Wishbook and Resource Guide*, by Bobbi McRae (see Bibliography).

The Herb Quarterly
P.O. Box 689
San Anselmo, CA 94960-0689
415/455-9540
quarterly, $24 a year for new subscriptions/$6 for a single copy

Nicely written and easy to use; articles about herb horticulture, garden designs, cooking, and individual herbs. No glossy photos but nice drawings and a pleasant, folksy feeling. The many ads from nurseries and suppliers provide useful, up-to-date sources for all kinds of products.

Herb Pharm
P.O. Box 116
Williams, OR 97544
503/846-6262
catalog free • medicinal herbs/herbal supplies • books

As the play on words in its name suggests, this company focuses on herbs for medicinal uses. The primary line is herbal tinctures, but they also sell tablets, dried herbs in bulk, and herbalist literature. All the products are made from herbs grown and harvested by the company.

Herb Society of America, Inc.
9019 Kirtland-Chardon Rd.
Mentor, OH 44060
publications list, free • publications/associations

The preeminent herb group in the country celebrated its sixtieth year in 1993. Publishes a magazine once a year, called *The Herbarist*, a quarterly newsletter (for members only), and some excellent small books. Membership is limited to those who meet certain qualifications and are sponsored by an existing member, but anyone can purchase the publications. They are also a mail-order source for many other fine books on herbs.

Herbally Yours
P.O. Box 26
Changewater, NJ 07831
908/689-6140
catalog $1.00 • herbal products • packaged herbs • medicinal herbs/herbal supplies • kitchen supplies • craft supplies

A small catalog with a rich selection of unusual herbal products: dried herbs in bulk, dried flowers and oils for potpourri, beauty products such as rosemary hair rinse, herb blends for cooking, teas and tea blends, tablets (medicinal), products for your pets—lots of interesting stuff.

Indiana Botanic Gardens
P.O. Box 5
Hammond, IN 46325
219/947-4040
catalog free • medicinal herbs/herbal supplies • herbal products

This company claims to be "America's oldest and largest supplier of herbs and herbal products." Reading the catalog is like visiting an old-fashioned drugstore: rheumatism ointment, chamomile shampoo, tonics for various ailments, and a very long list of herbal teas with medicinal claims, among the many, many items. But don't go looking for a garden to stroll through—it's not *that* kind of botanical garden.

International Herb Growers and Marketers Assoc.
1202 Allanson Rd.
Mundelein, IL 60060
708/566-4566
Annual dues $50–$200, • depending on type of membership

Primarily for those who are pursuing herbs as a business interest.

Le Jardin du Gourmet
P.O. Box 75
St. Johnsbury Center, VT 05863
802/748-1446
catalog 50 cents • seeds/plants • kitchen supplies/recipes

The name of the company means "The Gourmet's Garden," and that focus gives this company an intriguing and unusual collection of items: shallots, garlic, leeks, top-set onions, and almost 50 types of herb plants—mostly cooking herbs, as you might imagine. They also sell flowering perennials, a few books, and an impressive list of gourmet food products from around the world. But their main virtue, in my opinion, is their seeds: more than 200 varieties, including about 70 herbs. Best of all, they sell sample packets of all the seeds for 25 cents; what a good idea!

Johnny's Selected Seeds
Foss Hill Road
Albion, ME 04910
207/437-9294
catalog free • seeds/plants • gardening supplies

A general catalog for home gardeners—seeds, gardening tools and supplies, kitchen gadgets, and books. They have seeds for many varieties of vegetables, a basic collection of flowers, including edible flowers, everlastings, and wildflowers, and about 30 herbs. There are extensive growing instructions for each species, but color photos are limited to the flowers. The company emphasizes its extensive research and service orientation. They also have (for the 1992 catalog) the most stunning cover I've yet seen.

Dody Lyness Co.
7336 Berry Hill (MS)
Rancho Palos Verdes,
CA 90274-4404
310/377-7040
price list free with 2-stamp • SASE • craft supplies

A very complete selection of supplies for making potpourri: dried blossoms, herbs, and spices; fixatives; and fragrance oils. Also dried and pressed flowers for wreaths and other floral crafts. Dody Lyness is also the author/editor of a newsletter and book about potpourri; see entry under *The Flora-Line*.

McCormick & Co.
Consumer Affairs
211 Schilling Circle
Hunt Valley, MD 21031
packaged herbs • kitchen supplies/recipes

This well-known name in commercial herbs has produced a number of free brochures for home cooks, including two excellent charts, both chock full of good ideas: "Everyday Seasonings for Anytime Meals" and "Low-Sodium Spice & Herb Chart."

Mellinger's
2310 W. South Range Rd.
North Lima, OH 44452-9731
216/549-9861
catalog free • gardening supplies • seeds/plants

An all-around catalog for home gardeners, with trees, shrubs, flowering perennials, fruit trees, as well as seeds for vegetables and flowers. A good selection of seeds (about 30 types) and plants (also about 30) of the most popular herbs. Extensive range of garden tools and supplies.

Merry Gardens
P.O. Box 595
Camden, ME 04843
207/236-9064
catalog $2.00 • plants

Mary Ellen and Ervin Ross have been growing herbs, geraniums, fuchsias, and other plants for forty-five years. Their compact catalog lists almost 200 herbs and an astonishing variety of scented geraniums. Visitors are welcome to enjoy the greenhouse and the large eighteenth-century display herb garden.

Nichols Garden Nursery
1190 N. Pacific Highway
Albany, OR 97321
503/928-9280
seeds/plants • craft supplies • kitchen supplies • gardening supplies • packaged herbs • books

A family business now in its second generation, Nichols sells "herbs and rare seeds"—their slogan—along with lots of other useful goodies. Brief but complete descriptions tell how to grow and use each herb. Also unusual vegetable and flower seeds. Other items include dried herbs, tea blends, essential oils, potpourri ingredients, a good selection of gardening books, and kitchen and gardening aids. One unusual focus: advice for those interested in developing a small horticulture business.

Northwind Farm Publications
RR 2, Box 246
Shevlin, MN 56676
publications

Northwind Farm has three types of publications of interest to those who love herbs: *The Business of Herbs,* a newsletter for businesses involving herbs; $20/year (6 issues); $3.75 for sample issue. *The Herb Resource Directory,* a comprehensive where-to-find-it guide that is updated every other year; 1992–93 edition is $12.95. Books from Northwind Farms: a thoughtfully selected line of approximately 50 books about herbs; the booklist contains concise, personal, and very helpful descriptions of each book, all by Northwind owner Paula Oliver. Booklist free.

Geo. W. Park Seed Co.
Cokesbury Rd.
Greenwood, SC 29647-0001
catalog free • seeds/plants • gardening supplies

Well-known general garden catalog, with seeds for flowers and vegetables, plants, bulbs, and gardening supplies. One of the "majors."

Penn Herb Company, Ltd.
603 N. Second St.
Philadelphia, PA 19123-3098
215/925-3336
catalog $1.00, credited to first order • medicinal herbs • herbal products • craft supplies • kitchen supplies/recipes • seeds • books

Leafing through the pages of this densely packed catalog is like browsing in an incredibly well stocked health food store. Penn Herb carries teas, Chinese herbs, bath and personal care products, essential oils, food items, a long list of books, even herb seeds. But the main focus is the medicinal herbs: dried in bulk, in capsules, extracts, and various formulations for all sorts of disorders.

Potions & Lotions
Body and Soul, Inc.
10201 N. 21st Ave., Suite 8
Phoenix, AZ 85021
602/944-6642
catalog 50 cents • herbal products • craft supplies

This company, which has franchise retail operations in several states in addition to mail order, sells bath and beauty products that are custom scented with their own oils—almost 200 fragrance oils and 25 essential oils extracted from herbs. You can also buy the oils alone, for your own projects.

Rachel-Dee Herb Farm
40622 196th Ave. SE
Enumclaw, WA 98022
800/841-7534
price list, free • herbal products

A small line of gourmet food products: herbal vinegars and jellies (blueberry tarragon jam, for instance).

Rasland Farm
N.C. 82 at U.S. 13
Godwin, NC 28344-9712
919/567-2705
catalog free • seeds/plants • craft supplies • herbal products • books

A rather small catalog crammed with herbal goodies. Herb plants in almost 200 varieties, more than 70 types of scented geraniums, wreaths and other gift items, dried flowers and herbs to make your own dried arrangements, potpourri items, teas and herb blends, pet items, and a very nice selection of books. Guided tours offered to groups; annual Herb Fest early in June.

Redwood City Seed Co.
P.O. Box 361
Redwood City, CA 94064
415/325-SEED
catalog $1.00 • seeds/plants • books

Seeds for nearly 300 kinds of plants—most of them vegetables, but almost 40 kinds of herbs. Company specializes in what they call old-fashioned varieties: no hybrids.

Richters Herbs
357 Highway 47
Goodwood, Ontario
Canada LoC 1A0
416/640-6677
catalog $2.50 • seeds/plants • gardening supplies • herbal products • medicinal herbs/herbal supplies • craft supplies • books

One of Canada's leading herb nurseries, Richters carries hundreds of herbs in the form of seeds, plants, and sometimes dried herbs in bulk. The catalog is full of very useful information about growing and using the herbs, and is wonderfully organized: all herbs are listed in alphabetical order by common name, and all forms are grouped into one listing. Thus, under "Anise Hyssop," you will find a price for seeds in four different quantities, a price for the plant, and a price for dried leaves. Also essential oils and other potpourri supplies, gourmet food items, herbal remedies, gardening tools and supplies, organic pest controls, and an extensive selection of books. Richters ships all over North America, and welcomes visitors for free herb lectures.

Rocknoll Nursery
7812 Mad River Rd.
Hillsboro, OH 45133
513/393-5545
catalog free • plants

Rocknoll carries a modest selection of herbs among its ornamental plants—16 species, each with several varieties.

Jeanne Rose
New Age Creations
219 Carl St.
San Francisco, CA 94117
415/564-6785
catalog $2.50 • medicinal herbs

Jeanne Rose is a New-Age herbalist and author who offers a correspondence course in basic herbalism and a line of books by herself and others. She also offers The Herbal Information Line, 900/896-ROSE: recorded information at $1.49 per minute, or answers to specific questions for $3 per minute.

Rutland of Kentucky
P.O. Box 182
Washington, KY 41096
606/759-7815
catalog free • packaged herbs

This wholesale nursery also sells dried herbs and herb mixtures by mail order, and offers classes and monthly herb walks.

Sandy Mush Herb Nursery
Rt. 2, Surrett Cove Rd.
Leicester, NC 28748-9622
704/683-2014
catalog $4.00; free plant list • seeds/plants • books

An amazingly broad selection of hundreds of herb plants, with many unusual varieties: there are, for example, 10 sages, 38 thymes, 17 rosemarys, and 73 scented geraniums. Seeds for herbs, gourmet vegetables, and everlastings. Books and notecards. The calligraphed catalog (they call it a handbook) is a visual delight, and full of valuable information, far beyond the usual plant descriptions: lists to help you choose herbs, recipes, garden layouts, gardening hints, and a unique, concise growing guide. If you already know what the plants look like, write for their plant list and order form, which is free.

Shady Hill Gardens
821 Walnut St.
Batavia, IL 60510
catalog $2.00, refundable • seeds/plants

Shady Hill is the largest commercial grower of geraniums in the country—it's all they do. Among the hundreds of varieties is a nice selection of scented-leaf types.

Shepherd's Garden Seeds
6116 Highway 9
Felton, CA 95018
408/335-6919
catalog free • seeds/plants • gardening supplies • kitchen supplies/recipes

Seeds of vegetables, herbs, and flowers in several groupings: fragrant, everlasting, old-fashioned, bouquet—all thoroughly and enthusiastically described.

The catalog features delicate illustrations and is sprinkled generously with Renee Shepherd's recipes. The herbs are mostly those that can be grown from seeds, but four plants are offered: rosemary, tarragon, lemon thyme, and peppermint. One very nice feature is the many seed collections—scented basils, culinary herbs, container herbs, for crafters, for children, and more. Ask for brochure on herbal vinegars. Special focus on seeds and supplies for container gardening.

Sunnybrook Farms
9448 Mayfield Rd. P.O. Box 6
Chesterland, OH 44026
216/729-7232
catalog $1.00 • seeds/plants • packaged herbs • craft supplies

Sunnybrook Farms has sold herbs (plants and seeds) and perennial ornamentals for three generations. The herb list is extensive: 25 varieties of thyme, for example, and there are seven herb collections (the fragrance collection, dye plant collection, etc.). Also essential and fragrance oils, and dried herbs, spices, and flowers for potpourri.

Tom Thumb Workshops
Rt. 13, P.O. Box 357
Mappsville, VA 23407
804/824-3507
catalog $1.00 • craft supplies • packaged herbs • herbal products • books

Make your own potpourri from the extensive list of supplies: many kinds of intriguing dried flowers, herbs, spices, cones, and seed pods, fragrance oils, fixatives, wreath bases, potpourri containers, and craft accessories. Or choose one of the 40 blends already made up. Miscellaneous gift items, craft patterns, and a wide selection of floral craft books. This catalog is small but very packed.

Triple Oaks Nursery & Florist
P.O. Box 385
Franklinville, NJ 08322
609/694-4272
catalog free with SASE • craft supplies • seeds/plants

This company features herbs, fragrant plants, and potpourri supplies—dried flowers, herbs, spices, and fixatives. The catalog is really a plant list, with no descriptions, so you have to know already what things look like, but the selection is large. Triple Oaks also offers a range of classes and lectures at the greenhouse, and an annual Herb Festival in early June.

The Uncommon Herb
731 Main Street
Monroe, CT 06468
203/459-0716
catalog $1.00 • packaged herbs • herbal products • kitchen supplies • craft supplies

This manufacturer of packaged herbs (available in stores and by mail) has also assembled a delightful collection of home and personal products made from herbs: skin care, cosmetics, herbal soaps, pet care products, and many more. Also kitchen items, seasoning blends, and a nice line of books. Shop and greenhouse open to visitors.

Andre Viette, Farm and Nursery
Route 1, Box 16
Fishersville, VA 22939
703/943-2315
catalog $3.00 • plants

This company specializes in perennial flowers; there are a few herbs mixed in, but you must know the Latin name to find them.

White Flower Farm
30 Irene St.
Torrington, CT 06790
203/496-9600
catalog free • seeds/plants

This exquisite catalog, with beautiful layout and graceful writing, would be most suitable for herb lovers who also have large flower gardens, for flowering bulbs and perennials are the primary focus. The herb selection is small—8 types. The catalog features a very helpful planting guide: what types of plants do well in various conditions.

Craft Supplies

- Dorothy Biddle Service, Herb Dept.
- Caprilands Herb Farm
- Cherchez
- Curtis Woodward
- Dabney Herbs
- Essential Oil Co.
- Gourmet Gardener
- Harvest Health
- Herbally Yours
- Dody Lyness Co.
- Nichols Garden Nursery
- Penn Herb Co.
- Potions & Lotions
- Rasland Farm
- Richters Herbs
- Sunnybrook Farms
- Tom Thumb Workshops
- Triple Oaks Nursery & Florist
- The Uncommon Herb

Gardening Supplies

- Dorothy Biddle Service, Herb Dept.
- W. Atlee Burpee & Co.
- Cook's Garden
- Dabney Herbs
- Gardener's Supply Company
- Johnny's Selected Seeds
- Mellinger's
- Nichols Garden Nursery
- Geo. W. Park Seed Co.
- Richters Herbs
- Shepherd's Garden Seeds

Herbal Products

- Cherchez
- Common Scents
- Dabney Herbs
- Frontier Cooperative Herbs
- Garden Spot Distributors
- Gardeners' Supply Company
- Gourmet Gardener
- Herbally Yours
- Indiana Botanic Gardens
- Penn Herb Co.
- Potions & Lotions
- Rachel-Dee Herb Farm
- Rasland Farm
- Richters Herbs
- Tom Thumb Workshops
- The Uncommon Herb

Kitchen Supplies/Recipes

- Albertina's
- American Spice Trade Association
- Cook's Garden
- Dabney Herbs
- Gourmet Gardener
- Harvest Health
- Herbally Yours
- Le Jardin du Gourmet
- McCormick & Co.

Frontier Cooperative Herbs
Garden Spot Distributors
Gardener's Supply Company
Nichols Garden Nursery
Penn Herb Co.
Shepherd's Garden Seeds
The Uncommon Herb

Medicinal Herbs and Herbal Supplies

Elixir Farm Botanicals
Essential Oil Company
Garden Spot Distributors
Harvest Health
Herb Pharm
Herbally Yours
Indiana Botanic Gardens
Penn Herb Co.
Richters Herbs
Jeanne Rose

Packaged Herbs

Cherchez
Dabney Herbs
Frontier Cooperative Herbs
Garden Spot Distributors
Harvest Health
Herbally Yours
McCormick & Co.
Nichols Garden Nursery
Rutland of Kentucky
Sunnybrook Farms
Tom Thumb Workshops
The Uncommon Herb

Publications/Associations

American Botanical Council
American Spice Trade Association
Caprilands (books by Adelma Simmons)
The Flora-Line newsletter
Garden Way Publishing (books and booklets)
Goodwin Creek Gardens (book by Jim and Dotti Becker)
The Herb Companion magazine
The Herb Quarterly magazine
Herb Society of America
International Herb Growers and Marketers Association
Roberta Moffitt (books on dried flowers)
Northwind Farm Publications (*The Business of Herbs* newsletter and *Herb Resource Directory*)

Seeds/Plants

- Bluestone Perennials
- W. Atlee Burpee & Co.
- Caprilands Herb Farm
- Carroll Gardens Inc.
- Companion Plants
- Comstock, Ferre & Co.
- Cook's Garden
- Dabney Herbs
- Dutch Mill Herb Farm
- Elixir Farm Botanicals
- Fragrant Fields
- Gardener's Supply Co.
- Goodwin Creek Gardens
- Gourmet Gardener
- Gurney's Seed & Nursery Co.
- Heirloom Garden Seeds
- Le Jardin du Gourmet
- Johnny's Selected Seeds
- Mellinger's
- Merry Gardens
- Geo. W. Park Seed Co.
- Penn Herb Co.
- Rasland Farm
- Redwood City Seed Co.
- Richters Herbs
- Rocknoll Nursery
- Sandy Mush Herb Nursery
- Shady Hill Gardens
- Shepherd's Garden Seeds
- Sunnybrook Farms
- Triple Oaks Nursery & Florist
- Andre Viette Farm and Nursery
- White Flower Farm

BIBLIOGRAPHY

For Further Reading

The resurgence of interest in herbs has prompted a number of new books on the subject, some of them all-purpose treatments and many others focused on just one aspect. A few personal favorites are suggested here.

This list is highly subjective, not comprehensive by any means. In your favorite bookstore you will find many other fine books. Also, don't forget to check your local library. There you will find many excellent earlier works on herbs, books that are now out of print and thus not in bookstores, but chock full of timeless information.

General Books

Bremness, Lesley. *The Complete Book of Herbs.* New York: Viking, 1988.

An outstanding book, with comprehensive information: growing, cooking, medicinal, and household uses, along with full-page descriptions of more than 100 herbs. Excellent photographs, not just pretty pictures. Very highly recommended.

Rodale's Illustrated Encyclopedia of Herbs. Emmaus, Pa.: Rodale Press, 1987.

Rodale Press is also the publisher of *Organic Gardening* magazine, and the company's organic philosophy is evident throughout. The book is organized in alphabetical entries, which occasionally makes it difficult to find things, but the quality of information is superb. Very well written, with thorough and witty presentation of all the points you need to know, plus some you didn't know you needed. Black-and-white drawings for herb identification.

Books with a Specific Focus

Brooklyn Botanic Gardens, 1000 Washington Avenue, Brooklyn, N.Y. 11225.

This respected organization, one of the world's leading botanical gardens, publishes a series of booklets on gardening topics. Each is a collection of short articles, all on one subject. Three dealing with herbs are:

Culinary Herbs
Herbs and Cooking
Herbs and Their Ornamental Uses

Garden Way booklets. Storey Communications, Schoolhouse Road, Pownal, Vt. 05261.

This company publishes, among other products, the "Country Wisdom" bulletins, a series of small, inexpensive books on various home topics; each 32-page booklet deals with just one subject. All are packed tight with good, easy-to-use information. Four of interest for herb growers:

Grow 15 Herbs for the Kitchen
Salt-Free Herb Cookery
Growing and Using Basil
Making Potpourri

McRae, Bobbi. *The Herb Companion Wishbook and Resource Guide*. Loveland, Colo.: Interweave Press, 1992.

Published by the same folks who create that lovely magazine *The Herb Companion*, this delightful book is something like a catalog of catalogs. It gives access information and informed descriptions of mail-order companies, herb organizations, educational opportunities, public gardens, and much more. Large size soft-cover book with attractive layout.

The Magic and Medicine of Plants. Pleasantville, N.Y.: Reader's Digest Books, 1986.

A good all-around reference on the medicinal uses of herbs. Each plant description is enhanced with both color photos and color illustrations, giving a clear view of what the plants look like. Toxic plants are clearly marked with a red *X*.

Norris, Dorry Baird. *Sage Cottage Herb Garden Cookbook*. Chester, Conn.: Globe Pequot Press, 1991.

Recipes, gardening tips, and tidbits of herbal lore, all organized by month. Includes special menus and traditions for special occasions each month, such as Valentine's Day, Fourth of July, and Johnny Appleseed's Birthday. A delightful book.

Oster, Maggie. *Gifts and Crafts from the Garden*. Emmaus, Pa.: Rodale Press, 1988.

Excellent how-to drawings and very clear instructions for many craft projects based on herbs, dried flowers, and other plant materials.

Rogers, Jean. *Cooking with the Healthful Herbs*. Emmaus, Pa.: Rodale Press, 1983.

Subtitle says it all: "300 No-Salt Ways to Great Taste and Greater Health." The usual first-class job from Rodale.

Shaudys, Phyllis. *The Pleasure of Herbs* and *Herbal Treasures*. Pownal, Vt.: Garden Way Publishing, 1986 and 1990.

These two books, outgrowths of Phyllis Shaudys's newsletter, *Potpourri from Herbal Acres*, are enthusiastic collections of herbal hints. There is a wealth of information and ideas, on all aspects of growing and using herbs, organized by month. Like the newsletter, Mrs. Shaudys's own writings are supplemented with tips from expert gardeners, cooks, and craftspeople. There is some overlap between the two books, but I wouldn't be willing to give up either one.

Sheen, Joanna. *Herbal Gifts.* London: Ward Lock, 1991.

Includes a nice range of different kinds of projects; instructions are given in the text, without step-by-step illustrations.

Travelers' Guide to Herb Gardens. Herb Society of America, 9019 Kirtland-Chardon Road, Menton, Ohio 44060. $4.75.

There is no better way to learn about herbs than to visit herb gardens, and there are few activities more peaceful. This manual, compiled by the prestigious Herb Society, lists more than five hundred opportunities for restoring the soul—public and private gardens throughout the United States and Canada, organized by state and province. New edition was published in summer 1992.

Weiss, Gaea and Shandor. *Growing and Using the Healing Herbs.* Emmaus, Pa.: Rodale Press, 1984.

Both historical and present-day home remedies based on herbs, from the trustworthy Rodale organization; very elegant black-and-white drawings of the plants.

Index

Page numbers in **bold** indicate main listings in the Encyclopedia section.